sipri

AF771175

Stockholm International Peace Research Institute

SIPRI is an independent international institute for research into problems of peace and conflict, especially those of arms control and disarmament. It was established in 1966 to commemorate Sweden's 150 years of unbroken peace.

The Institute is financed mainly by the Swedish Parliament. The staff, the Governing Board and the Scientific Council are international.

The Governing Board and the Scientific Council are not responsible for the views expressed in the publications of the Institute.

Stockholm International Peace Research Institute
Pipers väg 28, S-170 73 Solna, Sweden
Cable: SIPRI
Telephone: 46 8/655 97 00
Telefax: 46 8/655 97 33

Cover design: *The scorpion is an arachnid with a long, slender, jointed tail ending in a curved poisonous sting. As an animal that is said to even sting and poison itself, it is analogous to mankind's use of chemical and biological weapons, which easily contaminate the users themselves.*

Control of Dual-Threat Agents: The Vaccines for Peace Programme

Control of Dual-Threat Agents: The Vaccines for Peace Programme

Edited by
Erhard Geissler and John P. Woodall

sipri

Stockholm International Peace Research Institute

OXFORD UNIVERSITY PRESS
1994

This book has been printed digitally and produced in a standard specification in order to ensure its continuing availability

OXFORD
UNIVERSITY PRESS

Great Clarendon Street, Oxford OX2 6DP

Oxford University Press is a department of the University of Oxford.
It furthers the University's objective of excellence in research, scholarship,
and education by publishing worldwide in

Oxford New York

Auckland Cape Town Dar es Salaam Hong Kong Karachi
Kuala Lumpur Madrid Melbourne Mexico City Nairobi
New Delhi Shanghai Taipei Toronto

With offices in

Argentina Austria Brazil Chile Czech Republic France Greece
Guatemala Hungary Italy Japan South Korea Poland Portugal
Singapore Switzerland Thailand Turkey Ukraine Vietnam

Published in the United States
by Oxford University Press Inc., New York

Reprinted 2008

ISBN 978-0-19-829172-5

Contents

Foreword *xi*
Preface *xiii*
Contributors *xiv*
Acronyms and abbreviations *xvi*

Part I. Introduction

1. Introduction 3
Erhard Geissler and John P. Woodall
I. Introduction 3
II. Vaccines for Peace 3
III. The Global Epidemiological Surveillance System proposal 4
IV. The Biesenthal Vaccine Initiative 4

2. The Vaccines for Peace programme: executive summary 6
Erhard Geissler and John P. Woodall
Table 2.1. Implications of the VFP programme 8

3. Arms control, health care and technology transfer under the Vaccines for Peace programme 10
Erhard Geissler
I. Introduction 10
II. Biological defence R&D raises suspicion of possible offensive intentions 10
III. Protection of civilians against dual-threat agents 16
IV. Vaccine R&D and production for military purposes need not necessarily be carried out by the military 21
V. The BWC lacks universal adherence 22
VI. The BWC is not free of loopholes 23
VII. Scientific and technological developments 24
VIII. Verification 25
IX. Prevention of proliferation vs. enhancement of co-operation 27
X. The technology gap between North and South increases 31
XI. Conversion of facilities involved in BW programmes 32
XII. Establishing the VFP programme 33
XIII. Conclusions 37
Table 3.1. Biological weapon status of selected countries, excluding Iraq 16
Table 3.2. Dual-threat agents known to have caused natural outbreaks of disease, 1985–88 17
Table 3.3. Putative anti-personnel biological warfare agents 29

Part II. Strengthening the Biological Weapons Convention

4. The missing link in implementation of the BWC: the war against pathogens 41
Félix C. Calderón
I. Introduction 41
II. The rights of States Parties 42
III. The Review Conferences 44
IV. Progress in the war against pathogens 46

5. Vaccines for Peace: a political scientist's critique 48
Oliver Thränert
I. Introduction 48
II. Does VFP lead to universality and prevent proliferation? 48
III. Is the threshold for VFP participation high enough? 51
IV. Biological defence and national sovereignty 52
V. Problems of establishing the VFP programme 54
VI. Conclusion 54

6. Control and co-operation in biological defence research: national programmes and international accountability 56
Nicholas A. Sims
I. Introduction 56
II. Return to earlier proposals 56
III. International accountability through greater openness 57
IV. International control 58
V. Transparency mechanisms 61
VI. Demonstrating compliance 63
VII. Civil–military co-operation 65

7. Verification of the BWC 67
Tibor Tóth, Erhard Geissler and Thomas Stock
I. Introduction 67
II. Identification of potential verification measures: VEREX I 69
III. Evaluation of possible verification measures: VEREX II–IV 72
IV. Lessons from the CWC negotiations 74
Table 7.1. Potential verification measures 70
Table 7.2. Illustrative examples of combinations of potential verification measures 73

8. The conversion of biological warfare research and development facilities to peaceful uses 77
Milton Leitenberg
I. Introduction 77
II. The conversion of the US biological warfare facilities 82
III. The biological warfare facilities of the former Soviet Union 89
IV. Conversion of the former Soviet biological warfare facilities 97
V. Prerequisites for conversion 102
Table 8.1. Destruction of US biological warfare agents 84

Part III. Vaccine R&D and production

9. Viral vaccines: their evolution and current trends 109
Florian Horaud
I. Introduction 109
II. Empiricism and efficacy 109
III. Safety of viral vaccines: the past 110
IV. Safety and efficacy of viral vaccines: the present 113
V. Recently licensed vaccines 115
VI. Making vaccines by new technology 117
VII. Desirable viral vaccines 118
Table 9.1. Human viral vaccines currently in use 111
Table 9.2. An historical account of viral vaccine development 112
Table 9.3. Examples of accidents induced by viral vaccines 113
Table 9.4. Main factors that contributed to the safety of viral vaccines 114

10. Human viral vaccines 120
Nizar Ajjan, Pierre Saliou and Louis Valette
I. Introduction 120
II. Measles vaccine 121
III. Rubella vaccine 121
IV. Mumps vaccine 122
V. Poliomyelitis vaccine 122
VI. Influenza vaccine 124
VII. Hepatitis vaccine 124
VIII. Rabies vaccine 125
IX. Haemorrhagic fever vaccines 126
X. Herpes virus vaccines 126
XI. Rotavirus vaccine 128
XII. Discussion 128
XIII. Conclusion 128

11. Viral vaccine research, development and production in the former Soviet Union: a brief review of the situation 129
Sergey G. Drozdov
I. Introduction 129
II. Poliovirus vaccine 129
III. Tick-borne encephalitis vaccine 130
IV. Hepatitis vaccines 131
V. Conclusion 132

12. The Scientific and Production Association Vector: the current situation 133
Sergey V. Netesov
I. Introduction 133
II. Basic research 133
III. Applied research 134
IV. Challenges and opportunities 135
Table 12.1. Main achievements of the Institute of Molecular Biology 134
Table 12.2. Basic research at the Institute of Molecular Biology 135
Table 12.3. Applied research at the Institute of Molecular Biology 136
Table 12.4. The Institute of Biologically Active Substances 137
Table 12.5. The Experimental Production Plant 137

13. Vaccines against dual-threat agents: regulation and quality, issues and constraints 139
Jack Melling
I. Introduction 139
II. Product licensing issues 140
III. Manufacture 145
IV. Conclusions 146

Part IV. Public health and biological defence

14. Vaccines for biological defence: defence considerations 151
Graham S. Pearson
I. Introduction 151
II. Why is biological defence important? 152
III. Elements of biological defence 154
IV. Medical countermeasures 156

V. The aim of biological defence 156
VI. The BWC 157
VII. Vaccines for biological defence 158
VIII. Vaccines for civil use 160
IX. International development and use of vaccines 160
X. Conclusions 161
Table 14.1. Comparison of conventional, chemical, biological and nuclear warheads 153
Table 14.2. Vaccines for public health and defence 161

15. Molecular aspects of the activity and design of antiviral agents 163
Peter Langen
I. Introduction 163
II. The current situation 163
III. Antiviral agents 164
IV. Antiviral agents and the Vaccines for Peace programme 166
Table 15.1. Proteins encoded by virus genomes as targets for antiviral compounds 164
Table 15.2. Current status of chemotherapy against cancer cells, bacteria and viruses 165

16. Vaccines for public health: can Vaccines for Peace help in the war against disease? 168
Stephen S. Morse
I. Introduction 168
II. Comparison of emerging diseases and BW agents 168
III. Is it possible to be prepared for emerging diseases? 170
IV. The need for preparedness 171
V. Possible defences against emerging diseases 172
VI. Constraints on developing vaccines for emerging diseases indicate a role for new programmes 173
Table 16.1. Some examples of 'emerging' viruses 169
Table 16.2. Some emerging viruses and probable factors in their emergence 171

17. The Global Epidemiological Surveillance System and Vaccines for Peace: complementary initiatives in public health and weapon control 176
Mark L. Wheelis
I. Global epidemiological surveillance 176
II. Relationship to the Vaccines for Peace programme 179
III. Conclusion and recommendations 181

Part V. International programmes for prevention of disease

18. The WHO global smallpox eradication programme: vaccine supply and variola virus stocks 185
Frank Fenner
I. Introduction 185
II. The early history of vaccination 186
III. The WHO Smallpox Eradication Programme, 1959–66 187
IV. The WHO Intensified Smallpox Eradication Programme, 1967–80 188
V. Assuring the quality of vaccine 188

VI. The WHO Reference Centres for Smallpox Vaccine 191
VII. Development of improved vaccines 193
VIII. Methods of vaccination 197
IX. Reasons for the success of the Intensified Smallpox Eradication Programme 197
X. The use of variola virus as a biological warfare agent 199
XI. Summary 202
Table 18.1. Countries believed to have endemic smallpox in 1959 and 1967: summary by continent 188
Table 18.2. Initial potency of three production lots of vaccine, 1967 192
Table 18.3. Heat stability (4 weeks at 37°C) of three production lots of vaccine, 1967 192
Table 18.4. Bacterial counts of three production lots of vaccine, 1967 192
Table 18.5. Testing of production batches by the International Reference Centres, 1967 193
Table 18.6. Results of quality-control testing by the International Reference Centres, 1967–80 195
Table 18.7. Smallpox vaccine production in densely populated endemic countries 195
Table 18.8. Biological and socio-political features of smallpox that made its global eradication possible 198
Table 18.9. Laboratories holding variola virus in 1975, and the reduction in numbers as of July 1977 200
Table 18.10. Laboratories holding variola virus stocks at the end of calendar years 1977–83 200
Figure 18.1. Locations of various categories of producers of freeze-dried smallpox vaccine, 1967–79; and of the WHO Reference Centre for Smallpox Vaccine for the Americas (Toronto, Canada) and the WHO International Reference Centre for Smallpox Vaccine (Bilthoven, the Netherlands) 194
Figure 18.2. Vaccination with the bifurcated needle 196

19. Options for the development and transfer of vaccine technology 203

Devaguptapu Subrahmanyam

I. Introduction 203
II. The role of the United Nations Industrial Development Organization 203
III. Health-care problems in developing countries 204
IV. International efforts for controlling infections through vaccination 204
V. The current vaccine-production scenario in the developing countries 205
VI. The need for a long-term strategy 206
VII. New research developments 206
VIII. Vaccine-production problems and possible solutions 207
IX. Technical support to vaccine-manufacturing centres 209
X. Biotechnology development in developing countries 209
XI. Conclusions 212

20. Funding and managing international programmes in biosciences and health care 213

John P. Woodall

I. Funding 213
II. Managing 215

Part VI. Final discussion

21. From BVI to VFP: towards a system of global biological security 219

Erhard Geissler, Félix C. Calderón and John P. Woodall

I. The Biesenthal Vaccine Initiative 219
II. VFP vs. Atoms for Peace 220
III. Conversion 222
IV. Dual-threat agents 223
V. Different vaccines for public health and military defence? 226
VI. Biological terrorism 228
VII. National vs. international biological defence 229
VIII. Production and stockpiling of vaccines 231
IX. Deterrence 231
X. Verification 232
XI. The Global Epidemiological Surveillance System proposal 233
XII. VFP and ProMED would avoid the need for definitions 235
XIII. Proliferation 235
XIV. Participation in the BWC 237
XV. Co-ordination 238
XVI. Funding 238
XVII. Conclusions and recommendations 239
Table 21.1. Diseases in developing countries ranked by total disease burden 224
Table 21.2. Putative BW agents that cause emerging diseases and their mode of transmission 225

Part VII. Annexes

Annexe A. The 1972 Biological Weapons Convention 243

Annexe B. Final Declaration of the Third Review Conference of the BWC 246

Annexe C. The Biesenthal Vaccine Initiative (Vaccines for Peace) Biesenthal Consensus 255

Annexe D. The Biesenthal Vaccine Initiative Mission Statement 258

Annexe E. Mission Statement of the Federation of American Scientists (FAS) Project on the Global Control of Emerging Infectious Diseases 259

Annexe F. US House of Representatives Resolution H.R. 5241 261

SIPRI publications on CBW 264

Foreword

For more than 20 years, the 1972 Convention on the Prohibition of the Development, Production and Stockpiling of Bacteriological (Biological) and Toxin Weapons and on their Destruction (BWC) and the category of weapons regulated by it have been areas of central concern to the Stockholm International Peace Research Institute (SIPRI).

There have been numerous proposals to strengthen the BWC by additional measures, including confidence-building measures (CBMs). A proposal to establish an international programme for the development and use of vaccines against 'dual-threat agents' (DTAs)—bacteria, viruses, fungi and toxins which are natural enemies of humans, animals and plants, and also putative BW and toxin weapon agents—was favourably acknowledged by the 1991 Third Review Conference of the BWC. This initiative, later called the Vaccines for Peace (VFP) programme, was proposed by Professor Erhard Geissler. It is especially interesting owing to its novel approach for addressing concerns about possible offensive military research and development (R&D) related to vaccines. The VFP programme proposes greater transparency combined with significant contributions to improving global health care and presents an opportunity to reduce the biotechnology gap between North and South. If implemented in the near future, the programme could strengthen the international norm against biological and toxin warfare. Transparency, large-scale production of vaccines for developing countries and conversion of BW facilities are admirable goals.

The VFP programme proposal was examined, modified and further developed at a 1992 workshop in Biesenthal, Germany, and resulted in a modified proposal, the Biesenthal Vaccine Initiative (BVI). The Biesenthal workshop and the project in its entirety were made possible by a generous grant from the German Volkswagen Foundation. This volume contains revised versions of the papers presented at Biesenthal. The contributors, who write in their personal capacities, are specialists in biological defence, health protection, conversion, prevention of proliferation, international law, international peaceful co-operation and vaccine research, development and use. The editors of the volume, Professor Geissler and Dr John P. Woodall, have accomplished the enormous task of co-ordinating and reviewing the contributions.

The VFP programme and the BVI, as envisaged and discussed here, could contribute to: (*a*) protection of both civilian and military personnel from diseases caused by DTAs, (*b*) improving transparency in the R&D and production of vaccines, including vaccines developed for military purposes, (*c*) reducing doubts about offensive military intentions of vaccine production, (*d*) conversion to peaceful use of BW and TW facilities, (*e*) enhancement of peaceful international co-operation and prevention of misuse of DTAs, (*f*) prevention of diseases, especially in developing countries, (*g*) increasing the world capacity to produce vaccines, and (*h*) expanding participation in the BWC and its CBMs.

In their discussion of the advantages and disadvantages of the proposed VFP programme, the contributors have focused on the question of whether or not the VFP programme would enhance or diminish common security as it relates to BW. They address such questions as: Can national biological defence be internationalized? Is conversion of former BW facilities feasible in countries like Russia under such a programme? Would the VFP programme promote international co-operation under Article X of the BWC? What are the vaccines which would need to be produced under such a programme, bearing in mind the needs of developing countries? What organizational and institutional aspects must be considered if the VFP programme is implemented? Would such a programme stop or promote proliferation of BW and related technology and knownow?

The VFP proposal is discussed and reviewed in detail in light of experience from World Health Organization (WHO) vaccination programmes. Funding for such programmes is in short supply, and this must be taken into account if the VFP programme is to be implemented in the near future. The interests of the industry involved in vaccine production, the advantages of establishing an international system where vaccines can be provided world-wide and the possible improvement of health care, especially in developing countries, must all be considered. If the VFP programme were combined with additional verification requirements it could also help to strengthen the BWC.

Special thanks go to Jetta Gilligan Borg for her diligent editorial work and her perseverance in preparing final camera-ready copy of the texts.

Dr Thomas Stock
Series Editor and
SIPRI CBW Project Leader

Dr Adam Daniel Rotfeld
Director, SIPRI
March 1994

Preface

The Max Delbrück Centre for Molecular Medicine (MDC) in Berlin-Buch is proud that one of its leading scientists, Professor Erhard Geissler, took the initiative to organize the September 1992 Biesenthal Workshop at which his proposal for an international Vaccines for Peace (VFP) programme was further developed and, together with Dr John P. Woodall, to edit its proceedings.

The ambivalent nature of scientific research and its application is particularly evident in genetics, biotechnology and molecular medicine, the main areas of MDC research. The MDC not only conducts research but also assesses its applications, especially those which may benefit society such as gene therapy, with an awareness that some applications may represent a threat to society or lead to abuse, such as the development of biological weapons (BW).

The Biological Weapons Convention outlawed some of the potentially most destructive weapons of war—toxins and infectious agents, including those produced by gene technology—but it does not remove the risk to nations or individuals of such weapons. The scientific community must do all it can to strengthen the BWC and to minimize risk. The MDC is proud to participate in these activities and thanks the Volkswagen Foundation for its generous support.

As in many areas of science and technology, the line between civilian and military is not easily drawn. Defensive research programmes can mask offensive military activities, and some such examples have recently been revealed. There have also been accusations that some countries have violated the BWC. Although various mechanisms, such as inspection, have been suggested to resolve such disputes, inspection can only go so far in verifying compliance with existing agreements. If nations conduct defensive research programmes it is perhaps inevitable that violations and abuses will occur. It is therefore logical to strengthen international programmes of vaccine development for the prevention of disease. The inclusion of scientific and technical personnel from developing countries in such programmes is particularly interesting.

The VFP programme is designed to undertake research on, and the production of, vaccines against pathogens and toxins that could be used for vaccination programmes to improve health throughout the world and as antidotes to putative biological weapons. Under the auspices of the United Nations and other similar organizations, such as the World Health Organization (WHO), the VFP programme could play an important role in the conversion of biological defence facilities to peaceful purposes. The Biesenthal workshop and this publication are major steps towards the goal of establishing the VFP programme. It is encouraging that the proposal has already received support from the Third Review Conference of the States Parties to the BWC.

I am extremely grateful that the MDC and Erhard Geissler have addressed these important issues, and I hope that our close co-operation with the Stockholm International Peace Research Institute (SIPRI) will continue and flourish.

Professor Detlev Ganten, MD, PhD
Scientific Director
Max Delbrück Centre for Molecular Medicine

Contributors

Dr Nizar Ajjan
Fondation Marcel Mérieux
17 rue Bourgelat
BP 2021
F – 69227 Lyon CEDEX 02
France

Dr Félix C. Calderón
Legal Adviser
Preparatory Commission for the Organisation for the Prohibition of Chemical Weapons
The Hague
The Netherlands

Professor Sergey G. Drozdov
Director
Institute of Poliomyelitis and Viral Encephalitides
142 782 Moscow Region
Russia

Professor Frank Fenner
John Curtin School of Medical Research
The Australian National University
PO Box 334
Canberra, ACT 2601
Australia

Professor Erhard Geissler
Head, Bioethical Research Group
Max Delbrück Centre for Molecular Medicine
Robert Rössle Strasse 10
D – 13122 Berlin
Germany

Professor Florian Horaud
President
International Association of Biological Standardization
Virologie Medicale
Institut Pasteur
28, rue du Dr Roux
F – 75724 Paris CEDEX 15
France

Professor Peter Langen
Co-ordinator,
Cell Biology/Growth Control Research Programme
Max Delbrück Centre for Molecular Medicine
Robert Rössle Strasse 10
D – 13122 Berlin
Germany

Milton Leitenberg
Senior Fellow
Center for International and Security Studies
University of Maryland
College Park, Maryland 20742 – 1811
USA

Professor Jack Melling
Director
Public Health Laboratory Service
Centre for Applied Microbiology and Research
Porton Down
Salisbury, Wilts. SP4 0JG
UK

Professor Stephen S. Morse
The Rockefeller University
1230 York Avenue, Box 2
New York, New York 10021 – 6399
USA

Dr Sergey V. Netesov
Senior General Director
Institute of Molecular Biology
Vector Scientific and Production Association
Koltsovo
633159 Novosibirsk Region
Russia

Dr Graham S. Pearson
Director General
Chemical & Biological Defence Establishment
Porton Down
Salisbury, Wilts. SP4 0JQ
UK

Professor Pierre Saliou
Medical Director
Pasteur Mérieux Sérums & Vaccins
3, avenue Pasteur
BP 10
F – 92430 Marnes-La-Coquette
France

Nicholas A. Sims
Senior Lecturer in International Relations
London School of Economics and Political Science
Houghton Street
London WC2A 2AE
UK

Dr Thomas Stock
Head, CBW Project
Stockholm International Peace Research Institute
Pipers väg 28
S – 171 73 Solna
Sweden

Dr Devaguptapu Subrahmanyam
United Nations Industrial Development Organization
Biotechnology and Genetic Engineering Unit
PO Box 300
A – 1400 Vienna
Austria

Dr Oliver Thränert
Senior Researcher
Foreign Policy Research Division
Friedrich Ebert Stiftung
Godesberger Allee 149
D – 53175 Bonn
Germany

Ambassador Tibor Tóth
Chairman
Ad Hoc Group of Governmental Experts to Identify and Examine Potential Verification Measures
Permanent Representative of the Republic of Hungary
81, avenue de Champel
CH – 1206 Geneva
Switzerland

Dr Louis Valette
Scientific Director
Fondation Marcel Mérieux
17 rue Bourgelat
BP 2021
F – 69227 Lyon CEDEX 02
France

Dr Mark L. Wheelis
Head, Department of Microbiology
University of California
College of Letters and Science
Davis, California 95616
USA

Dr John P. Woodall
Division of Epidemiological Surveillance and Health Situation & Trend Assessment
World Health Organization
CH – 1211 Geneva 27
Switzerland

Acronyms and abbreviations

ACIH	Agency for Cooperation in International Health
BCG	Bacille dilié de Calmette-Guérin (tuberculosis vaccine)
BSE	Bovine spongiform encephalopathy
BTW	Biological and toxin weapon
BVI	Biesenthal Vaccine Initiative
BW	Biological weapon
BWC	Biological Weapons Convention
CBDE	Chemical & Biological Defence Establishment (British)
CBM	Confidence-building measure
cDNA	Complementary DNA
CFE	Conventional Armed Forces in Europe
CIS	Commonwealth of Independent States
CNS	Central nervous system
CVI	Children's Vaccine Initiative
CW	Chemical weapon
CWC	Chemical Weapons Convention
DHF	Dengue haemorrhagic fever
DNA	Deoxyribonucleic acid
DOD	Department of Defense (US)
DPT	Diphtheria, pertussis and tetanus (vaccine)
DSS	Dengue shock syndrome
DTA	Dual-threat agent
EEE	Eastern (equine) encephalitis
EPI	Expanded Programme on Immunization
FAO	Food and Agriculture Organization of the United Nations
FAS	Federation of American Scientists
FDA	Food and Drug Administration (US)
GESS	Global Epidemiological Surveillance System
GLP	Good laboratory practice
GMO	Genetically modified organism
GMP	Good manufacturing practice
HAV	Hepatitis A virus
HBs-Ag	Hepatitis B virus soluble antigen
HBV	Hepatitis B virus
HIV	Human immunodeficiency virus (AIDS virus)
IAEA	International Atomic Energy Agency
IBMA	International Biological Monitoring Agency
ICGEB	International Centre for Genetic Engineering and Biotechnology
ID_{50}	Median infective dose
IND	Investigational new drug
IOE	International Office of Epizootics
IPV	Inactivated poliomyelitis vaccine
MRE	Microbiological Research Establishment (British)
NBC	Nuclear, biological and chemical (warfare, weapons)
NCTR	National Center for Toxicological Research (US)
NGO	Non-governmental organization
NIH	National Institutes of Health (US)
NPT	Non-Proliferation Treaty
OPCW	Organisation for the Prohibition of Chemical Weapons

OPV	Oral poliomyelitis vaccine
PAHO	Pan American Health Organization
ProMED	Global Program for Monitoring Emerging Diseases
PVD	Programme for Vaccine Development
R&D	Research and development
rDNA	Recombinant DNA
RNA	Ribonucleic acid
TBE	Tick-borne encephalitis
TW	Toxin weapon
UN	United Nations
UNDP	United Nations Development Programme
UNEP	United Nations Environment Programme
UNESCO	United Nations Educational Scientific & Cultural Organization
UNGA	United Nations General Assembly
UNICEF	United Nations Children's Fund
UNIDO	United Nations Industrial Development Organization
UNSCOM	United Nations Special Commission on Iraq
USAMRIID	US Army Medical Research Institute of Infectious Diseases
VEE	Venezuelan (equine) encephalitis
VFP	Vaccines for Peace
VP(1)	Viral protein (no. 1)
WEE	Western (equine) encephalitis
WEU	Western European Union
WHO	World Health Organization
WIPO	World Intellectual Property Organization

Part I. Introduction

1. Introduction

ERHARD GEISSLER and JOHN P. WOODALL

I. Introduction

Numerous bacteria, viruses and toxins that are naturally dangerous to people, animals and plants are also putative biological weapon (BW) and toxin weapon (TW) agents that may be used deliberately for hostile purposes to cause disease or death in humans, animals or plants.

The BW and TW agents thus far under consideration are not artificial products of research but products of biological evolution which are dangerous to other living organisms, including human beings to a greater or lesser extent, owing to their nature and characteristics. They can therefore be described as 'dual-threat agents' (DTAs). Research on the structure and function of DTAs as well as research and development (R&D) related to measures for their detection, differential diagnosis and for the prevention and treatment of diseases caused by them, including R&D about vaccines and their use, is thus necessary for both civilian and military purposes. However, military R&D on DTAs, especially R&D on vaccines against DTAs, frequently creates suspicion of possible offensive intentions. In particular the disclosures about the offensive BW R&D programmes in the former Soviet Union and in Russia, which were carried out not only in more or less secret facilities but also in several nominally civilian research institutes, make it clear that such concern is justified.

II. Vaccines for Peace

To counter reservations about military R&D on vaccines and the production of vaccines, and to facilitate the needed provision of vaccines, it was proposed that an 'international program of development and use of vaccines against dual-threat agents' be established[1] following the model of the World Health Organization (WHO) Intensified Smallpox Eradication Programme.[2] The programme, which was subsequently called Vaccines for Peace (VFP),[3] would be administered by the WHO. The VFP programme would *inter alia:* (*a*) provide transparency in the R&D and production of vaccines, including vaccines developed for military purposes; (*b*) help to prevent the development and use of biological and toxin weapons for offensive purposes; (*c*) contribute to the conversion of BW and TW facilities, especially in the former Soviet Union; (*d*) contribute to health protection, particularly in developing countries; and (*e*) promote peaceful international co-operation in the biosciences, especially between industrialized and developing countries.

[1] Geissler, E., *Biological and Toxin Weapons: The Renewed Threat*, with comments by Stefan Noreen of the Swedish Mission to the UN NGO Committee on Disarmament Forum at the United Nations, 2 Feb. 1989, transcript (NGO Committee on Disarmament: New York, 1989); 'The international control of biological weapons' (interview), *geneWATCH*, vol. 6, no. 1 (1989), pp. 1–4.

[2] Fenner, F. *et al.*, *Smallpox and its Eradication* (World Health Organization: Geneva, 1988).

[3] Geissler, E., 'Vaccines for Peace: an international program of development and use of vaccines against dual-threat agents', *Politics and the Life Sciences*, vol. 11, no. 2 (Aug. 1992), pp. 231–43.

The proposal to establish an international programme to develop and use vaccines against DTAs was favourably acknowledged by the Third Review Conference of the States Parties to the 1972 Convention on the Prohibition of the Development, Production and Stockpiling of Bacteriological (Biological) and Toxin Weapons and on their Destruction (BWC).[4] Article X of the Convention specifically commits States Parties to the 'exchange of equipment, materials and . . . information for the use of bacteriological (biological) agents and toxins for peaceful purposes'. In its Final Declaration, the conference welcomed the effort:

> to elaborate an international programme of vaccine development for the prevention of diseases involving scientific and technical personnel from developing countries which are States Parties to the Convention. The Conference recognizes that such a programme might not only enhance peaceful international cooperation in biotechnology but also will contribute to improving health care in developing countries and provide transparency in accordance with the Convention.[5]

The Final Declaration was adopted by consensus, with none of the countries participating in the conference expressing any objections to the proposal. This offers some hope that the programme can be established.

III. The Global Epidemiological Surveillance System proposal

Essentially independently of the VFP proposal, Dr Mark Wheelis, Professor Stephen S. Morse and others recommended the establishment of the Global Epidemiological Surveillance System (GESS)[6] which would also promote increased international efforts to fight against pathogens and toxins, including DTAs. The proposal to create the GESS was also welcomed by the participants of the Third Review Conference as another possible means to implement the obligations of Article X of the BWC.[7] A Steering Committee has been formed to launch the Global Epidemiological Surveillance System. [8]

IV. The Biesenthal Vaccine Initiative

In order to evaluate the VFP proposal experts in biotechnology, defence, diplomacy, international development, medicine, molecular biology and vaccinology from Australia, France, Germany, Hungary, India, Peru, Russia, Sweden, the United Kingdom and the United States as well as representatives or observers from the WHO, the United Nations Industrial Development Organization

[4] For the text of the BWC, see annexe A in this volume.

[5] Final Document of the Third Review Conference of the Parties to the Convention on the Prohibition of the Development, Production and Stockpiling of Bacteriological (Biological) and Toxin Weapons and on their Destruction, part II, *Final Declaration*, BWC/CONF.III/23, 27 Sep. 1991, p. 23.

[6] Wheelis, M., 'The role of epidemiology in strengthening the Biological Weapons Convention', eds E. Geissler and R. H. Haynes, *Prevention of a Biological and Toxin Arms Race and the Responsibility of Scientists* (Akademie Verlag: Berlin, 1991), pp. 277–85; Morse, S. S., 'Epidemiologic surveillance for investigating chemical or biological warfare and for improving human health', *Politics and the Life Sciences*, vol. 11, no. 1 (Feb. 1992), pp. 28–29; Wheelis, M., 'Strengthening biological weapons control through global epidemiological surveillance' (with commentaries and responses), *Politics and the Life Sciences*, vol. 11, no. 2 (Aug. 1992), pp. 179–97.

[7] See note 5.

[8] See annexe E in this volume.

(UNIDO) and the United Nations Office for Disarmament Affairs met in Biesenthal near Berlin, Germany, on 9–14 September 1992. The meeting was organized by the Max Delbrück Centre for Molecular Medicine (MDC), Berlin-Buch and the Stockholm International Peace Research Institute (SIPRI) and was supported by the Volkswagen Foundation.

The proposed VFP programme was examined, modified and further developed at the meeting. In the Biesenthal Consensus[9] the participants of the workshop agreed that a modified Vaccines for Peace programme should be established and that a Steering Committee which had been formed during the meeting should set up the agreed programme and establish a schedule for its implementation. Subsequently, the Steering Committee decided to designate the modified programme the Biesenthal Vaccine Initiative.[10]

This volume is a compilation of the majority of the papers which were presented at the Biesenthal meeting. They have been revised to reflect the results of the discussions on the Vaccines for Peace proposal and are presented here for further consideration by those involved in biological defence, health protection, conversion, prevention of proliferation, international peaceful co-operation and vaccine research, development and use. However, they have generally not been revised with respect to other developments in biological arms control. This volume also includes a chapter written by Nicholas A. Sims who was unable to participate in the Biesenthal workshop.

The opinions expressed in the chapters are those of the authors. They do not necessarily reflect the positions of either their institutes, their governments, of SIPRI or of the editors of this volume.

[9] See annexe C in this volume.
[10] See annexe D in this volume.

2. The Vaccines for Peace programme: executive summary

ERHARD GEISSLER and JOHN P. WOODALL

Infectious diseases threaten more people world-wide, including military personnel, than cancer, cardiovascular diseases or weapons. In all wars throughout history infectious diseases have been the major cause of military casualties.

Numerous infectious diseases and intoxinations (i.e., diseases caused by toxins) are caused by dual-threat agents (DTAs). DTAs are those viruses, bacteria, fungi and arthropods as well as toxins which are not only naturally dangerous to living organisms but which can be deliberately used for hostile purposes as biological weapon (BW) or toxin weapon (TW) agents to cause disease or death in humans, animals or plants.

Most DTAs are endemic in developing countries (some even world-wide) and at least some cause natural disease outbreaks with very high morbidity and/or mortality rates. Moreover, several DTAs also threaten people in industrialized countries as causative agents of 'emerging diseases' (i.e., diseases caused by pathogens that have recently appeared in the population or which are rapidly expanding their range). In addition, civilians are also increasingly threatened world-wide by the possible hostile dissemination of DTAs in low-intensity conflicts or undeclared wars or in the event of their use by terrorists. Civilians would be more endangered by the hostile use of DTAs than would troops since troops are protected by equipment and prophylactic measures.

The development, production, stockpiling and use of BW and TW are forbidden by one or more of the following: the 1925 Geneva Protocol, the 1972 Biological Weapons Convention (BWC) and the 1993 Chemical Weapons Convention (CWC). Nevertheless the danger that DTAs might be used for hostile purposes has increased since the end of the cold war, thereby threatening both military personnel and the civilian population. The development of measures for the prevention and treatment of diseases caused by DTAs is therefore necessary.

The development, production and use of vaccines are the primary measures needed to prevent infectious diseases and intoxinations, including diseases caused by DTAs, since immunization has been shown to be the most cost-effective health intervention.

While several activities are under way, co-ordinated mainly by the World Health Organization (WHO), to prevent *major* infectious disease threats such as diphtheria, measles, pertussis, poliomyelitis, tetanus and tuberculosis, insufficient efforts have been made thus far to prevent diseases caused by DTAs, mainly because such vaccines would not be commercially profitable.

Activities to develop and produce vaccines against DTAs are essentially restricted to military programmes as protective activities permitted under the BWC and the CWC. However, it is not the primary goal of military vaccine programmes to provide vaccines for the protection of the civilian population.

Moreover, military research and development (R&D) related to DTAs, especially R&D on vaccines and the production of vaccines against DTAs, frequently raise suspicion of possible offensive intentions. In particular the disclosures about the offensive BW R&D programmes in the former Soviet Union, which were carried out not only in basically secret facilities but also in several nominally civilian research institutes as well as in declared facilities, have revealed that such concern is justified.

To meet reservations about such military use and to facilitate the needed research on and development and production of vaccines against DTAs, a proposal was made to establish a Vaccines for Peace (VFP) programme as an international programme for the development and use of vaccines against DTAs.

Following the model of the WHO's Intensified Smallpox Eradication Programme, which through international co-operation eradicated one of mankind's most serious plagues, the VFP programme is envisaged as being administered by the WHO in close co-operation with the Programme for Vaccine Development (PVD) run by the WHO and the United Nations Development Programme (UNDP) with the financial assistance of the Rockefeller Foundation and other donors. The VFP programme would contribute to (see table 2.1):

(*a*) protecting both civilians and military personnel from diseases caused by DTAs independently of whether the DTAs are causing natural outbreaks of disease or are being disseminated during hostile activities;

(*b*) providing transparency in the R&D and production of vaccines, including vaccines developed for military purposes, hence reducing doubt about the possible offensive intentions of such programmes;

(*c*) further prevention of the development and use of biological and toxin weapons for offensive purposes, since the existence of prophylaxis and the availability of stockpiles of vaccines would reduce the effectiveness of such weapons;

(*d*) narrowing the (bio)technology gap between North and South as called for in Article X of the BWC, without increasing the danger of proliferation of biological and toxin weapons and of related know-how and technology;

(*e*) the conversion to peaceful uses of BW and TW facilities, especially in the former Soviet Union; and

(*f*) making the BWC more attractive to at least some of the approximately 65 states which have not yet acceded to the Convention.

The proposal to establish an international programme of development and use of vaccines against DTAs was favourably acknowledged by the 1991 Third Review Conference of the States Parties to the BWC.

The VFP proposal was examined, modified and further developed at a September 1992 workshop held in Biesenthal near Berlin, Germany. According to the so-called Biesenthal Consensus[1] the participants at the workshop agreed that a modified VFP programme, now designated the Biesenthal Vaccine Initiative (BVI),[2] should be established. Implementation of the BVI should be the first step in the establishment of the VFP programme. Immediate action should be taken to use BVI and the VFP programme to implement Article X and to assist in the conversion of BW facilities, especially in the former Soviet Union.

All other facilities world-wide which are suitable for participation in the VFP

[1] See annexe C in this volume.
[2] See annexe D in this volume.

Table 2.1. Implications of the VFP programme

Area of concern	Consequences of establishment of the VFP programme	Consequences of rejection of the VFP programme
Lack of universal adherence to the BWC	Overcome by providing an incentive to accede to the BWC	Not overcome
Major loopholes in the BWC	Would be sealed	Would continue to weaken the BWC
Misuse of permission to conduct peaceful activities	Restricted, at least as regards vaccines	Still possible, especially as regards vaccines
Development of vaccines to protect military personnel	Could be done without creating suspicion	Would still create suspicion of offensive intentions
CBMs are not legally binding	Not of concern since major activities directly related to the BWC would be carried out under international supervision	Still of concern because of incomplete participation which restricts the value of submitted reports
Implementation of Article X of the BWC	Would be accomplished, at least to some extent	Would not occur (unless ProMED were to be established)
Contradiction between Articles III and X of the BWC	Would cease to exist since prophylactic activities with DTAs and dual-use techniques would be carried out under international supervision	Would still exist (export controls attempt to reduce proliferation but interfere with the obligation of peaceful co-operation)
Danger of proliferation	Would be reduced because legitimate wish to have access to DTAs and dual-use techniques for peaceful purposes would be allowed under conditions of transparency	Would remain unchanged as it is incompletely addressed by export controls
Conversion of former BW facilities	Would be greatly facilitated and allows use of existing facilities, equipment, personnel and skills to develop urgently needed vaccines	Is thus far not specifically addressed
Lack of verification	Would be addressed by the establishment of a specific VFP verification regime which could simultaneously provide input for development of a comprehensive BWC verification system	Would still be of concern and is dependent on the impact of the results of the 1994 special conference to evaluate the results of VEREX
Attempts to obtain access to DTAs and BW technology for hostile use	Could not be prevented by VFP but could be restricted since activities prohibited by the BWC could no longer be labelled 'peaceful' if conducted outside the VFP regime	Could not be prevented by rejection of the VFP programme

Area of concern	Consequences of establishment of the VFP programme	Consequences of rejection of the VFP programme
Information on DTA vaccines and related technology	Could deter a possible attacker from using such agents	Might be available to a possible attacker from the open literature or intelligence sources
Protection of civilians from hostile attack with DTAs	Would be provided to the extent possible	Would not be provided
Absence of vaccines against 'exotic agents' endemic in the South and/or causing emerging diseases in the North	Would be addressed	Situation would remain unchanged
New strategies necessary to protect against emerging diseases	Would be introduced	Would still be needed
Increased health protection in the South	Would be provided	Would not be provided and would remain limited by export controls and the like
Global biological security from both natural pathogens and BW attack	Would be provided to the extent possible and would deter potential BW proliferators and users	Would not be provided despite increasing vulnerability to emerging diseases and biological attack, including terrorism

programme should be invited to do so on the condition that the country responsible for them is a State Party to the BWC and participates actively in the confidence-building measures (CBMs) agreed upon by the Second and the Third BWC Review Conferences.

To prevent misuse of the VFP programme, including 're-conversion', participation in it requires readiness to participate in a verification system. The specific conditions of this system should be established as soon as possible, particularly as a comprehensive verification system for the BWC has not yet been agreed upon. The VFP programme would thus contribute to further confidence building by providing at least partial verification.

In order to establish a system of common biological security, states should reconsider their biological defence policies. This should be done by transferring all of the *biological* activities permitted by the BWC to international programmes such as the Vaccines for Peace programme and the Global Epidemiological Surveillance System (now called the Program for Monitoring Emerging Diseases, ProMED), which would assume the task of abolishing the distinction between defence against natural outbreaks of diseases and diseases caused by the hostile use of DTAs. It would also abolish the difference between protection of the civilian population and of troops.

The UN Secretary-General is therefore asked to consider whether support could be given to the Vaccines for Peace programme and the Program for Monitoring Emerging Diseases as components of the discussion and examination of means to improve the implementation of Article X of the BWC, as was requested by the Third Review Conference.

3. Arms control, health care and technology transfer under the Vaccines for Peace programme

ERHARD GEISSLER*

I. Introduction

Infectious diseases are the major cause of mortality, 'causing more deaths than either cardiovascular diseases or cancer'.[1] Numerous bacteria and viruses causing infectious diseases are not only naturally dangerous to people, animals and plants, especially in developing countries, but can also be used for hostile purposes as biological weapon (BW) agents.[2] The same holds true for numerous toxins which not only cause natural intoxinations but which can also be used as toxin weapon (TW) agents.[3] Such bacteria, viruses and toxins can therefore be described as 'dual-threat agents' (DTAs).[4]

Vaccines are the most effective and cost-effective means to prevent infectious disease and intoxinations.[5] Research on and development of (R&D) and production of vaccines against DTAs is necessary for both civilian and military purposes, but military research into vaccines against DTAs frequently raises suspicion of possible offensive intentions.

II. Biological defence R&D raises suspicion of possible offensive intentions

The development, production, transfer, acquisition, stockpiling and use in war of BW and TW agents are prohibited by the Convention on the Prohibition of the Development, Production and Stockpiling of Bacteriological (Biological)

[1] National Institutes of Health (NIH), *NIH Strategic Plan: Panel Report on Immunology and Vaccines*, Final Draft, 7 Sep. 1992, p. 16.

[2] Biological weapons are living organisms and viruses (BW agents) that may be deliberately used, sometimes in combination with special means of delivery, for hostile purposes to cause disease or death in humans, animals or plants.

[3] TW agents are poisonous chemical compounds originally derived from living organisms that also may be used for hostile purposes. Because they are non-living, TW agents are chemical weapon (CW) agents.

[4] Geissler, E., 'Vaccines for Peace: an international program of development and use of vaccines against dual-threat agents', *Politics and the Life Sciences*, vol. 11, no. 2 (Aug. 1992), pp. 231–43.

[5] Lederberg, J., Shope, R. E. and Oaks, Jr, S. C. (eds), *Emerging Infections: Microbial Threats to Health in the United States* (National Academy Press: Washington, DC, 1992), p. 150; see also National Institutes of Health (note 1), p. 16.

* The author was supported by a grant from the Volkswagen Foundation and by the Stockholm International Peace Research Institute and is grateful for advice and comments from Félix C. Calderón, Eileen R. Choffnes, Jonathan Dean, Rolf Ekéus, Duane J. Gubler, Elisa D. Harris, Donald Ainslie Henderson, Darryl Howlett, Winfried Lang, Joshua Lederberg, Milton Leitenberg, S. Johan Lundin, Herbert Marcovich, Jack Melling, Joseph Melnick, Robert Mikulak, Stephen S. Morse, Graham S. Pearson, James A. Poupard, P. K. Ramachandran, Suryanarayan Ramachandran, Brad Roberts, Julian P. Perry Robinson, Barbara Rosenberg, Jonas Salk, Victor W. Sidel, Nicholas A. Sims, Robert L. Sinsheimer, Thomas Stock, Jonathan B. Tucker, Victor Utgoff, Mark L. Wheelis, John P. Woodall and Raymond A. Zilinskas.

and Toxin Weapons and on their Destruction, otherwise known as the Biological Weapons Convention (BWC); by the Protocol for the Prohibition of the Use in War of Asphyxiating, Poisonous or Other Gases, and of Bacteriological Methods of Warfare, the 1925 Geneva Protocol; and by the Chemical Weapons Convention (CWC).

However, Article I of the BWC explicitly permits the development, production, acquisition and stockpiling of DTAs 'for prophylactic, protective or other peaceful purposes'.[6] In response to the perceived renaissance of a BW and TW threat[7] and of continuing offensive BW and TW activities in the former Soviet Union,[8] extensive biological defence research programmes (BDRPs) were established in the United States and other countries from the early 1980s. The US BDRP is described as follows:

> The mission objectives of the program provide for:
>
> (*a*) medical protection and treatment capabilities such as vaccines, drugs, and patient management, and test procedures and reagents for biological agent identification in clinical specimens,
>
> (*b*) physical protective measures such as protective masks, clothing and shelters,
>
> (*c*) decontamination capability and
>
> (*d*) reconnaissance, detection and identification methods, particularly detection capabilities for environmental specimens in battlefield settings . . .
>
> Medical defense constitutes approximately two-thirds of the [US] BDRP.[9]

The main focus of the medical defence programme is the production of vaccines.

Nevertheless, many experts are convinced that 'the great difficulty of separating what constitutes "defensive research", particularly for biological weapons, from "offensive research"'[10] might raise suspicion: 'To mount a program specifically for medical "defense" against such [dual-threat] agents would appear to others in the world to be simply a continuation of an arms race in these weapons'.[11] It is therefore easy to agree with US Congressman Wayne Owens that 'growing expenditures on biological defense programs will continue to provoke international suspicion and, in the process, escalate the proliferation of biological weapons'.[12] This is especially true with regard to vaccine R&D and production and to threat analysis.

[6] See Article I of the BWC, annexe A, in this volume.

[7] See section VII below.

[8] See section VIII below.

[9] Huxsoll, D. L., then Commander of USAMRIID, testimony on 'Germ wars: biological weapons proliferation and the new genetics', 17 May 1989, in *Global Spread of Chemical and Biological Weapons*, Hearings before the Committee on Governmental Affairs and its Permanent Subcommittee on Investigations, US Senate (US Government Printing Office: Washington, DC, 1990), pp. 464–73, see especially pp. 465–66.

[10] Sidel, V., past President of the American Public Health Association, testimony on 'Assessing challenges and responses', 9 Feb. 1989, in *Global Spread of Chemical and Biological Weapons* (note 9), pp. 42–55, 512–18, see especially p. 51.

[11] See Sidel (note 10); see also MacLean, D., 'Ethics and biological defense research', ed. R. A. Zilinskas, *The Microbiologist and Biological Defense Research: Ethics, Politics, and International Security*, Annals of the New York Academy of Sciences, vol. 666 (New York Academy of Sciences: New York, 1992), pp. 100–11, see especially pp. 102–4.

[12] Owens, W., testimony in *Global Spread of Chemical and Biological Weapons* (note 9), pp. 180–82, see especially p. 181.

Threat analysis

Threat analysis is a component of the BDRPs. As early as 1942 the Canadian biological warfare expert committee M-1000 reported to the Ministry of Defence that 'Bacterial warfare . . . defence depends absolutely on a complete knowledge and understanding of the nature and the possible methods of using biological agents of disease and pests as offensive weapons'.[13] This assessment still holds true. In 1987, for example, the *Ad Hoc* Subgroup on the BDRP of the US Army Science Board concluded that the 'development, testing and evaluation of tactical and strategic doctrine and training in BD [biological defence] cannot be accomplished without adequate knowledge of potential threats'.[14]

How can adequate knowledge of potential threats be gained? One obvious way is by the improvement and testing of existing BW and TW agents, or the creation of new agents and their testing. If this is done ostensibly for defensive purposes such activities would not be prohibited by the BWC, even though they might lead to the development of new weapons. Thus threat analysis raises suspicion of possible offensive intentions, and such activities potentially pose tremendous danger for the personnel involved and for the environment, even without hostile activity, owing to the possibility of unintentional release of the agents under study.[15]

On the other hand, genetic manipulation of pathogenic agents and toxins, including DTAs, might be justified and necessary for non-military purposes such as the development of strategies to fight emerging viruses[16] or the development of immunotoxins or other novel drugs. Hence, prohibition of such dual-purpose activities is not possible. The only way of ensuring that such activities are carried out without creating suspicion of possible underlying offensive intention is to conduct them in a climate of complete transparency and openness.

Vaccines

R&D and production of vaccines against DTAs can also cause suspicion especially if carried out by the military and/or military contractors, since the incentives of those who develop and produce such vaccines are subject to interpretation.[17]

[13] *Second Report of the [Canadian] Committee M.1000*, 12 June 1942, National Archives of Canada, Record Group 77, 87-88/104, box 69, 36-5-0-9, quoted in Bryden, J., *Deadly Allies: Canada's Secret War 1937–1947* (McClelland & Stewart: Toronto, Ontario, 1989), p. 106.

[14] US Army Science Board, *Final Report of the Ad Hoc Subgroup on Army Biological Defense Research Program* (Department of the Army: Washington, DC, 1987), p. 3.

[15] This danger notwithstanding, participants at the Third Review Conference *did not* follow proposals forwarded by Peru and other delegations, as well as by numerous non-governmental experts, to emphasize that 'the creation, by any means, of biological agents or toxins with altered properties that might increase their usefulness as weapons agents is not justified under the BWC for any military purpose'. See Chile, Panama, Peru and Venezuela, 'Proposals for action by the Third Review Conference of the Biological Weapons Convention', Working Paper BWC/CONF.III/ COW/WP.2, 16 Sep. 1991. It is to be hoped that further measures to strengthen the BWC—to be adopted, for example, by the Fourth Review Conference—will address this important topic.

[16] See Morse, chapter 16, in this volume; Lederberg *et al.* (note 5).

[17] Strauss, H. and King, J., 'The fallacy of defensive biological weapon programmes', ed. E. Geissler, SIPRI, *Biological and Toxin Weapons Today* (Oxford University Press: Oxford, 1986), pp. 66–73; Woodall, J., 'An exceptional window of opportunity: comments on "Vaccines for Peace"', *Politics and the Life Sciences*, vol. 12, no. 1 (Feb. 1993), pp. 91–92.

Vaccines can be described as having a 'quadruple-capability'.[18] They are necessary: (*a*) to protect both civilians and troops against biological agents in peacetime, (*b*) to protect serviceman in conventional or other non-biological war, (*c*) to protect against biological attack, and (*d*) to prepare biological and toxin warfare and to provide a biological first-strike capability.

Infectious diseases have been the major cause of casualties among troops in all wars throughout history.[19] For example, US soldiers who served in Viet Nam were hospitalized more frequently because of infectious diseases than as a result of hostile action. Some of these diseases were caused by DTAs that are endemic in South-East Asia such as chikungunya virus, dengue virus and Japanese B encephalitis virus.[20] Another DTA, Korean haemorrhagic fever (Hantaan) virus, was first noted by Western physicians as a cause of troop loss during the Korean War when at least 3000 troops suffered from it.[21]

Military leaders therefore have legitimate reasons for providing vaccines which will protect their troops from naturally occurring infectious diseases, independently of whether these diseases are caused by DTAs or by pathogens not considered to be BW agents.

In addition, military leaders claim that vaccines must be developed to protect troops against biological and toxin warfare. The author shares the view of many experts that not even small contingents of troops can be effectively protected through vaccination against a *surprise* attack involving BW or TW agents. Vaccines act specifically against only one or a few agents, and they have to be provided weeks or even months before they generate their protective effects.[22] Of course, if vaccines are available, they should be used if military leaders anticipate a BW threat. US and British troops were vaccinated during the 1991 Persian Gulf War against anthrax and botulism.[23]

On the other hand, vaccines might also be used to protect personnel involved in offensive BW and TW R&D. For example, 'the program on medical defense against biological warfare was initiated at Fort Detrick, MD, in the 1950s primarily to protect the workers in the offensive program'.[24] Moreover, vaccines might be used to protect troops in advance of an intended attack, thereby providing a BW or TW first-strike capability, especially if vaccines are devel-

[18] Geissler, E., 'Contribution of confidence-building measures to greater transparency in activities directly related to the Biological Weapons Convention', ed. S. J. Lundin, *Views on Possible Verification Measures for the Biological Weapons Convention*, SIPRI Chemical & Biological Warfare Studies, no. 12 (Oxford University Press: Oxford, 1991), pp. 10–25, see especially p. 12.

[19] Poindexter, J. S., 'Responsible uses of microorganisms and microbiological products', in eds P. DeForest *et al.*, *Biotechnology, Professional Issues and Social Concerns* (American Association for the Advancement of Science (AAAS): Washington, DC, 1988), pp. 51–71.

[20] Boyles, C. A., DeCoufle, P. and O'Brien, T. R., 'Long-term health consequences of military service in Vietnam', *Epidemiologic Reviews*, vol. 11 (1989), pp. 1–32.

[21] Fields, B. N. (ed.), *Virology* (Raven Press: New York, 1985), pp. 1074–75; LeDuc, J. W. *et al.*, 'A retrospective analysis of sera collected by the Hemorrhagic Fever Commission during the Korean conflict', *Journal of Infectious Diseases*, vol. 162 (1990), pp. 1182–84.

[22] Strauss and King (note 17); Yamamoto, K. R., testimony in *Global Spread of Chemical and Biological Weapons* (note 9), pp. 485–97.

[23] '28 December 1990', Institute for Defense and Disarmament Studies, *Arms Control Reporter* (IDDS: Brookline, Mass.), sheet 701.B.65, Jan. 1991; '6 January 1991', sheet 701.B.67, Feb. 1991; '16 July 1991', sheet 701.B.77, Sep. 1991; Boatman, J., 'Biological vaccine for US troops', *Jane's Defence Weekly*, vol. 15, no. 2 (12 Jan. 1991), p. 44; *Biological Warfare: Role of Salk Institute in Army's Research Program*, Report to the Chairman, Committee on Governmental Affairs, US Senate, GAO/NSIAD-92-33 (US General Accounting Office: Washington, DC, Dec. 1991).

[24] Huxsoll, D. L., Patrick, III, W. C. and Parrott, C. D., 'Veterinary services in biological disasters', *Journal of the American Veterinary Association*, vol. 190, no. 6 (1987), pp. 714–22.

oped that are effective in protecting against a variant genetically modified agent constructed secretly in violation of the international norm against biological weapons. In fact in World War I, a major in the Medical Corps of the German Army proposed to attack London and the British seaports with plague bacteria (*Yersinia pestis*) and to protect from a British counterattack by producing '(in all secrecy) . . . sufficient quantities of plague serum'.[25] For such reasons even deterrence measures may include offensive aspects.[26]

Confidence-building measures

To counter reservations about the intent of military vaccine programmes, proposals were made—by a group of experts[27] prior to the Second Review Conference of the States Parties to the BWC, by Finland during the Conference,[28] and by Austria and Ireland[29] at the *Ad Hoc* Meeting of Scientific and Technical Experts—that States Parties provide information on the vaccination programmes of their armed forces. At the Second Review Conference, France also proposed that countries be invited to supply proof that the staff of high-containment facilities and military personnel have not been vaccinated against presumed BW agents.[30] These proposals were not accepted. Similar proposals made during the Third Review Conference[31] were also not accepted.

However, the Third Review Conference agreed on an additional confidence-building measure (CBM) requesting States Parties to provide declarations of vaccine production facilities 'producing vaccines licensed by the State Party for the protection of humans'.[32] This declaration is of limited value because parties are requested to provide information only on facilities producing vaccines already licensed, information which is usually general knowledge. More important in this context is the decision taken by the Third Review Conference to

[25] Winter, (–), 'The past and the future: reflections on the pros and cons of bacterial warfare', Dec. 1942, English trans. in *Intelligence Report: Translation of German Folder of Official Directives and Correspondence on B.W.*, MIS, War Department, ALSOS Mission, Washington, 31 July 1946, Secret, declassified 26 July 1983, pp. 54–63.

[26] As Stephenson and Weal point out, 'if one side could effectively shield itself from attack (or at least greatly reduce the effects of a nuclear [or biological, E. G.] exchange) while at the same time could increase its ability to take our enemy weapons and command posts, then a clear war-winning chance would have been created'. See Stephenson, M. and Weal, J., *Nuclear Dictionary* (Longman: Harlow, Essex, 1985), pp. 47–48. A similar situation exists with respect to the availability of vaccines against putative BW agents.

[27] Geissler, E. *et al.*, 'Conclusions and recommendations', in ed. E. Geissler, *Biological and Toxin Weapons Today* (note 17), pp. 121–29, see especially p. 128.

[28] Second Review Conference of the Parties to the Convention on the Prohibition of the Development, Production and Stockpiling of Bacteriological (Biological) and Toxin Weapons and on their Destruction, *Summary Record of the 5th Meeting,* BWC/CONF.II/SR.5, 19 Sep. 1986, p. 5.

[29] *Ad Hoc* Meeting of Scientific and Technical Experts from States Parties to the Convention on the Prohibition of the Development, Production and Stockpiling of Bacteriological (Biological) and Toxin Weapons and on their Destruction, *Report*, BWC/CONF.II/EX/2, Attachment, 'Proposal by Ireland and Austria on agenda item 4 (a)', 21 Apr. 1987, p. 30.

[30] Second Review Conference (note 28), *Summary Record of the 8th Meeting*, BWC/CONF.II/ SR.8, 22 Sep. 1986, p. 7.

[31] Third Review Conference of the Parties to the Convention on the Prohibition of the Development, Production and Stockpiling of Bacteriological (Biological) and Toxin Weapons and on their Destruction, *Final Document*, part III, Report of the Committee of the Whole, Annex I, 'Proposals put before the Committee of the Whole', BWC/CONF.III/23, part III, 'Confidence-building measures proposed by France', 13 Sep. 1991, p. 79; Finland, 'Proposal for a confidence-building measure: military vaccination programmes', 13 Sep. 1991, p. 93.

[32] *Final Document* of the Third Review Conference (note 31), Annex to Final Declaration on Confidence-Building Measures, BWC/CONF.III/23, part II, annex, pp. 46–47.

amend the CBM (already agreed by the Second Review Conference) on exchange of data on research centres by the request for detailed information on national biological defence R&D programmes. Some of the 'areas to be addressed shall include: prophylaxis, studies on pathogenicity and virulence',[33] (i.e., information on military R&D programmes).

To make vaccine R&D and production for military purposes and other biomedical activities directly related to the BWC more transparent, shifting such activities from military to civilian institutions, such as the US National Institutes of Health (NIH), has been proposed.[34] 'Any biological research that can be effectively conducted by a civilian agency should be removed from military supervision in order to defuse unnecessary suspicion about our [i.e., US] objectives'.[35] The openness gained by such a decision would have 'advantage(s) that far outweigh any risk. It makes US policy [and that of other states participating] credible. It helps in recruiting and keeping the most talented investigators and in exposing shoddy work or misguided lines of research. Openness accelerates progress through the kind of scientific interchange characteristic of the health sciences'.[36]

The proposal to establish an International Program of Development and Use of Vaccine (IPDUV)[37] focused on countering reservations about military misuse of R&D and production of vaccines and facilitating the provision of vaccines urgently needed in many countries, including developing nations. The proposal was initiated for two reasons. First, it was based on an assumption that a shift of vaccine R&D and other permitted activities from military to civilian facilities might provide the transparency needed to inspire confidence in BWC compliance, but might not function as a CBM in the approximately 11 countries suspected of, or known to be interested in, gaining access to biological weapons (see table 3.1).[38] Iraq's BW preparations, for example, were conducted not in a military institution but at the so-called National Center for Technical Research. Hence, national actions are insufficient; international measures are needed. The second reason for proposing the IPDUV emerged from a panel discussion with David L. Huxsoll, then Commander of the US Army Medical Research Institute for Infectious Diseases (USAMRIID), Fort Detrick, Maryland.[39] Huxsoll had explained that *one* of the reasons for the USAMRIID to develop vaccines against exotic pathogens and toxins was to serve civilians in underdeveloped

[33] See note 32, p. 31.

[34] 'A bill to require that all federal research, development, testing, and evaluation of the use of biological agents in the development of defenses against biological warfare be conducted by the Director of the National Institutes of Health, and for other purposes', H.R. 5241, introduced in the House of Representatives by Congressman Wayne Owens, Washington, DC, 11 Aug. 1988 (see annexe F in this volume).

[35] See Owens (note 12).

[36] Meselson, M., testimony in *Global Spread of Chemical and Biological Weapons* (note 9), pp. 207–11, pp. 498–505, see especially p. 209.

[37] Geissler, E., '"Biological and toxin weapons: the renewed threat", with comments by Stefan Noreen of the Swedish Mission to the UN', NGO Committee on Disarmament Forum at the UN on 2 Feb. 1989, transcript (NGO Committee on Disarmament: New York, 1989); Geissler, E., 'The international control of biological weapons' (interview), *geneWATCH*, vol. 6, no. 1 (Aug. 1989), pp. 1–4.

[38] *Countering the Chemical and Biological Weapons Threat in the Post-Soviet World*, Report of the Special Inquiry into the Chemical and Biological Threat of the Committee on Armed Services, US House of Representatives, 102nd Congress, 2nd session, 23 Feb. 1993 (US Government Printing Office: Washington, DC, 1993), p. 11.

[39] Huxsoll, D., 'Defensive biological and toxin weapons research in the United States and the Soviet Union', AAAS Annual Meeting, San Francisco, Calif., 17 Jan. 1989.

Table 3.1. Biological weapon status of selected countries, excluding Iraq[a]

State	Status
Algeria	No ambitions evident
Belarus	Capable
China	Potential possessor
Cuba	Remote threat
Egypt	Unlikely possessor
India	Potential possessor
Iran	Potential developer
Israel	Potential possessor
Jordan	Unlikely to seek capability
Kazakhstan	Unlikely possessor
North Korea	Potential possessor
South Korea	Possibly capable
Libya	Developer
Pakistan	Potentially capable
Russia	Possessor
South Africa	Potential possessor
Syria	Potential possessor
Taiwan	Potential developer
Ukraine	Capable(?)/unlikely possessor

[a] Iraq is subject to the obligations of United Nations Security Council Resolution 687 (the so-called Persian Gulf War cease-fire resolution) of 3 Apr. 1991. The text of Resolution 687 is reproduced in *SIPRI Yearbook 1992: World Armaments and Disarmament* (Oxford University Press: Oxford, 1992), pp. 525–30.

Source: Based on Reed, J., *Defence Exports: Current Concerns*, A Jane's Special Brief (Jane's Consultancy Services: Coulsdon, Surrey, Apr. 1993).

countries owing to a lack of interest in such vaccines on the part of the pharmaceutical industry.

As a consequence of several discussions the proposal was subsequently designated Vaccines for Peace (VFP), because it would contribute not only to strengthening the BWC but also to health care in and to technology transfer to developing countries—thus also indirectly acting as a peace-keeping measure by reducing tension between countries. The VFP programme should be administered by the World Health Organization (WHO), following the model of the WHO's Intensified Smallpox Eradication Programme, which through international co-operation eradicated one of the most serious plagues previously affecting humanity.[40]

III. Protection of civilians against dual-threat agents

Although they can be used for hostile purposes, current BW and TW agents originated and occur naturally (see table 3.2). Many of them are endemic in developing countries, though they occur less frequently than other pathogenic agents. Yellow fever, a disease caused by a DTA, ranks among the most frequent infectious and parasitic diseases and is the thirteenth most frequent such

[40] See Fenner, chapter 18, in this volume; see also Fenner, F. *et al.*, *Smallpox and its Eradication* (World Health Organization: Geneva, 1988).

Table 3.2. Dual-threat agents known to have caused natural outbreaks of disease, 1985–88

Bacillus anthracis[a]
Chikungunya virus[a]
Coxiella burnetti[a]
Crimean-Congo haemorrhagic fever virus[a]
Dengue virus[a]
Domoic acid (an algal neurotoxin)
Eastern encephalitis virus
Francisella tularensis[a]
Hantaan (Korean haemorrhagic fever) virus[a]
Hepatitis A virus
Japanese encephalitis virus
Rift Valley fever virus[a]
Tick-borne encephalitis virus[a]
Trichothecene mycotoxins[a]
Western encephalitis virus
Yellow fever virus[a]

[a] Indicates that a vaccine against this agent is developed by the US Army (*Biological Defense Research Program: Final Programmatic Environmental Impact Statement* (US Army Medical Research and Development Command: Frederick, Md., Apr. 1986), pp. A4-3–A4-4.

Source: Based on Woodall, J. P. and Geissler, E., 'Information on outbreaks of infectious diseases and intoxinations', ed. E. Geissler, *Strengthening the Biological Weapons Convention by Confidence-Building Measures*, SIPRI Chemical & Biological Warfare Studies, no. 10 (Oxford University Press: Oxford, 1990), pp. 105–24.

disease.[41] Other frequently occurring diseases caused by DTAs include dengue and dengue haemorrhagic fever, which now occur in most of the tropical world, Japanese encephalitis, which is endemic in Asia from India to Japan, and Korean haemorrhagic fever.[42]

Though mainly endemic to developing countries, DTAs potentially threaten industrialized countries, too, as causative agents of 'emerging diseases' (i.e., of diseases that are rapidly expanding their range with a corresponding increase in the number of cases of the disease).[43] DTAs might cause emerging diseases if introduced, for example, as a result of the steadily increasing international traffic and eroding borders, or by refugees. Therefore, in addition to vaccines against frequently occurring pathogens, vaccines against DTAs are also necessary for protecting civilians, in both industrialized and underdeveloped countries, against locally endemic diseases or outbreaks of exotic diseases.

Vaccine programmes

After successful completion of the Smallpox Eradication Programme in 1974,[44] the WHO, in co-operation with the United Nations Children's Fund (UNICEF),

[41] *Global Health Situations and Projections: Estimates* (World Health Organization: Geneva, 1992).

[42] *Implementation of the Global Strategy for Health for All by the Year 2000: Second Evaluation and Eighth Report on the World Health Situation* (World Health Organization: Geneva, in press); see also Calderón, chapter 4, Woodall, chapter 20, and Geissler, Calderón and Woodall, chapter 21, in this volume.

[43] Lederberg *et al.* (note 5); Morse, S. S., 'Viruses, emerging', ed. J. Lederberg, *Encyclopedia of Microbiology*, vol. 4 (Academic Press: San Diego, 1992), pp. 347–62; see also Morse, chapter 16, in this volume.

[44] Fenner (note 40).

launched the Expanded Programme on Immunization (EPI). The aim of the EPI is to immunize 60 million children annually against six major causes of mortality: diphtheria, measles, pertussis, poliomyelitis, tetanus and tuberculosis. By the end of 1991 some 80 per cent of the world's children had been immunized against the six diseases, thus saving millions of young lives.[45]

In addition, the Children's Vaccine Initiative (CVI) was launched in 1991 by the WHO, UNICEF, the United Nations Development Programme (UNDP), the World Bank and the Rockefeller Foundation with the support of over 100 representatives of UN organizations, public and private foundations, private industry and bilateral aid programmes.[46] The immediate goals of the CVI are to develop convenient measles, poliovirus and tetanus vaccines. The ultimate goal is the development of means of immunizing children with a single procedure at birth against all important disease threats.

In addition, a Programme for Vaccine Development (PVD) was launched by the WHO and the UNDP. Its goal is 'to employ newly developed technology to produce contemporary vaccines which are efficient in a developing world setting, and less expensive'.[47] The PVD funds research in transdisease vaccinology (i.e., those aspects of vaccine development common to more than one vaccine, for example, thermostability, slow release and adjuvants), research on dengue and Japanese encephalitis vaccines, as well as research in other priority areas.

Industrialized countries

In industrialized countries, new strategies may be necessary to protect people from emerging infectious diseases. The only major institutions engaged in R&D and production of vaccines against DTAs are military ones. Currently, vaccines against the marked agents listed in table 3.2 and against Argentinian and Bolivian haemorrhagic fever viruses, *Clostridium botulinum*, Lassa virus, Venezuelan encephalitis virus and several toxins are developed by the US Army and its contractors within the BDRP.[48] In 1988, the US Department of Defense (DOD) funded vaccine projects for roughly 25 viruses, 12 toxins and 4 species of bacteria.[49]

However, the US BDRP 'is a military program designed and focused to protect military personnel'.[50] Though military experts realize that there is also a

[45] Ransome-Kuti, O., 'Introductory remarks', in *Children's Vaccine Initiative: Report of the First Meeting of the Consultative Group*, Geneva, 16–17 Dec. 1991, WHO CVI/91.5 (World Health Organization: Geneva, 1991), pp. 15–16.

[46] 'New Children's Vaccine Initiative launched: better vaccines promised for the children of the world', *Press Release*, WHO/63 (World Health Organization: Geneva, 17 Dec. 1991); 'The Children's Vaccine Initiative', *World Health*, 46th year, no. 2 (Mar./Apr. 1993).

[47] WHO/UNDP Programme for Vaccine Development, *MIM/PVD/Priorities* (World Health Organization: Geneva, 1992).

[48] *Biological Defense Research Program: Final Programmatic Environmental Impact Statement* (US Army Medical Research and Development Command: Frederick, Md., Apr. 1989), pp. A4-3–A4-4; *Biological Warfare: Better Controls in DOD's Research Could Prevent Unneeded Expenditures,* Report to the Chairman, Committee on Governmental Affairs, US Senate, GAO/NSIAD-91-68 (US General Accounting Office: Washington, DC, Dec. 1990).

[49] Wright, S. and Ketcham S., 'The problem of interpreting the U.S. Biological Defense Research Program', ed. S. Wright, *Preventing a Biological Arms Race* (MIT Press: Cambridge, Mass., 1990), pp. 178–79; Burck, G. M., 'Biological, chemical, and toxin warfare agents', ed. S. Wright, pp. 352–67, see especially p. 366.

[50] Huxsoll (note 9), p. 471.

BW threat to the civilian population,[51] the BDRP is not designed or intended to provide protection for civilians. The responsibility for medical protection of the civilian population lies with the US Department of Health and Human Services.[52] However, civilians—both in industrialized countries and world-wide—are threatened not only by emerging pathogens but also by biological and toxin weapons. Civilians may be endangered even more than military personnel because they are not trained in nuclear, biological and chemical (NBC) defence, and they lack masks and protective suits. In biological warfare, as in chemical warfare, the ratio between civilian and military casualties is therefore estimated to be approximately 20: 1. If vaccines are developed with the declared intention of protecting against BW attack, they should be made available both to military personnel and to civilians, particularly because the US NIH, like other civilian institutions, has not thus far considered developing 'orphan vaccines'.[53]

It is obvious that the existing means for the provision of vaccines are not sufficient to protect against outbreaks of infectious diseases, be they caused by emerging pathogens or by the hostile dissemination of BW agents. Stockpiles of orphan vaccines are needed whether or not they will ever be used. This cannot be accomplished by traditional commercial vaccine R&D and production because, currently, a market for such vaccines does not exist. Until now the decision to develop a vaccine has been based *inter alia* on estimated development costs and market analysis, including the potential for liability problems.[54] In the USA the number of manufacturers of human vaccines decreased by 50 per cent during the 1980s, from 10 to 5 manufacturers.[55] Considering the importance of vaccines in combating emerging diseases, the US Committee on Emerging Microbial Threats to Health expects 'potentially catastrophic consequences if the [vaccine] development process is left entirely to free enterprise'.[56]

Developing countries

The situation in developing countries is even worse, particularly with regard to vaccines against DTAs. The majority of developing countries are not able to produce vaccines, nor is the pharmaceutical industry in developed countries interested in producing vaccines against exotic agents. Only a few vaccines now at the field-trial stage have been developed or produced by developing nations, partially in co-operation with other countries.[57] Vaccines against the DTAs dengue virus, Japanese encephalitis virus, Korean haemorrhagic fever (Hantaan) virus and yellow fever virus have been developed in Thailand,[58] India and Thai-

[51] Richardson, B., Acting Deputy Assistant Secretary for Chemical Matters, US DOD, testimony in *Global Spread of Chemical and Biological Weapons* (note 9), pp. 177–79, p. 196.

[52] Huxsoll (note 9), p. 471.

[53] The term 'orphan vaccines' is used to designate vaccines that have no significant market in the industrialized countries. See Morehouse, W., *Vaccine Production in the Third World: the Search for Alternatives, Report to UNIDO*, CLT 89/225, 12 Nov. 1989, p. 15.

[54] Lederberg *et al.* (note 5), p. 152.

[55] Lederberg *et al.* (note 5), p. 155.

[56] Lederberg *et al.* (note 5), pp. 155–56.

[57] Subrahmanyam, chapter 19, in this volume; see also Subrahmanyam, D., 'Development and transfer of vaccine technology: long-term challenges and strategies', unpublished, 1992.

[58] *Background Document on New Scientific and Technological Developments Relevant to the Convention on the Prohibition of the Development, Production and Stockpiling of Bacteriological (Biological) and Toxin Weapons and on their Destruction*, BWC/CONF.III/4, 26 Aug. 1991, pp. 18–33, see especially p. 20.

land,[59] Korea[60] and Nigeria,[61] respectively. However, even if some developing countries are able to produce their own vaccines, the production capacity may be insufficient for that country.[62] In addition, the development and production of vaccines often rely heavily on equipment, raw materials, media and the like imported from industrialized countries. The proportion of imported supplies can be as high as 80 per cent,[63] thereby posing a severe economic burden.

Until at least the late 1980s, the US Army Medical Research and Development Command said that one reason for developing vaccines against exotic pathogens was to benefit developing countries.[64] Indeed, vaccines and other medical supplies produced and stockpiled by the US Army Medical Research and Development Command have been used successfully for non-military medical needs in the USA and abroad, including in developing countries[65] and the former USSR.[66] It should be noted, however, that concern is sometimes expressed by developing countries that they might by used as a testing ground for vaccines and drugs developed in industrialized countries.[67] In fact, from the perspective of a DOD investigator 'the importance of this *field efficacy phase of vaccine testing* cannot be overemphasized' (emphasis added).[68]

Recommendations

To satisfy the demand for orphan vaccines, especially in developing countries, Robbins and Freeman[69] proposed *inter alia* that the UN create a special international institute: 'Such an institute could pursue new technologies that are particularly appropriate to Third World public health needs without having to earn rapid profits'. As 'the creation of such a center would be both costly and time-consuming, and the politics of international cooperation are brutal', Robbins and Freeman conclude, however, that the importance of vaccine development and production 'is too critical to the health of the world to rely at the start on an international center alone'. They suggest the additional establishment of vaccine development and production units in developing countries.

Taking into account the problems inherent in Robbins and Freeman's recommendations, Morehouse[70] proposed creating a Consultative Group for International Vaccine Research (CGIVR) to stimulate and co-ordinate R&D on new and improved vaccines for diseases of major importance in developing coun-

[59] McKinney, J., Private communication with the author, 1991.

[60] Moon, H. M., Private communication with the author, 1992.

[61] Ransome-Kuti (note 45).

[62] Freeman, P., 'Vaccines for Latin America: an innovative regional system', *geneWATCH*, vol. 6, no. 2-3 (1989), pp. 6–9.

[63] Roustai, M. H., 'Concerns and views of a vaccine producer of the developing countries', Paper submitted to the *Ad Hoc* Group of Governmental Experts to identify and examine potential verification measures, Geneva, 3 Apr. 1992.

[64] Huxsoll (note 39).

[65] Dasey, C. F., 'Medical benefits of the Biological Defense Research Program', *Politics and the Life Sciences*, vol. 9, no. 1 (1990), pp. 77–84.

[66] Dalrymple, J. M., 'DoD-sponsored virus vaccine development: an investigator's perspective', Zilinskas (note 11), pp. 202–17, see especially p. 210.

[67] Jayaraman, K. S., 'India and the United States agree on vaccine programme', *Nature*, vol. 332, no. 6161 (1988), p. 198.

[68] Dalrymple (note 66).

[69] Robbins, A. and Freeman, P., 'Obstacles to developing vaccines for the Third World', *Scientific American*, vol. 259, no. 5 (Nov. 1988), pp. 90–95.

[70] Morehouse (note 53), p. 30.

tries as well as an International Vaccine Corporation (IVC), a 'transnational enterprise for vaccine production and distribution'.

To overcome limitations in supplying orphan vaccines on a national basis, the Committee on Emerging Microbial Threats to Health recommended 'that the United States develop a means for generating stockpiles of selected vaccines and a "surge" capacity for vaccine development and production that could be mobilized to respond quickly to future infectious disease emergencies [which capacity] would require development of an integrated national process'.[71] The NIH Panel on Immunology and Vaccines also proposed establishment of a Human Vaccine Project, consisting of 5 to 10 national co-operative vaccine development consortia which would be multi-institution collaborations between academia, industry and the US federal government.[72]

The VFP programme would achieve some of the major goals of these proposals while simultaneously meeting the protection needs of both the civilian population and the military via its production of some orphan vaccines, namely those against DTAs. Hopefully, there would be less political objection to the VFP programme since it would not only solve health problems, but also contribute to arms control and peaceful international co-operation.

IV. Vaccine R&D and production for military purposes need not necessarily be carried out by the military

The proposal to shift biomedical research activities from military to civilian institutions[73] was rejected by representatives of the US DOD as an 'extremely bad recommendation'[74] because 'the provision of defensive materials is the responsibility of the Secretary of Defense, and that responsibility should not be divided. Moving the function elsewhere would increase costs, decrease program effectiveness, and would not result in any more openness than exists today'.[75] In addition, it is argued that 'the NIH is primarily concerned with disease threats to the United States. We [the Army] must be concerned with global threats and the prioritization of those threats'. [76]

The argument is also sometimes made that military vaccines have to be designed specifically and—in contrast to vaccines for civilian use—must protect, for example, from agents disseminated by aerosols.[77] However, as argued above, such vaccines should first be made available so that the civilian population can also be protected from a BW attack. Second, as the Assistant to the US Secretary of Defense explained, 'the development of protective vaccines and drugs requires the development of experimental animal models of diseases caused by various biological threat agents. Validation of such models requires that the baseline information on parameters such as the dose required for infection, severity, and pathogenesis of infection be identified. *These scientific*

[71] Lederberg *et al.* (note 5), pp. 158–59.

[72] National Institutes of Health (note 1), p. 47.

[73] See section II, subsection 'confidence-building measures'.

[74] Richardson, B., testimony in *Global Spread of Chemical and Biological Weapons* (note 9), pp. 177–79, see especially p. 179.

[75] Hinds, J., Deputy Assistant to the Secretary for Negotiations Policy, US DOD, testimony in *Global Spread of Chemical and Biological Weapons* (note 9), pp. 174–77, see especially p. 176.

[76] Richardson (note 74).

[77] See Pearson, chapter 14, in this volume.

efforts are largely common with those used in the civilian biomedical research' (emphasis added).[78]

Finally, it has been claimed that military facilities are more efficient at developing and producing vaccines against exotic agents than civilian institutions.[79] However, the experiences of the Persian Gulf War would indicate that the US BDRP is not as efficient as it could be.[80] For example, the vaccines provided to US military personnel involved in Operations Desert Shield and Desert Storm were not produced by the Army's contractor for biological warfare vaccines, but had to be purchased on the open market.[81] Senator John Glenn, Chairman of both the US Governmental Affairs Committee and the Armed Services Subcommittee on Manpower and Personnel, therefore felt it necessary to work 'with the Department of Defense to make sure that they follow the law and stop wasting taxpayers' money on research questions that could be better addressed by the National Institutes of Health or the *World Health Organization*' (emphasis added).[82]

As discussed above, the shift of activities directly related to the BWC from military institutions to civilian facilities appears to be confidence-building only in open societies. It is reasonable that military and political leaders in such countries are therefore reluctant to accept such unilateral recommendations. However, international actions such as the proposed VFP programme and the Global Epidemiological Surveillance System (GESS) might provide a means of satisfying the demand for vaccines, including the military demand, without raising suspicion of offensive intentions and without creating global instability in the field of BW and TW defence.

V. The BWC lacks universal adherence

The development, production, transfer and stockpiling of BW and TW agents are prohibited by the BWC, which now has 126 States Parties,[83] leaving approximately 65 countries that have not yet ratified or acceded to it.[84] The overwhelming majority of countries that have not yet ratified the BWC are developing countries, including nations in geopolitically sensitive regions. It is therefore important that participation in the BWC be expanded, but how can those states be convinced to renounce possession of the so-called 'poor man's

78 Barker, R. B., Assistant to the US Secretary of Defense, '1989: Questions [and answers] on the Biological Defense Research Program', in *Global Spread of Chemical and Biological Weapons* (note 9), pp. 474–84, see especially p. 478.

79 Huxsoll (note 39).

80 *Biological Warfare: Better Controls in DOD's Research Could Prevent Unneeded Expenditures*, Report to the Chairman, Committee on Governmental Affairs, US Senate, GAO/NSIAD-91-68 (US General Accounting Office: Washington, DC, Dec. 1990).

81 Letter dated 25 March 1991 from Richard Davis, Director, Army Issues, US GAO, National Security and International Affairs Division, addressed to the Hon. John Glenn, Chairman, Committee on Governmental Affairs, US Senate; *Biological Warfare: Role of Salk Institute in Army's Research Program* (note 23); Harsanyi, Z. P., 'Biological defense and industry', Zilinskas (note 11), pp. 219–29, see especially p. 225.

82 Glenn, J., 'Glenn faults Pentagon for misuse of research funds', *News Release*, Washington, DC, 11 Feb. 1992.

83 'Major multilateral arms control agreements', *SIPRI Yearbook 1993: World Armaments and Disarmament* (Oxford University Press: Oxford, 1993), annexe A, pp. 759–91.

84 *Arms Control: US and International Efforts to Ban Biological Weapons*, Report to the Hon. Albert Gore, Jr, US Senate, GAO/NSIAD-93-113 (US General Accounting Office: Washington, DC, Dec. 1992), p. 15.

atomic bombs'?[85] Nigeria pointed out during the Third Review Conference that implementation of Article X of the Convention (which calls for peaceful international co-operation, see below) could serve as an incentive to non-parties to become parties to the Convention.[86]

The Vaccines for Peace programme might provide such an incentive to ratify the Convention at least for those developing countries which are not regarded as 'key non-members',[87] because only States Parties to the Convention would be invited to participate in the programme and to share bioscientific and biotechnological progress with industrialized nations.

VI. The BWC is not free of loopholes

The BWC has been referred to as a 'milestone agreement—the first international binding instrument to prohibit and prevent the development, production and stockpiling of an entire category of weapons of mass destruction'.[88] Nevertheless, 'the Convention has not been effective in stopping the development of biological weapons'.[89] The BWC may not be able to eliminate the BW and TW threat because it contains serious loopholes, some of which became obvious only after the rapid scientific progress caused by the introduction of molecular biotechnology.[90] This continues to be the case in the new geopolitical situation resulting from the peaceful end of the cold war.

For example, the BWC does not restrict research on potential BW and TW agents. In addition, it prohibits only the development, production and stockpiling of types and quantities of agents 'that have no justification for prophylactic, protective, and other peaceful purposes'.[91] It is easy to agree with the Permanent Select Committee on Intelligence of the US House of Representatives that 'these provisions . . . contain important gaps: it would be hard to name a biological agent that could not be produced under the rationale of "prophylactic, protective or other peaceful purposes". Even the production of quantities of anthrax might not necessarily be a breach of the Convention'.[92]

[85] *Countering the Chemical and Biological Weapons Threat in the Post-Soviet World* (note 38), p. 9; see also Carus, W. S., *The Poor Man's Atomic Bomb? Biological Weapons in the Middle East*, Washington Institute Policy Papers, no. 23 (Washington Institute for Near East Policy: Washington, DC, 1991).

[86] Statement by Ambassador I. C. Olisemeka, Nigeria, to the Third Review Conference of the Biological Weapons Convention, 12 Sep. 1991.

[87] 'Key non-members' are several Middle Eastern and North African countries with significant military capabilities, including Algeria, Egypt, Israel, Morocco and Syria. They have linked membership to the BWC to regional security interests. See *Arms Control* (note 84), pp. 15–16.

[88] 'Message to the participants at the XIIth Kühlungsborn Colloquium from Mr Yashushi Akashi, Under-Secretary General for Disarmament Affairs, United Nations', eds Geissler, E. and Haynes, R. H., *Prevention of a Biological and Toxin Arms Race and the Responsibility of Scientists* (Akademie-Verlag: Berlin, 1991), pp. xv–xvi.

[89] *Arms Control* (note 84), p. 2.

[90] See section VII below.

[91] See Article I of the BWC, annexe A, in this volume.

[92] *Soviet Biological Warfare Activities*, Permanent Select Committee on Intelligence, US House of Representatives, June 1980, p. 2, quoted by Leitenberg, M., 'Soviet activities related to biological weapons', *Arms Control*, vol. 12, no. 2 (Sep. 1991), pp. 161–90, see especially p. 168.

VII. Scientific and technological developments

Participants at the Second and Third Review Conferences of the BWC[93] and numerous governmental and non-governmental experts expressed concern that the rapid progress in many areas of molecular biotechnology, including genetic engineering, could contribute to increasing the danger of biological and toxin warfare.[94] 'Genetic engineering' or 'gene technology' is a complex of methods whereby genetic material is directly analysed and modified. Together with new techniques such as cell technology, protein engineering, immune technology and classical (fermentation) biotechnology, it forms 'molecular biotechnology'.

One of the military implications of molecular biotechnology is that new methods of vaccine development have arisen. Concern has therefore been raised that 'an increased protection capability might be an inducement to use biological warfare, since the instigator has a decreased risk of being harmed by his own actions'.[95] The expertise gained and the techniques used in the course of developing genetically engineered vaccines[96] might also be used to construct consummate, novel BW and TW agents. Single or even multiple foreign genes, including toxin genes, can be inserted into the genetic material of some viruses. Highly contagious viruses armed with additional toxin genes could be very efficacious combinations of BW and TW agents. Such types of agents would represent pathogens not found in nature but created in the laboratory (in contrast to 'classical' BW and TW agents); the present author has proposed that they be designated 'second-generation biological weapons'.[97]

For these and other reasons, participants at the Third Review Conference shared the view of the United States that the 'confidence derived from the belief that certain technical problems would make biological weapons unattractive for the foreseeable future has eroded'.[98] Consequently, the USA and other nations established extensive biological research programmes involving more than 200 military and non-military facilities.

Concern was raised following the establishment of these programmes, since even clear-cut defensive activities might require the handling of highly infectious pathogens and super-toxic toxins. Work with pathogens and toxins poses

[93] Final Document of the Second Review Conference of the Parties to the Convention on the Prohibition of the Development, Production and Stockpiling of Bacteriological (Biological) and Toxin Weapons and on their Destruction, Part II, *Final Declaration*, BWC/CONF.II/13, 30 Sep. 1986; Final Document of the Third Review Conference of the Parties to the Convention on the Prohibition of the Development, Production and Stockpiling of Bacteriological (Biological) and Toxin Weapons and on their Destruction, Part II, *Final Declaration*, BWC/CONF.III/23, 1991.

[94] For reasons summarized, for example in Piller, C. and Yamamoto, K. R., *Gene Wars: Military Control over the New Genetic Technologies* (Beech Tree Books, William Morrow: New York, 1988); Geissler, E., 'New assessments of the potential value of BW and TW agents', ed. E. Geissler, *Strengthening the Biological Weapons Convention by Confidence-Building Measures*, SIPRI Chemical & Biological Warfare Studies, no. 10 (Oxford University Press: Oxford, 1990), pp. 15–31; Wright (note 49); Geissler, E., 'Molecular biotechnology and the Third Review of the Biological Weapons Convention', eds H. G. Brauch *et al.*, *Controlling Military Research & Development and Exports of Dual Use Technologies as a Problem of Disarmament and Arms Control Policy in the 1990s* (VU University Press: Amsterdam, 1992), pp. 95–108.

[95] *Summary of the Genetic Engineering Expert Panel*, Submitted to Assistant Secretary of State James Malone, 26 May 1981 (US Department of State: Washington, DC, 1981), p. 4.

[96] See Horaud, chapter 9, in this volume.

[97] Geissler, E., 'Biological and toxin weapons and the responsibility of scientists', Geissler and Haynes (note 88), pp. 3–28, see especially p. 7.

[98] See note 58, pp. 27–33, see especially p. 33.

a threat both to the personnel involved and to the public.[99] There would be an additional threat if R&D activities involving putative BW and TW agents were carried out under conditions of insufficient technical competence and responsibility. This is another reason to request both universal adherence to the BWC and the complete transparency of all R&D programmes involving pathogenic biological agents and toxins, including biological defence programmes. The author of this chapter strongly agrees with the notion that the 'development and production of biological weapons by countries of insufficient technical competence, outside maximum containment facilities, is a universal threat even without their actual use'.[100]

VIII. Verification

Progress in molecular biotechnology and the provisions of the BWC for 'peaceful' activities cause additional concern because the BWC and the Geneva Protocol both lack verification measures. The difficulties of verification, particularly in the BW and TW areas, are well known. During the Third Review Conference many delegations pointed out that verification would be highly advisable but difficult to achieve since 'activities necessary for the development of a BW offensive arsenal are virtually identical to most legitimate activities in the field of microbiology'.[101] It is impossible, for example, to be certain that genetic engineering of viral vectors has been conducted in order to develop a second-generation BW agent[102] or a vaccine against a DTA, and whether the latter activity has been done for defence purposes or with the intention of acquiring a first-strike capability. Complete verification will thus not be possible. Hence the US Government, convinced that incomplete verification is worse than no verification, argued that 'the Convention is not effectively verifiable and we do not know any way to make it so'.[103]

This is exemplified most dramatically by the successful attempts of the former Soviet Union to hide its offensive BW programme and to mislead large factions of BW analysts,[104] and by the inability of the USA and its allies to prove these violations. Beginning in 1980[105] the USA repeatedly claimed that the Soviet Union was conducting an offensive BW programme and that a 1979 outbreak of anthrax in the city of Sverdlovsk (now Ekaterinburg) had been caused by an accident in a BW facility.[106] However, 10 years later the US Gov-

[99] Experience gained in experimentation with pathogenic micro-organisms has demonstrated an average of one to five infections per 10^6 working hours. See Israeli, E., 'Biosafety in biotechnological, processes', *Advances in Biotechnological Processes*, vol. 6 (1986), pp. 1–30. This means that up to five infections take place per 500 persons involved per year.

[100] Ezz, E. A., 'Development and production of biological weapons by countries of insufficient technical competence, outside maximum containment facilities, is a universal threat even without their actual use', Paper presented at Pugwash Meeting no. 178, 16th Workshop of the Pugwash Study Group on Chemical Warfare. Geneva, 26–27 Jan. 1991.

[101] Statement by Ambassador Gerard Errera, France, to the Third Review Conference, 12 Sep. 1991.

[102] See section VII above.

[103] Statement by Ambassador Ronald F. Lehman, II, USA, to the Third Review Conference, 10 Sep. 1991.

[104] Including not only this author.

[105] See Leitenberg, chapter 8, in this volume.

[106] Zilinskas, R. A., 'Anthrax in Sverdlovsk: epidemic or BW?', *Bulletin of the Atomic Scientists*, vol. 39, no. 6 (1983), pp. 24–27; Meselson, M., 'The Biological Weapons Convention and the Sverdlovsk anthrax outbreak of 1979', *F.A.S. Public Interest Report*, vol. 41, no. 7 (Sep. 1988), pp. 1–6; see also Abramova, F. A. *et al.*, 'Pathology of inhalational anthrax in 42 cases from the Sverdlovsk outbreak of

ernment still lacked conclusive evidence of a violation of the BWC by the former Soviet Union. During a US Senate Committee on Governmental Affairs hearing in 1989 the following dialogue took place (emphasis added):[107]

Chairman Glenn.[108] We have, under Article VI of the [BW] Convention, a complete right to lodge officially complaints when there are violations of the BWC. Why didn't we lodge those complaints on the Soviet Union . . . ?

. . .

Why didn't we file an official complaint?[109]

Ambassador Holmes.[110] We have, Mr. Chairman, under Article V of the treaty, sought bilateral consultations with the Soviets to seek explanations on all these questions. And we also have, in the review conferences—in the 5-year review conferences, we have also sought answers to these violations. . . .

Chairman Glenn. But we can file an official complaint with the UN under this. Why don't we do that when we know there are violations, instead of bilateral talks and discussions at other meetings and things like that? Why don't we file them?

If we are really as concerned as all your statements indicate we are concerned, it would seem to me we would be taking tougher action than we are taking.

Ambassador Holmes: Our basic approach is *to try to get the facts* before we go public with accusations of violations.

Chairman Glenn. *Have we lacked the facts*?

Ambassador Holmes: *Yes*.

Chairman Glenn: Have we lacked sufficient evidence in these cases that we could not file an official complaint?

Ambassador Holmes: To my understanding, we have never been able to get sufficient information to establish the facts on these violations, and so we have pursued the question through bilateral contacts.

We are continuing—we have never gotten, for example, a satisfactory explanation on the 1979 outbreak of pulmonary anthrax at Sverdlovsk. But what we are now trying to do is to get more information on the facility, the biological facility at Sverdlovsk, and we are pursuing that.

In the meantime Russia's President Boris Yeltsin admitted that the epidemic was caused by an accident in a military facility. He also acknowledged that the former Soviet Union had carried out an offensive BW programme which continued until early 1992. Likewise, the Russian Ambassador to the Conference on Disarmament (CD) informed members of the US National Security and International Affairs Division 'that Russia admitted having an offensive BW program from the 1940s to March 1992'.[111] Yeltsin contended in this connection that Soviet military leaders obviously even misled leaders of the Soviet

1979', *Proceedings of the National Academy of Sciences, USA*, vol. 90 (Mar. 1993), pp. 2291–94; Meselson, M., 'New evidence on the 1979 Soviet anthrax epidemic', *ASA Newsletter*, 93-2, no. 35 (8 Apr., 1993), pp. 1, 5.

[107] *Global Spread of Chemical and Biological Weapons* (note 9), pp. 190–91.

[108] Senator John Glenn, Chairman of the Committee on Governmental Affairs and Vice Chairman of the Permanent Subcommittee on Investigations, US Senate.

[109] Lodging a complaint with the Security Council as established by Article VI of the BWC is currently the only formal mechanism for addressing a suspected violation of the Convention.

[110] H. Allen Holmes, Assistant Secretary for Politico-Military Affairs, US Department of State.

[111] *Arms Control* (note 84), p. 53.

Government and the Communist Party with respect to secret offensive BW activities.[112] Hence, verification may be difficult even within a country.

The VFP programme would contribute to confidence-building and verification because its implementation would require specific verification measures: (*a*) to ensure that all vaccine R&D and production activities within the programme would be in accordance with the provisions of the BWC, and (*b*) to prevent misuse of the programme for proliferation purposes. These measures are discussed in section XI below and in section X of chapter 21. The VFP programme would additionally contribute to verification because it includes the establishment of priority lists of DTAs.[113] According to the US Department of State,[114] establishment of a list of micro-organisms for the purpose of export controls (i.e., of DTAs) would be the first step towards a verification regime.

IX. Prevention of proliferation vs. enhancement of co-operation

The BWC contains loopholes and is also weakened by an obvious contradiction between Articles III and X. Article X requests States Parties to participate in peaceful co-operation and exchange in microbiology (and biotechnology),[115] while Article III urges States Parties not to transfer BW and TW agents, equipment or means of delivery.[116]

Though contradictory both obligations are necessary. The intention of Article III is to reduce the dangerous proliferation of BW and TW agents and corresponding equipment and technology. Proliferation is a real problem as the results of the United Nations Special Commission on Iraq (UNSCOM) investigations of Iraq's BW and TW preparations *inter alia* have demonstrated.[117] In addition, during the 20 years of the existence of the BWC 'the number of countries considered to be developing or recently engaged in offensive BW programs has risen from 4 in 1972 to at least 10 in 1992'.[118] For these reasons, it is easy to agree with a statement by the Director of the US Arms Control and Disarmament Agency, that the 'most urgent arms control tasks are related less to the traditional questions of the East–West military balance and more to ensuring that weapons of mass destruction and their means of delivery do not proliferate . . . Our expanded agenda must ensure that weapons of mass destruction do not come under the control of irresponsible entities'.[119]

[112] Yeltsin, B., interview, Komsomol'skaya *Pravda*, 27 May 1992; Smith, R. J., 'Soviet germ caused epidemic in '79', *Los Angeles Times*, 16 June 1992; see also Leitenberg, chapter 8, in this volume.

[113] See section XII, subsection 'vaccines covered', below.

[114] As quoted in *Arms Control* (note 84), pp. 17–18.

[115] See Article X of the BWC, annexe A, in this volume.

[116] See Article III of the BWC, annexe A, in this volume.

[117] 'Second UN biological weapons inspection team concludes mission to Iraq', *UN Press Release*, 31 Oct. 1991; see also *Countering the Chemical and Biological Weapons Threat in the Post-Soviet World* (note 38), pp. 18–22; Ekéus, R., 'The United Nations Special Commission on Iraq: activities in 1992', *SIPRI Yearbook 1993* (note 83), pp. 691–703.

[118] *Arms Control* (note 84), p. 16; see also *Countering the Chemical and Biological Weapons Threat in the Post-Soviet World* (note 38), pp. 9–25.

[119] 'Arms control in a post cold war era', UNIDIR 10th Anniversary Public Lecture Series, Speech by Ronald F. Lehman, II, Director, US Arms Control and Disarmament Agency, Geneva, 12 Sep. 1991.

One means to prevent BW, CW and TW proliferation is through the implementation of export controls.[120] BW and TW controls have been instituted by Germany,[121] Norway,[122] the USA[123] and recently also by Russia.[124] Finland and Sweden have established controls on high-level biological containment facilities, and Switzerland has instituted controls on certain dual-use equipment.[125] The DTAs included on the lists developed by the Australia Group and used by Germany, Norway and the USA for export control purposes and those on the Russian list are reproduced in table 3.3. Nevertheless the efficacy of export controls for prevention of proliferation is limited, as discussed below, quite apart from the fact that they hamper peaceful international co-operation.

Lists of DTAs

Export controls usually rely on lists. A prerequisite for the establishment of lists of DTAs is a definition of BW and TW agents,[126] but such definitions do not exist. The negotiators of the BWC refused to agree on definitions and lists because they were aware that progress in microbiology would lead to the discovery of new agents that might be suitable for biological and toxin warfare, and because there was no apparent agreement on a supervisory body or on the involvement of international agencies, such as the WHO, that would monitor scientific progress and revise such lists.[127]

There are, of course, national definitions and national lists. The US DOD, for example, 'defines a "biological warfare threat" as a biological agent that is assessed (or "validated") by the intelligence community [the Armed Forces Medical Intelligence Center, in conjunction with other intelligence agencies] as being developed or produced as a weapon'. The US list of validated BW threat agents 'includes biological agents that are in various stages of research and development . . . The list also indicates the degree of certainty of the threat based on available intelligence information . . . The list is then used by the [US Army] Academy of Health Sciences . . . to establish *vaccine requirements*

[120] Harris, E. D., 'Chemical and biological weapons: preventing the spread of the "poor man's atomic bomb"?', ed. J.-F. Rioux, *Limiting the Proliferation of Weapons* (Carlton University Press: Ottawa, Canada, 1992), pp. 75–97.

[121] 'Prevention of BW proliferation: tightening of the foreign trade and payments controls since the beginning of 1989', in 'Working paper: legislation in the Federal Republic of Germany on the prohibition of biological weapons', submitted to the Third Review Conference, BWC/CONF.III/7, 10 Sep. 1991, pp. 5–11.

[122] 'Biological agents and dual use biological equipment: Norwegian export control', Paper submitted to the *Ad Hoc* Group of Governmental Experts to Identify and Examine Potential Verification Measures from a Scientific and Technical Standpoint, BWC/CONF.III/VEREX/ NONE 33, 24 Nov. 1992.

[123] *Arms Control* (note 84), pp. 5–6, 29–37.

[124] Presidential Directive, 'On the introduction of controls on the export from the Russian Federation of pathogens, their genetic variations, and fragments of genetic material, which could be used in the creation of bacteriological (biological) and toxic weapons', Russian Federation President's directive no. 711-rp, 17 Nov. 1992, *Rossiyskiye Vesti* (Moscow), 5 Dec. 1992, p. 3 (in Russian).

[125] According to an Australian Embassy official quoted in *Arms Control* (note 84), p. 36. See also Stock, T., 'Chemical and biological weapons: developments and proliferation', *SIPRI Yearbook 1993* (note 83), pp. 259–92.

[126] For a discussion of the problems of defining BW and TW agents, see Geissler, E., 'Introduction', ed. E. Geissler, *Biological and Toxin Weapons Today* (note 17), pp. 1–20, see especially pp. 4–5.

[127] Kischlat, W.-D., *Das Übereinkommen über das Verbot der Entwicklung, Herstellung und Lagerung bakteriologischer (biologischer) Waffen und von Toxin-Waffen sowie über die Vernichtung solcher Waffen* (Haag & Herchen Verlag: Frankfurt am Main, 1976), p. 123.

Table 3.3. Putative anti-personnel biological warfare agents[a]

	WHO[b]	A&K[c]	BDP[d]	GER[e]	AU[f]	RUS[g]
Bacillus anthracis	+	+	+	+	+	+
Brucella spp.	+			+	+[h]	+[h]
Chikungunya virus	+	+	+	+	+	+
Chlamydia psittaci				+	+	+
Clostridium botulinum					+	+
Coxiella burnetti	+	+	+	+	+	+
Crimean-Congo haemorrhagic fever virus		+	+		+	+
Dengue virus	+	+		+	+	+
Eastern encephalitis virus		+	+	+	+	+
Ebola virus		+	+	+	+	+
Francisella tularensis	+	+	+	+	+	+
Hantaan (Korean haemorrhagic fever) virus		+	+		+	+
Influenza virus	+			+		
Japanese encephalitis virus	+				+	+
Junin (Argentinian haemorrhagic fever) virus		+	+	+	+	+
Lassa fever virus		+	+	+	+	+
Legionella pneumophila				+		+
Lymphocytic choriomeningitis virus		+			+	+
Machupo (Bolivian haemorrhagic fever) virus		+	+	+	+	+
Marburg virus		+		+	+	+
Monkeypox virus				+	+	+
Pseudomonas mallei				+	+	+
Pseudomonas pseudomallei				+	+	
Rickettsia prowazekii	+			+	+	
Rickettsia rickettsii	+			+	+	
Rift Valley fever virus	+	+	+	+	+	+
Salmonella typhi	+			+	+	+
Shigella dysenteriae					+	+
Smallpox virus	+	+	+	+	+	+
Tick-borne encephalitis virus[i]	+	+	+		+	+
Venezuelan encephalitis virus	+	+	+	+	+	+
Vibrio cholerae				+	+	+
Western equine encephalitis virus		+	+		+	+
White pox virus					+	+
Yellow fever virus	+	+	+	+	+	+
Yersinia pestis	+			+	+	+

[a] Agents listed only by one of the references (i.e., o'nyong-nyong virus, covered only by the WHO list) are not included in this table. Several additional agents are covered in the Russian list, including 'Genetically altered micro-organisms producing the following toxins: botulinum, gas gangrene, *Staphylococcus* enterotoxin, ricin, saxitoxin, dysentery toxin, conotoxin, tetrodotoxin, verotoxin, abrin, cholera toxin, tetanus toxin, trichothecene mycotoxins'. See Presidential Directive, 'On the introduction of controls on the export from the Russian Federation of pathogens, their genetic variations, and fragments of genetic material, which could be used in the creation of bacteriological (biological) and toxic weapons', Russian Federation President's directive no. 711-rp, 17 Nov. 1992, *Rossiyskiye Vesti* (Moscow), 5 Dec. 1992, p. 3 (in Russian).

[b] Agents considered to be BW agents in the 1970 WHO study *Health Aspects of Chemical and Biological Weapons,* Report of a WHO Group of Consultants (WHO: Geneva, 1970).

[c] Agents considered to be BW agents by Anderson, III, W. C. and King, J. M., *Vaccine and Antitoxin Availability for Defense against Biological Threat Agents,* US Army Health Care Studies Division, report no. 83-002 (US Army Health Services Command: Fort Sam Houston, Tex., 1983).

Table 3.3 *cont.*

[d] Agents considered in the US BDRP, see *Biological Defense Research Program: Final Programmatic Environmental Impact Statement* (US Army Medical Research and Development Command: Frederick, Md., Apr. 1989), pp. A4-3–A4-4.

[e] Agents considered to be BW agents by Germany, see 'Kriegswaffenliste. II. Biologische Waffen', in 'Gesetz über die Kontrolle von Kriegswaffen', *Bundesgesetzblatt*, Teil 1, no. 64 (1990), pp. 2506–19, see especially pp. 2515–16.

[f] Agents considered by the Australia Group and by the USA for export control, see *Arms Control: US and International Efforts to Ban Biological Weapons*, Report to the Hon. Albert Gore, Jr, US Senate, GAO/NSIAD-93-113 (US General Accounting Office: Washington, DC, Dec. 1992), p. 15.

[g] Presidential Directive (note *a*).

[h] *Brucella abortus, B. melitensis* and *B. suis.*

[i] Russian spring–summer encephalitis virus.

needed to counter biological warfare threat agents'[128] (emphasis added). Although the list is secret,[129] it can be concluded from a US General Accounting Office (GAO) report[130] that it includes *Coxiella burnetti*, eastern (equine) encephalitis virus, *Francisella tularensis*, smallpox virus, Venezuelan (equine) encephalitis virus and western (equine) encephalitis virus. More comprehensive lists of putative BW and TW agents have been compiled previously by non-governmental experts[131] from the open literature.[132]

At the Third Review Conference numerous countries recommended the creation of *agreed* official lists of microbiological or other biological agents and toxins that have potential as weapons. In this context Germany mentioned that the decision of the negotiators of the BWC to refrain from defining biological agents 'is no longer consistent with the standard we should now expect, especially in the light of our experience in negotiating a ban on chemical weapons'.[133] A step forward has been taken by the Australia Group[134] which developed lists on which other export control lists (e.g., that of the USA) are based (see table 3.3).

Although such lists are useful, the proliferation of BW and TW agents and of corresponding technology cannot be prevented by regulating the transfer of agents, technology and information. This is because of the dual-threat character of the agents and the dual-use character of the related know-how and technology. Restriction of the transfer of DTAs and of corresponding know-how

[128] *Biological Warfare* (note 23), pp. 2–3.

[129] Welch, T. J., *Biological Warfare Testing*, Hearing before the Subcommittee on Arms Control, International Security and Science of the Committee on Foreign Affairs and the Subcommittee on Energy and Military Installations and Facilities of the Committee on Armed Services, House of Representatives, 3 May 1988 (US Government Printing Office: Washington, DC, 1988), p. 32.

[130] *Biological Warfare* (note 23), p. 14.

[131] See, for example, Geissler, E., 'A new generation of biological weapons', ed. E. Geissler, *Biological and Toxin Weapons Today* (note 17), pp. 21–35, see especially pp. 22–23; Burck (note 49); *Proposals for the Third Review Conference of the Biological Weapons Convention*, Report of the Federation of American Scientists Working Group on Biological and Toxin Weapons Verification, revised, Oct. 1990, reprinted in Geissler and Haynes (note 88), pp. 485–505.

[132] *Biological Defense Research Program* (note 48); Anderson, III, W. C. and King, J. M., *Vaccine and Antitoxin Availability for Defense Against Biological Threat Agents*, US Army Health Care Studies Division, report, no. 83-002 (US Army Health Services Command: Fort Sam Houston, Tex., 1983).

[133] Statement by Ambassador Dr Adolf Ritter von Wagner, Federal Republic of Germany, to the Third Review Conference of the BWC, 10 Sep. 1991.

[134] The 26-country Australia Group, which was formed in 1984, includes the NATO countries (except Iceland and Turkey), the Commission of the European Communities, and Argentina, Australia, Austria, Hungary, Ireland, Japan, New Zealand, Sweden and Switzerland.

and technology might also conflict with the obligations laid down in Article X of the BWC. The same holds true with respect to the danger of 'human proliferation' (see section XI below).[135] A 'brain drain' from North to South is essential for peaceful international co-operation but is extremely dangerous if it supports weapon development.

The Vaccines for Peace programme, if possible in connection with the GESS programme, might contribute to enhancing peaceful international co-operation in biotechnology and microbiology in a manner so transparent that concern about possible proliferation would be lessened. A prerequisite would be that all participants in these programmes provide full information on all of their activities to the bodies supervising the programmes, and that their facilities would be open to inspections carried out under these programmes.

X. The technology gap between North and South increases

Proliferation of weapons of mass destruction and of corresponding technology cannot be prevented by restricting technology and information transfer as the Iraqi case demonstrates; 'the gap between developed and developing countries, even in the availability of information on the use of biotechnology and genetic engineering for peaceful purposes, has further widened',[136] even though protection against infectious and toxic agents requires 'global cooperative efforts'.[137]

Then UN Secretary-General Javier Perez de Cuellar noted in his message to the Third Review Conference that 'it is essential . . . to ensure that, on the one hand, the Convention is implemented in a manner that does not hamper the economic and technological development of States Parties, as called for in the Convention itself, and that, on the other hand, the Convention is not outpaced or its effectiveness weakened by scientific and technological advances'.[138]

Accordingly, the participants of the Second and the Third Review Conferences agreed that the provisions of Article III 'should not be used to impose restrictions and/or limitations on the transfer for purposes consistent with the objectives and the provisions of the Convention of scientific knowledge, technology, equipment and materials' under Article X.[139]

Nevertheless, since the danger of proliferation exists, the joint establishment of the VFP and GESS programmes might provide a realistic means by which industrialized countries could share progress in the biosciences with developing countries which are States Parties to the BWC. This kind of sharing should

[135] Opening statement by Senator Sam Nunn, 5 Feb. 1992, in *Assisting the Build-Down of the Former Soviet Military Establishment*, Hearings before the Committee on Armed Services, US Senate, 102nd Congress, 2nd session (US Government Printing Office: Washington, DC, 1992), pp. 1–4, see especially p. 2.

[136] Statement by Ambassador Prakash Shah, India, at the Third Review Conference of the BWC, 11 Sep. 1991.

[137] 'Because these [BW] agents do not respect national borders and constitute universal threat to the health of the humans all over the world their combat requires global cooperative efforts. Research work on biological agents for peaceful and humanitarian purposes . . . should not be monopolized, but shared with all nations and should have no commercial value', see Ezz (note 100).

[138] 'Message of the Secretary-General of the United Nations to the Third Review Conference of the Parties to the Biological Weapons Convention, Geneva, 9–27 September 1991', *Press Release*, DC/1744 (UN Information Service: Geneva, 9 Sep. 1991).

[139] Final Document of the Second Review Conference (note 93), p. 4; Final Document of the Third Review Conference (note 93), p. 12.

raise fewer concerns about military misuse of the specialists, information, biological agents, equipment, skill and technology transferred.

XI. Conversion of facilities involved in BW programmes

A new situation evolved in the early 1990s as a result of world-wide efforts to reduce arms production and enhance conversion, and especially as a consequence of the disintegration of the former Soviet Union. The problem of conversion has replaced many traditional issues on the security agenda.[140]

Conversion is usually discussed in terms of nuclear weapons and nuclear specialists, but similar problems are raised by chemical and biological weapons and the corresponding specialists. What can be done to contribute to the conversion of the unknown number of facilities[141] in the former USSR that were involved in the offensive BW and TW programme of the former USSR and of Russia until March 1992[142] to facilities engaged in exclusively peaceful pursuits? How can the transfer of BW and TW (defence) technology and/or equipment be prevented? How can the scientists and technicians of these and other microbiological research and production facilities be employed so that their skills are used only for national and international health care purposes? Finally, how can a 'brain drain' be prevented from former military institutions and their contractors to countries still interested in BW programmes? The Director of the CIA estimated that 'a few thousand [Soviet scientists] have the knowledge and the marketable skills to develop and produce biological weapons'.[143] The US Assistant Secretary of Defense for International Security Policy also expressed concern that 'highly skilled workers with sensitive expertise now face the prospect of losing relatively well-paying and very prestigious jobs . . . [so] that these individuals could become receptive to offers of high pay and other inducements to sell their knowledge and capabilities to those nations that might threaten international security'.[144]

Fortunately, thanks to the dual-threat nature of BW and TW agents and of corresponding technology and facilities, conversion seems easier in this field than in other areas of concern. Special centres were established to retrain nuclear physicists and other specialists in the former Soviet Union, but the VFP programme, and if possible the GESS programme, would provide an inexpensive means of preventing the emigration of BW mercenaries and of converting BW programmes, facilities and specialists—not only in the former Soviet Union.[145]

The facilities which would undergo comprehensive conversion under the VFP programme would be fully converted. It would be not sufficient, for example, to involve single laboratories or units of military institutions or their

[140] Tromp, H., 'After the cold war: conversion?', *Peace and the Sciences* (Vienna), Dec. 1991, pp. 1–3.

[141] During an international meeting in 1990, a Soviet representative informally mentioned that approximately 70 facilities were then involved in the Biological 'Defence' Research Program of the USSR.

[142] *Arms Control* (note 84), p. 53; Stock (note 125); Leitenberg, chapter 8, in this volume.

[143] Gates, R., testimony, US Senate, 15 Jan. 1992, quoted in *Chemical Weapons Convention Bulletin*, no. 15 (Mar. 1992), p. 13.

[144] Hadley, S. J., Statement, *Assisting the Build-Down* (note 135), pp. 19–26, see especially p. 25.

[145] A proposal to make use of the VFP programme for conversion of former Soviet BW facilities and funded by the International Science and Technology Centre has since been forwarded to the Commission of the European Communities (1 Apr. 1993).

contractors in the VFP and GESS programmes while other parts of a facility remained under military control.[146]

Under the VFP programme assurance would have to be given that the converted facilities could not be reconverted to offensive biological warfare facilities and that their personnel would not become involved in proliferation. Verification of the non-military use of a facility after conversion could be achieved at least partially by the presence of several international scientists and technicians working at the facility for a period of time. On the one hand, they would serve as vaccine production experts assisting the local staff to adopt good manufacturing practices (GMP) and to initiate the research and production programme. On the other hand, trainees could be sent from developing countries to learn how to carry out research on vaccines and how to implement good laboratory practices (GLP) and GMP.[147] It would be difficult to hide prohibited activities with international visiting scientists given the run of the facility and working alongside the national staff. Furthermore, a transfer of know-how and technology would take place, a process much desired by the developing countries that are States Parties to the BWC. Additional measures might be necessary to prevent 'counter-conversion' and proliferation. Until such time as a general BWC verification regime has been adopted, annual declarations might be required from converted facilities, and a verification regime could be introduced to verify the contribution of the VFP programme to conversion.

XII. Establishing the VFP programme

Co-ordination

The United Nations system could co-ordinate the Vaccines for Peace programme. The United Nations Organization itself and the following UN agencies and other international organizations could be involved in running the VFP programme: the United Nations Educational, Scientific & Cultural Organization (UNESCO), the United Nations Industrial Development Organization (UNIDO), the WHO, the Food and Agriculture Organization (FAO) and the International Office of Epizootics (IOE).

UNESCO would be involved because the VFP programme promotes scientific collaboration among nations; UNIDO's involvement would relate to the VFP programme's contribution to biotechnology transfer and the consequent narrowing of the gap between industrialized and developing countries. The WHO, the FAO and the IOE would be involved because the VFP programme deals with the development, production and distribution of vaccines against pathogens, a large number of which are anti-personnel and anti-animal agents.

The creation of a BWC Verification Organization[148] could be useful. Vaccines for Peace deals with activities covered by the BWC and is intended to

[146] Development of drugs under military supervision might easily be shifted to civilian programmes (see Langen, chapter 15, in this volume) so that there would no longer be a need to carry out biological and medical R&D under military control except for the development of physical protective measures such as masks, protective suits, etc. The biological testing required for such activities can be conducted with non-pathogenic simulants.

[147] See Horaud, chapter 9, and Melling, chapter 13, in this volume.

[148] Sims, N. A., 'Endogenous development of the multilateral treaty regime (MTR) flowing from the BWC: proposals for special conferences and for a continuous central capability', Geissler and Haynes

strengthen the BWC in various ways, including enhancement of participation, provision of confidence-building transparency regarding permitted activities, prevention of proliferation and implementation of Article X. In addition, the establishment of the VFP programme depends on agreement on lists of putative BW and TW agents, one of the necessary components of a BWC verification regime.

The primary incentive for proposing the VFP programme was to strengthen the BWC. While the FAO and the IOE probably cover more vaccines against DTAs than does the WHO, the WHO would be the organization most suited to the VFP programme owing to its focus on vaccines and human health protection. The WHO could establish Vaccines for Peace as a programme independent of its currently existing vaccine programmes but one conducted in close co-operation with one or more of them.

Launching

A proposal 'to elaborate an international programme of vaccine development' was introduced by Peru at the Third Review Conference and was welcomed by the Conference.[149] There thus appears to be support among States Parties to the BWC for the VFP programme. As a next step, a draft resolution to establish the Vaccines for Peace programme might be forwarded to the UN General Assembly either by a member state, a group of member states or by the Secretary-General as requested by the Third Review Conference.[150]

The resolution might include language establishing the Vaccines for Peace programme, specifying that it be run by the WHO (or another specialized agency of the UN) in close co-operation with the other agencies affected by the programme, and calling for funding from member states and other sources.[151]

Structure

The VFP programme would require a Secretariat, a Management Advisory Committee and a Scientific Advisory Committee. The Scientific Advisory Committee should have as members governmental and non-governmental experts with expertise in a variety of fields, including epidemiology, biotechnology, medical microbiology and biological defence. The committees should act in close co-operation with similar bodies already active within the Children's

(note 88), pp. 443–69; Sims, N. A., 'Organizational aspects with regard to possible verification tasks under the Biological Weapons Convention', in Lundin (note 18), pp. 37–48.

[149] 'The Conference welcomes efforts to elaborate an international programme of vaccine development for the prevention of diseases which would involve scientific and technical personnel from developing countries which are States Parties to the Convention. The Conference recognizes that such a programme might not only enhance peaceful international cooperation in biotechnology but will also contribute to improving health care in developing countries and provide transparency in accordance with the Convention', Final Document of the Third Review Conference (note 93), p. 23.

[150] The Third Review Conference emphasized the increasing importance of Article X of the BWC, noted with concern the increasing gap between developed and developing countries, and called upon the Secretary-General of the UN 'to propose for inclusion on the agenda of a relevant United Nations body, not later than 1993, a discussion and examination of the means of improving institutional mechanisms in order to facilitate the fullest possible exchange of equipment, materials and scientific and technological information regarding the use of bacteriological (biological) agents and toxins for peaceful purposes', Final Document of the Third Review Conference (note 93), p. 22.

[151] Funds for that part of the VFP programme proposed to be involved in conversion of former Soviet BW facilities might be, at least in part, provided by the International Science and Technology Centre (see note 145).

Vaccine Initiative, the Expanded Programme for Immunization and the Programme for Vaccine Development.

Vaccines covered

The proposed Scientific Advisory Committee for the VFP programme should compile lists of DTAs for which vaccines are needed for both civilian and military purposes.

The Scientific Advisory Committee should elaborate lists of possible biological and toxin warfare agents against which vaccination is necessary for civilian and military purposes, and it should supervise all activities under the VFP programme. The establishment of lists of putative BW and TW agents is a critical aspect of the VFP programme and additionally, an important side-benefit of the programme, since such lists are indispensable for verification purposes.

Governmental experts have hesitated to negotiate internationally agreed lists of BW and TW agents[152] because such lists are subject to change. This argument is less convincing as regards the VFP programme since a number of years would elapse from a decision to add a vaccine against a special agent to the VFP programme list and the completion of work on such a vaccine. The Scientific Advisory Committee would also represent a body qualified to correct the lists as needed.

The Scientific Advisory Committee should compile three priority lists:

List 1—potential BW and TW agents against which vaccines should be produced (other agents—such as the AIDS virus HIV, which are not regarded as putative or possible warfare agents, or agents which are covered by other international immunization programmes—should be not covered by the VFP programme);[153]

List 2—agents on List 1 for which production and use of vaccines is technically possible and should be initiated; and

List 3—agents on List 1 for which vaccines are not available but are urgently needed, towards which end research should be focused. In order to avoid interference with existing vaccine programmes, the VFP programme should cover only vaccines against DTAs.[154]

In consultation with military medical experts, the VFP Scientific Advisory Council should also decide whether vaccines to protect troops against 'natural infection' caused by pathogens not regarded as DTAs should be covered by the VFP programme or by another programme. As of 1985, US military personnel are immunized against adenovirus types 4 and 7, influenza, measles, *Meningococcus*, poliomyelitis, rubella, tetanus/diphtheria and smallpox. In addition, alert forces are immunized against typhoid and yellow fever and, if required, against cholera and plague. 'High risk occupational groups' are immunized against hepatitis B, rabies and special agents such as those causing Q-fever and

[152] See section IX, subsection 'lists of DTAs' above.

[153] The list should be open for additions. If a state wants to include additional agents on the list for security and/or health reasons, it should be possible with the approval of the Scientific Advisory Committee on the condition that the state requesting (an) additional vaccine(s) fund this additional activity.

[154] The target diseases of the EPI are diphtheria, measles, poliomyelitis, tetanus, tuberculosis and whooping cough. The target diseases of the CVI are measles, poliomyelitis and tetanus.

Rocky Mountain spotted fever.[155] Some of these vaccines are covered by the EPI, namely diphtheria, measles, poliomyelitis and tetanus. As the causative agents of these serious diseases are naturally dangerous to humans, they should be included in one of the purely 'BW-independent' vaccine programmes. The VFP programme should help create a situation similar to that described in a bill proposed in 1988 in the USA[156]—'all functions and personnel of the Biological Defense Research Program[s] conducted by . . . the Army [should be] transferred to [civilian] Health . . . Services', with the exception of activities which are purely military in nature. The transparency which the VFP programme could provide and its function as a CBM would be seriously compromised if it did not lead to a complete shift of *all* biomedical R&D from military institutions and their contractors to civilian control.

Vaccine R&D and production

First, the decision must be taken as to which DTAs should be studied and which vaccines against DTAs should be developed and produced in the national and international research centres, enterprises and other facilities of countries which are States Parties to the BWC, including facilities in the Commonwealth of Independent States and in other successor states of the former Soviet Union. These states should then be encouraged to: (*a*) produce vaccines recommended by the Scientific Advisory Committee, or (*b*) conduct research on the development of necessary vaccines which are not produced because of scientific or technical limitations. All R&D and production would be supervised by the VFP's Scientific Advisory Committee.

In order to encourage peaceful international co-operation and to make the BWC more attractive to developing countries, facilities participating in the VFP programme would be obliged to involve scientists and technical personnel from developing countries *that are States Parties to the BWC*. The vaccines produced would be available to all States Parties for civilian and permitted military purposes under the supervision of the Scientific Advisory Committee. Vaccines would also be provided at low cost to developing countries.

The research and production activities of the VFP programme could start immediately by using existing microbiology and biotechnology facilities, especially those which previously were involved in activities directly related to the BWC.[157] These facilities would include both the facilities of Western states, such as the US Government Services Division at Swiftwater, Pennsylvania,[158] and those of the former Soviet Union. Facilities involved in the VFP programme might also include UNIDO's International Centre for Genetic Engineering and Biotechnology (Trieste and New Delhi[159]) and its 17 affiliated

[155] Kirkpatrick, J. W., *Military Immunization Policy*, Information Paper, DASG-PSP-D (Office of the Surgeon General, US Army, HQDA: Washington, DC, 3 May 1985).

[156] See note 34.

[157] See Geissler (note 4), appendix II.

[158] See Geissler, E. and Brunius, G., 'Information on high-risk laboratories', ed. E. Geissler, *Strengthening the Biological Weapons Convention by Confidence-Building Measures* (note 94), pp. 80–104, tables 7.2, 7.3.

[159] See Subrahmanyam, chapter 19, in this volume. When the Third Review Conference urged the United Nations and States Parties 'to take specific measures . . . for the promotion of the fullest possible international cooperation', 'active association with United Nations institutions, including the International Centre for Genetic Engineering and Biotechnology' was explicitly mentioned; see Final Document of the Third Review Conference (note 93), p. 21.

centres, and the Regional Vaccinology Centers planned by the Pan American Health Organization in Latin America.[160] Additional facilities such as the proposed International Research Centre, planned to support developing countries,[161] could also participate in the VFP programme.

All R&D and production activities under the programme would be supervised by the VFP Scientific Advisory Committee and a technical body of this Committee, possibly in close co-operation with National Authorities similar to or even identical with the National Authorities to be established under Article VII of the CWC.[162]

Declarations

After implementation of the VFP programme and the GESS,[163] the States Parties to the BWC should declare in an additional protocol (or in another document dealing with measures to strengthen the BWC) that they will cease further biological and medical R&D activities under national military control when the VFP and the GESS programmes have begun functioning, and that they will provide available vaccines for diagnostic and similar purposes. Participants in these programmes should further agree that such activities will be carried out only under the supervision of the Scientific Advisory Committees of the VFP and the GESS.

XIII. Conclusions

Vaccines for Peace would contribute to health care, to peaceful international co-operation in microbiology and biotechnology, to strengthening the BWC and to implementing major obligations assumed by States Parties under the BWC. The VFP programme, if possible together with the GESS, would make it unnecessary to carry out biological and medical R&D activities under military control, leaving no room for suspicion about the intention of such activities.

The VFP programme would contribute to: (*a*) provision of orphan vaccines needed for both civilian and military purposes; (*b*) expanding participation in the BWC; (*c*) sealing loopholes which have weakened the BWC; (*d*) removing the suspicion caused by biological defence research as regards possible offensive intentions; (*e*) verification of compliance with the Geneva Protocol and the BWC; (*f*) enhancing international co-operation in biotechnology without increasing the danger of weapon proliferation; (*g*) conversion of facilities and scientists previously involved in offensive BW R&D and production; and (*h*) narrowing the technology gap between industrialized and developing nations.

[160] Subrahmanyam, 'Development and transfer of vaccine technology: long-term challenges and strategies' (note 57).

[161] Labini, P. S ., 'Reflections on the constitution of an International Research Centre connected with the United Nations', International Security in a Transformed World, 5th International Amaldi Conference of Academies of Sciences and National Scientific Societies, Report and Documentation, Heidelberg, 1–3 July 1992, pp. 361–64.

[162] 'In order to fulfil its obligation under this Convention, each State Party shall designate or establish a National Authority to serve as the national focal point for effective liaison with the Organization [for the Prohibition of Chemical Weapons] and other States Parties', Conference on Disarmament document CD/1170, 24 Aug. 1992, appendix, p. 24.

[163] See Morse, chapter 16, and Wheelis, chapter 17, in this volume.

Part II. Strengthening the Biological Weapons Convention

4. The missing link in implementation of the BWC: the war against pathogens

FÉLIX C. CALDERÓN*

I. Introduction

Although the fact is frequently ignored, any arms control or disarmament agreement embodies basic obligations which provide for specific prohibitions or restrictions associated with certain complementary rights. There are indeed exceptions to this rule, namely the 1925 Geneva Protocol, the 1963 Partial Test Ban Treaty (PTBT), the 1971 Seabed Treaty and the 1981 'Inhumane Weapons' Convention. However, other agreements would hardly have been achieved if convergent rights, requested mainly by developing countries, had not been added to the originally proposed undertakings.

That is particularly true of the 1968 Non-Proliferation Treaty (NPT), where the rights of States Parties to use nuclear energy for peaceful purposes and to participate in the fullest possible exchange of equipment, materials and scientific and technological information emerged as the logical and unavoidable quid pro quo to the basic undertakings aimed at stopping the horizontal proliferation of nuclear weapons and other nuclear explosive devices. It is also the case with the 1972 Biological and Toxin Weapons Convention (BWC), as is shown below, and the 1993 Chemical Weapons Convention (CWC), where chemical disarmament and the non-proliferation of chemical weapons are closely tied to Article XI devoted to economic and technological development.[1]

The basic obligations of any arms control or disarmament agreement are naturally fully consistent with its object and purpose, and their implementation undoubtedly deserves priority once such an agreement enters into force, particularly the obligation of States Parties to demonstrate compliance. That is not the case with the implementation of complementary rights which seems to be left to the goodwill of States Parties, some of whom are unjustifiably reluctant to allow transfers of relevant dual-use technology among States Parties.

It has been said that the universality of any agreement can be achieved if it is made more attractive to potential States Parties. The implementation of complementary rights would do precisely that, owing to the wide range of opportunities which would be opened up in the area of non-prohibited activities thereby fostering co-operation and assistance among States Parties. It is equally important that non-States Parties be aware that their refusal to adhere to any particular agreement would imply their discrimination against it. The fact that this is not always so has aroused some misgivings because the business practices of some

[1] For the text of the CWC, see SIPRI, *SIPRI Yearbook 1993: World Armaments and Disarmament* (Oxford University Press: Oxford, 1993), pp. 735–56.

* Until November 1992 the author was deputy head of the Peruvian delegation to the Conference on Disarmament. Among other responsibilities, he was acting head of the Peruvian delegation to the Third Review Conference of the BWC and participated directly in the negotiations on the CWC from 1986 to August 1992. The views expressed here are those of the author and do not necessarily represent the position of Peru.

supplier States Parties sometimes take precedence over the object and purpose of the basic obligations which they have assumed under an agreement.

The NPT is again a case in point, since peaceful applications of nuclear energy have favoured either expensive or supposedly strategic projects not necessarily of highest priority for the populations of developing countries. For example, small- and medium-size power reactors, badly needed in the South, received little interest at the International Atomic Energy Agency (IAEA) during the 1970s because the profits for suppliers were not as great as those for larger power reactors which were obviously much more expensive. The same is true of technology transfers which are not closely related to the improvement of agricultural and medical techniques, though considered useful by the technical élite of the importing countries for other reasons. Of course, some efforts were made during the NPT Review Conferences to meet the concerns of the less developed States Parties. Nevertheless these efforts were primarily focused not on assistance and co-operation but on trade, and they failed to adequately address the demands of developing countries.

The BWC is another striking example of the lack of interest shown by the most advanced States Parties in assisting and co-operating with States Parties from the developing world, at least in the development and application of scientific discoveries in the field of bacteriology (biology) for prevention of disease, or for other peaceful purposes. Despite the political commitments of States Parties attending the three Review Conferences, not surprisingly almost nothing has been done to implement Article X.[2]

Based on the above discussion, this chapter examines, first, the rights of States Parties as stipulated in the BWC. Second, attention is drawn to the commitments made at the three Review Conferences, in particular those related to combating pathogens. Finally, some comments are made on two proposals for the enhancement of health care and the prevention of disease in developing countries as a way to make the BWC more attractive to non-States Parties.

II. The rights of States Parties

Nicholas Sims has aptly written that the BWC: 'unite[s] the world's intellectual and economic resources in making war *on* germs rather than *with* germs'.[3] In the view of this author, that phrase summarizes the philosophy of the BWC. Indeed, security benefits were the primary gains expected from the BWC—to ban bacteriological (biological) war—but public health benefits were inescapably linked to them as the altruistic side of the coin.

This complementary character of public health benefits to the States Parties emanates from Article I of the BWC, where microbial or other biological agents are prohibited so long as they 'have no justification for prophylactic, protective or other peaceful purposes'. In other words, all endeavours related to pathogens should, in principle, be for the benefit of mankind—the protective activities being the inevitable by-product of the need to protect against the

[2] For the text of the BWC, see annexe A in this volume.

[3] Sims, N., 'Biological and toxin weapons: the 1972 Convention and the reinforcement of its disarmament treaty regime (DTR) through the Review Conferences of 1980, 1986 and 1991', Paper presented at Inter-Faculty Seminar, Vrije Universiteit Brussels, 28 Nov. 1991, p. 17.

threat posed by the possible hostile use of those agents. It is in this perspective that Article X should be understood.

Article X of the Convention stipulates three types of States Parties rights: (*a*) the right 'to participate in the fullest possible exchange of equipment, materials and scientific and technological information for the use of bacteriological (biological) agents and toxins for peaceful purposes'; (*b*) the right 'to the further development and application of scientific discoveries in the field of bacteriology (biology) for prevention of disease or other peaceful purposes' through the co-operation of States Parties in a position to do so individually or together with other states or international organizations; and (*c*) the right not to be hampered in the 'economic or technological development . . . or international cooperation in the field of peaceful bacteriological (biological) activities, including the international exchange of bacteriological (biological) agents and toxins and equipment for the processing, use or production of bacteriological (biological) agents and toxins for peaceful purposes in accordance with the provisions of the Convention'.[4]

Although one of the unwritten goals of Article X is the narrowing of the biotechnology gap between North and South, it seems indisputable that the prevention of diseases continues to be the most urgent task directly emanating from Article X of the BWC. As Sims rightly noted: 'Here, if anywhere, inspiration can surely be found. Medical, immunological and therapeutic personnel could be exchanged and research fellowship established . . . South and North are more likely to find a common interest in fighting diseases, which are notoriously no respecters of national frontiers, than in any other putative application of Article X'.[5]

With the end of the cold war and the collapse of communism, States Parties now have a golden opportunity to take advantage of the unprecedented co-operation between East and West to defeat pathogens which continue to be the scourge of mankind, particularly in the poor countries. The lack of adequate verification measures under the BWC should not leave the door open for the creation by genetic engineering of new types of biological agents which could be used for biological warfare.

Today no one questions the role biotechnology should play in fostering economic and social development as well as international co-operation in biomedical R&D directly related to the BWC. However, this option freely implemented is not free from the risk of latent or open BW proliferation.

Narrowing the scope of Article X to purely systematic transfers and assistance in biotechnology does not help to strengthen the BWC. The current revolution in biotechnology makes a credible verification system an expensive, if not impossible, exercise given the imprecise borders between offensive and defensive BW programmes and the ambiguities of some scientific research, where small amounts of pathogens are sufficient for effective weapons. In addition, discrepancies still exist as regards the sometimes over-emphasized right of states to self-defence.

[4] United Nations, *Status of Multilateral Arms Regulations and Disarmament Agreements* (United Nations: New York, 1988), pp. 117–32.

[5] See Sims (note 3), p. 17.

III. The Review Conferences

Thus far there have been three Review Conferences which took place in Geneva in 1980, 1986 and 1991, and which concluded satisfactorily with the adoption by consensus of a Final Declaration. The growing expectations of developing countries concerning the implementation of Article X have been reflected in those documents; the last Final Declaration being, in the opinion of the present author, the finest achievement.

The First Review Conference

At the time of the First Review Conference in 1980, Article X failed to attract much attention since the commitments attached to it were very modest. Expectations concentrated basically either on compliance with the main obligations of Article X (which could be seen as additional proof of the tendency to neglect the full exercise of complementary rights), or States Parties felt there was simply not much expected of them under the article.

The Final Declaration candidly recognized the principle, then à la mode, of the relationship between disarmament and development but did not express clear awareness of the rather expensive nature of true disarmament.[6]

States Parties were called upon to increase their scientific and technological co-operation, particularly with developing countries, including the transfer and exchange of information, training of personnel and transfer of materials and equipment on a more systematic and long-term basis. However, since no indication was given of how this was to occur, the result was not much more than wishful thinking.

A request was also addressed to the United Nations Secretariat to provide information on the implementation of Article X by States Parties. Those efforts have subsequently proven useful.

The Second Review Conference

In 1986 the States Parties began to focus their interest on Article X, the paragraphs devoted to it taking up almost two pages of the Final Declaration. However, this change of mood, mainly evident in the developing countries, did not adequately address the war against pathogens, but rather concentrated on how to narrow the increasing gap between the developed and the developing countries 'in the field of biotechnology, genetic engineering, microbiology and other related areas'.[7]

The interest in promoting economic and social development, and scientific and technological progress, was certainly not wrong. Nevertheless, its emphasis and priority seemed biased, since public health and disease control did not

[6] First Review Conference of the Parties to the Convention on the Prohibition of the Development, Production and Stockpiling of Bacteriological (Biological) and Toxin Weapons and on their Destruction, BWC/CONF.I/10, 1980, p. 7.

[7] Second Review Conference of the Parties to the Convention on the Prohibition of the Development, Production and Stockpiling of Bacteriological (Biological) and Toxin Weapons and on their Destruction, BWC/CONF.II/13, 1986, pp. 8–9.

awaken similar interest despite the provisions of Article X and the crying need to fight epidemic diseases in the developing world.

The Second Review Conference *inter alia* urged States Parties to provide wider access to their scientific and technological knowledge on biotechnology, bacteriological agents and toxins with peaceful applications on an equal and non-discriminatory basis and encouraged the sharing of such information, in particular with developing countries. Furthermore, it suggested some specific measures to foster the fullest possible international co-operation in these areas.

The Conference also urged the use of existing institutional means within the UN system, as well as those provided by the specialized agencies and other international organizations, to pursue co-operation under Article X. To that end, it requested the UN Secretary-General to propose for inclusion on the agenda of a relevant UN body the discussion and examination of the means for improving institutional mechanisms in order to facilitate the fullest possible exchange of equipment, materials and scientific and technological information for the use of bacteriological (biological) agents and toxins for peaceful purposes. Additionally, it urged the specialized agencies—namely, the Food and Agriculture Organization (FAO), the WHO, the UN Educational Scientific & Cultural Organization (UNESCO), the World Intellectual Property Organization (WIPO) and the UN Industrial Development Organization (UNIDO)—to participate in this discussion and fully co-operate with the Secretary-General of the United Nations.[8]

This last decision was, in the view of some experts, by far the most concrete example of how to implement Article X in a reasonable way, trying to take advantage of inter-agency co-operation. However, nothing was done in the five years which followed the Second Review Conference, despite UN General Assembly (UNGA) Resolution 41/58A,[9] which requested the Secretary-General to render the necessary assistance and to provide the services required for implementation of relevant parts of the Final Declaration.

Finally, the Conference restated the relationship between disarmament and development but then buried the concept, owing to the open opposition of some developed countries to this vague objective.[10]

The Third Review Conference

Generally speaking, the 1991 Third Review Conference was the most successful of the Review Conferences. The compliance regime was considerably strengthened after the adoption by consensus of a set of confidence-building measures (CBMs) and the establishment of an *Ad Hoc* Group of Governmental Experts, open to all States Parties, to identify and examine potential verification measures from a scientific and technical standpoint. It was also the first time that, under Article X, States Parties agreed upon concrete measures, chiefly

[8] This proposal was actively negotiated by the present author at that Conference on behalf of Peru.
[9] United Nations General Assembly (UNGA) document A/RES/41/58, 3 Dec.1986.
[10] Deger, S., 'The United Nations International Conference on the Relationship between Disarmament and Development', SIPRI, *SIPRI Yearbook 1988: World Armaments and Disarmament* (Oxford University Press: Oxford, 1988), pp. 523–25.

related to public health and the prevention of disease, so as to render possible, at last, true implementation of the article.[11]

Besides the emphasis put on the promotion of international co-operation and exchange among States Parties of the peaceful uses of biotechnology, three proposals set up a framework in which one of the main provisions of Article X could be fully implemented. The first proposal, introduced by France, addressed co-operation in providing information on national epidemiological surveillance and data-reporting systems, and the provision of assistance, bilaterally or in conjunction with the WHO, for epidemiological surveillance with a view to improving the identification and timely reporting of significant outbreaks of human and animal diseases.[12]

The second proposal, introduced by Peru, called upon the UN Secretary-General to propose for inclusion on the agenda of a relevant UN body, not later than 1993, a discussion and examination of the means of improving institutional mechanisms in order to facilitate the fullest possible exchange of equipment, materials and scientific and technological information regarding the use of bacteriological (biological) agents and toxins for peaceful purposes.[13]

The third proposal, suggested to the Peruvian delegation by Erhard Geissler, welcomed efforts to set up an international programme of vaccine development for the prevention of diseases that would involve scientific and technical personnel from developing countries which are States Parties to the BWC. It was recognized that such a programme might not only enhance peaceful international co-operation in biotechnology but would also contribute to improving health care in developing countries and provide transparency in accordance with the BWC.

The scope and benefits of Geissler's idea are such that, together with the other proposals, it constitutes the best chance for States Parties to implement Article X, through converging the objectives of biological defence applications and the prevention of disease to fight pathogenic agents (and possibly toxins) which cause so much devastation and death.

IV. Progress in the war against pathogens

Nothing appears more logical than the idea of converting the BWC into an effective tool which could be used against pathogens. By so doing, a workable relationship could be found between disarmament and better conditions of living, and it is thus the BWC could additionally contribute to international co-operation for the sake of mankind.

The Final Declaration of the Third Review Conference offers States Parties an opportunity to take advantage of the existing institutional means within the UN system to establish an unprecedented programme for saving lives, while simultaneously reducing the risk of clandestine BW production. As mentioned above, action needs to be taken by the Secretary-General of the United Nations[14] to discuss and examine inter-agency co-operation in order to facilitate

[11] Third Review Conference of the Parties to the Convention on the Prohibition of the Development, Production and Stockpiling of Bacteriological (Biological) and Toxin Weapons and on their Destruction, BWC/CONF.III/23, 1991, pp. 21–23.

[12] See BWC/CONF.III/23 (note 11), part III, p. 153.

[13] See BWC/CONF.III/23 (note 11), part III, p. 154. The meeting was originally envisaged for 1992.

[14] See note 13; see also BWC/CONF.III/23 (note 11), part II, p. 22.

the implementation, at the lowest possible cost, of concrete proposals such as Geissler's Vaccines for Peace programme[15] and the Global Epidemiological Surveillance System (GESS) suggested by Mark Wheelis.[16]

Although funding would be needed to implement these new programmes—which would involve the WHO, the FAO, UNESCO and UNIDO *inter alia* (under the aegis of the WHO)—the net dividends are obvious, particularly as regards health care in developing countries. In addition, such programmes would facilitate the establishment of focal centres in the developing regions in collaboration with the specialized agencies, either as completely new structures or as extensions of existing ones.

The Vaccines for Peace programme represents a very specific and transparent approach which is intended to neutralize agents that originate naturally and which are endemic in many developing countries. It also aims to fill the void created by the lack of interest on the part of the pharmaceutical industries in developed countries to produce vaccines against diseases endemic in developing countries. It would certainly discourage the temptation of BW proliferation.

As for the GESS, it can be seen as a CBM because it would increase the likelihood of early detection of both suspicious outbreaks of diseases and of emerging diseases occurring outside their natural boundaries.

In order to begin the process of implementing these two initiatives, the UN General Assembly should provide guidance based on the 1991 consensus resolution, UNGA Resolution 46/35A.[17] The Secretary-General is called upon to render the necessary assistance and provide the required services for a meeting, as agreed in the 1991 Final Declaration of the Third Review Conference. A proposal should now be presented for a concrete project to facilitate decision-making on the design of an appropriate programme—particularly its structure, funding, inter-agency liaison and priorities.

In the view of the present author, such a programme can be put into practice now without prejudicing its final endorsement by the next BWC Review Conference scheduled for 1996. The value of the various programmes currently being implemented by the WHO should not be underestimated, but the uniqueness of the new programme would lie in its direct relationship to pathogens relevant to the BWC and to which Article X is clearly applicable. In addition, the search for better or new vaccines against bacteria should receive special attention, paralleling current efforts related to vaccines against viruses. Today bacteria constitute the greatest threat to vast segments of the population in the developing world owing to poor sanitary conditions. The recent cholera epidemic in Latin America and the world-wide spread of tuberculosis are blatant examples of the new priorities in public health.

[15] Geissler, E., 'Vaccines for Peace: an international program of development and use of vaccines against dual-threat agents', *Politics and the Life Sciences*, vol. 11, no. 2 (Aug. 1992), pp. 231–43.

[16] Wheelis, M. L., 'Strengthening biological weapons control through global epidemiological surveillance', *Politics and the Life Sciences*, vol. 11, no. 2 (Aug. 1992), pp. 179–89; see also Wheelis, chapter 17, in this volume.

[17] UNGA document A/RES/46/35, 27 Dec. 1991.

5. Vaccines for Peace: a political scientist's critique

OLIVER THRÄNERT

I. Introduction

The Vaccines for Peace (VFP) programme as originally proposed by Erhard Geissler is intended to strengthen the Biological Weapons Convention (BWC).[1] The growing importance of strengthening the BWC speaks for looking closely at every proposal aimed at achieving this goal. Looking closely at the VFP programme has led the author of this chapter to believe it will not strengthen the BWC. It may, however, help developing countries acquire vaccines for civilian purposes.

These remarks should be qualified by pointing out that, from the point of view of a political scientist, it is not possible to discuss in detail the development and production of vaccines or to judge which vaccines should or could be developed against the various pathogens.[2] This chapter therefore focuses not on the scientific substance of the Vaccines For Peace proposal, but rather concentrates on the prospects for success of such a programme in view of current developments in international politics. By prospects of success is meant the degree to which it can strengthen the BWC and prevent both the proliferation of biological weapons (BW) and the development of new or improved agents designed to improve their use in combat.[3] Such a political goal is undoubtedly worthy of pursuit. Therefore, the following critique of the VFP programme should be taken not as destructive, but as constructive criticism.

II. Does VFP lead to universality and prevent proliferation?

The VFP proposal proceeds from the assumption that those developing countries that have not yet signed the BWC have refrained from doing so because they have seen no advantage in taking such action. The VFP programme is now intended to offer them such an advantage. Indeed, it does seem that most developing countries view the BWC from an economic rather than an arms control perspective. They intend to use this Convention to narrow the gap between the industrial and the developing countries in the area of biotechnology by demanding that technical support be offered in return for acceptance of improved veri-

[1] Geissler, E., 'Vaccines for Peace: an international program of development and use of vaccines against dual-threat agents', *Politics and the Life Sciences*, vol. 11, no. 2 (Aug. 1992), pp. 231–43.

[2] See the contributions by Ajjan, Saliou and Valette, chapter 10, and Horaud, chapter 9, in this volume.

[3] There are various publications dealing with both the problems of biological proliferation and improvement of putative biological warfare agents and proposals to strengthen the BWC; the following deserve special mention: Geissler, E. and Haynes, R. M. (eds), *Prevention of a Biological and Toxin Arms Race and the Responsibility of Scientists* (Akademie-Verlag: Berlin, 1991); ter Haar, B., *The Future of Biological Weapons*, Center for Strategic and International Studies, Washington Papers, no. 151 (Praeger: London, 1991); Wright, S. (ed.), *Preventing a Biological Arms Race* (MIT Press: Cambridge, Mass., 1990); Lundin, S. J. (ed.), *Views on Possible Verification Measures for the Biological Weapons Convention*, SIPRI Chemical & Biological Warfare Studies, no. 12 (Oxford University Press: Oxford, 1991); Thränert, O. (ed.), *The Verification of the Biological Weapons Convention: Problems and Perspectives* (Friedrich Ebert Foundation: Bonn, 1992).

fication measures. The VFP programme could, in fact, be of benefit in this case and thereby offer a means of strengthening the BWC. This is particularly true with regard to the Third Review Conference of the BWC which took place in Geneva in September 1991. During the conference numerous developing countries presented proposals with a view to the required implementation of Article X of the Convention, which refers to co-operation of the States Parties in the field of biotechnology. As a consequence, in their final declaration, the states participating in the Review Conference noted, in reference to Article X, that the gap between industrialized and developing countries in terms of biotechnology should be narrowed. In order to achieve this, all States Parties were called upon to engage in international co-operation and technological transfer on an equal and non-discriminatory basis. In addition, a list of specific measures was provided.[4] On the other hand, over the course of the BWC Review Conferences, a number of countries including the People's Republic of China, Cuba, India and Pakistan have appeared either to view the BWC from a political and strategic perspective (i.e., from the perspective of the conflicts in their regions), or have wished to avoid granting foreign inspectors access to sensitive facilities. For both reasons, these countries remain very reluctant when it comes to verification issues. Consequently, these countries are unlikely to support the strengthening of the BWC as a consequence of the implementation of the VFP programme. Access to vaccines is simply not their most important concern with regard to the BWC.[5]

In most cases, the reasons for non-participation in the BWC are not those assumed by the VFP programme. Looking at the Middle East—one of the most pressing problem areas in this context—it can be concluded that the refusal of Israel to sign the BWC is of great significance to those states in the region, such as Syria, which also refuse to join the BWC. Israel has not signed the BWC because it does not participate whatsoever in international disarmament and arms control. There may or may not be political reasons for this, but these clearly do not arise from Israel's expectation that the BWC should provide support for the development of vaccines. It is Israel's political and strategic considerations that are decisive. Yet these are not even touched upon by the VFP programme. Thus, the signing of the BWC by Israel and other states of the Middle East as a result of the initiation of the VFP programme should not be expected. In other words, the VFP programme cannot achieve one of its most important goals, namely to make the BWC effective world-wide. With this programme, black African states like the Sudan, Uganda or Zambia might be convinced that joining the Convention would be advantageous. However, these countries are truly not the problem cases where the problem of proliferation of biological warfare agents is concerned.

For two reasons the VFP programme can hardly be expected to hinder the proliferation of biological warfare agents: those states, which as parties to the BWC may be interested to keep open their option of an offensive biological warfare programme, can hardly be encouraged by the VFP programme to contribute to the strengthening of the BWC. Those states not States Parties to the

[4] Bernauer, T., 'Verification of compliance with the Biological Weapons Convention: developing countries between passive participation and obstruction', Thränert (note 3), pp. 55–67. See also the contribution of Calderón, chapter 4, in this volume. The document referred to is BWC/Conf.III/22/ Add.2.

[5] Bernauer, T. (note 4).

BWC which also would like to keep their options open in terms of biological programmes are not likely to enter the BWC regime as a consequence of implementation of the VFP programme. Only those states not interested in biological warfare affairs but at the same time interested in acquiring access to vaccines for civilian purposes could be encouraged by the VFP programme not only to participate in the BWC, but also to contribute to its strengthening.

On the contrary, the VFP programme might even promote proliferation. Undoubtedly, the VFP programme would familiarize a great number of people with the potential of what Geissler calls dual-threat agents (DTAs).[6] If it is true—and this is one of Geissler's arguments in promoting the VFP programme—that even the development of vaccines might lead to a first-strike BW capability because soldiers and even the population could be vaccinated against a particular pathogen, and that this pathogen could then be used as a biological warfare agent, with only a small risk of causing the disease on the aggressor's side, then the knowledge and skills needed to develop and produce vaccines against DTAs should definitely not be shared with all of the current 126 States Parties to the BWC, some of which are suspected of conducting an offensive biological research programme. In any case, a potential aggressor should not know—to put it the other way round—which pathogens the defender can vaccinate his soldiers against, because this knowledge would offer the potential aggressor the option of using exactly those pathogens against which the defender has no vaccines.

This problem becomes even worse if the fact is taken into account that States Parties to the BWC can, under Article XIII, withdraw at any time. This article states that any State Party is allowed to withdraw if it decides that extraordinary events have jeopardized its supreme interests. The withdrawal should be announced to all other States Parties and to the United Nation's Security Council three months in advance.[7] Therefore, in theory it is possible that a State Party to the BWC might also participate in the VFP programme, gaining the knowledge of how to develop certain vaccines, and leave the BWC afterwards in order to pursue a secret offensive BW programme. Such a case might be unlikely, but it cannot be ruled out entirely.

The VFP programme might even promote proliferation more directly, as the following case illustrates. In 1988, Iraq—which at that time had signed but not yet ratified the BWC—bought tularaemia strains from the American Type Culture Collection (ATCC) in the United States. However, according to the Director of the ATCC, Robert Stevenson, the tularaemia strain purchased by Iraq was a weakened strain commonly used to develop vaccines. On the other hand, Stevenson said it is possible to obtain a far stronger strain simply by catching a rabbit or squirrel.[8] This would mean that the Iraqis achieved the capability to vaccinate their personnel working in laboratories, where they now could develop and produce tularaemia as a biological warfare agent.[9] Indeed, it appears that

[6] See the contribution by Pearson, chapter 14, in this volume.

[7] For the text of the BWC, see annexe A in this volume.

[8] Ottaway, D., 'Probe begins on whether Iraq got deadly bacteria from U.S.', *Washington Post*, 29 Jan. 1989, p. A34.

[9] I would like to thank Dr Gunnar Sandström of the Swedish National Defence Research Establishment (FOA) for this hint.

Iraq worked on tularaemia as part of its biological warfare programme prior to the 1991 Persian Gulf War.[10]

III. Is the threshold for VFP participation high enough?

The VFP's threshold for participation in its programme is actually quite low. Becoming a State Party to the Convention is all that is required. Yet the fundamental issue is the difficulty of verifying the BWC under current conditions. This does not, however, mean it is inevitably unverifiable.

For years, the former Soviet Union, one of the initial signatories of the BWC, violated at least the spirit if not the letter of the Convention. For instance, the anthrax outbreak in Sverdlovsk in 1979 apparently was not—as all Soviet governments had claimed—caused by contaminated meat sold on the black market, but by an accident in a military laboratory. Whether the programme conducted in this laboratory violated the BWC is still unclear, because the amounts of anthrax bacteria that were used are still unknown. However, the strategy of all Soviet governments—including that of Mikhail Gorbachev—of providing the Western public with this false account might be an indication that what went on in Sverdlovsk was unlikely to have been a defensive research programme.[11] In addition, for many years the Soviet Union also ran a BW test and evaluation installation on the island of Vozrozhdeniya in the Aral Sea. Whether or not real pathogens were tested there also remains unclear,[12] but not only the Soviet Union as a State Party to the BWC apparently was in violation of the Convention. Other states that are suspected of conducting offensive BW programmes like Iran and Libya are also States Parties to the BWC.[13]

This means that an increase in the number of States Parties to the BWC in no way implies an automatic strengthening of the Convention. The minimum condition for participation in the VFP programme should thus go beyond acceding to the BWC to include the implementation of the confidence-building measures (CBMs) agreed to at the 1986 and 1991 Review Conferences. These various CBMs are aimed at producing more openness between the States Parties to the BWC regarding those biological programmes not prohibited by the Convention. Participation in these CBMs is on a voluntary basis. As a consequence, only 14 States Parties took part in every annual round of information exchange between 1987 and 1991. In particular the participation of developing countries was insufficient.[14]

To make participation in the CBMs mandatory for all States Parties to the BWC would certainly deter states like Israel or Syria from entering the BWC regime. These states are not interested in providing access to any information on their defence programmes and policies. This is the case even though these

[10] Ekéus, R., 'The United Nations Special Commission on Iraq', SIPRI, *SIPRI Yearbook 1992: World Armaments and Disarmament* (Oxford University Press: Oxford, 1992), pp. 509–24; see especially p. 517.

[11] Leitenberg, M., 'Soviet activities related to biological weapons', *Arms Control*, vol. 12, no. 2 (Sep. 1991), pp. 161–90.

[12] The Soviet BW test site was already mentioned in a US Defense Intelligence Agency brochure; see *Soviet Biological Warfare Threat* (US Defense Intelligence Agency: Washington, DC, 1986), p. 1. See also the contribution by Leitenberg, chapter 8, in this volume.

[13] 'U.S. seeks successful outcome at NPT talks in Geneva', (excerpts from Clarke Senate testimony), *U.S. Policy Information and Texts*, no. 93 (13 July 1990), p. 13.

[14] Geissler, E., 'Contribution of confidence-building measures to greater transparency in activities directly related to the Biological Weapons Convention', Lundin (note 3), pp. 10–25.

CBMs are a long way from a decisive strengthening of the BWC in terms of verification measures. Moreover, it is possible that if the VFP programme or the BWC, respectively, required participating states to implement the CBMs, the process of improving them—which is urgently required—might even be hindered. Were participation in confidence-building to be mandatory, this would likely increase opposition to stronger CBMs during future BWC Review Conferences.

IV. Biological defence and national sovereignty

In general, it cannot be assumed that the States Parties to the BWC would be willing to transfer practically their entire biological defence research from national to international control. Even after the end of the cold war, and despite new perspectives for East–West co-operation, the inclination persists to be prepared for all eventualities. This is especially true of active and powerful states like the United States. The Persian Gulf War as well as the war in the former Yugoslavia have demonstrated that after the end of the East–West confrontation, war has become not less likely, but more likely. The powerful states of the state system, in particular, continue to reserve for themselves the right to intervene militarily in conflicts, and if necessary without a mandate from the United Nations. Again, this applies primarily to the United States, but increasingly also to the states which are members of the Western European Union (WEU). Both remain interested in holding open the option of intervening in military conflicts without the mandate of the United Nations, should such a mandate not be forthcoming.

As far as the WEU is concerned, this is particularly true after its June 1992 Petersberg Declaration.[15] This declaration states that troops under WEU Command could be engaged in peace-enforcement operations outside the original WEU area as long as these operations are in accordance with the UN Charter (i.e., as long as they comply with Article 51, collective self-defence). In other words, a UN mandate like the one that allowed UN members to undertake all necessary measures to expel Iraq from Kuwait would not necessarily be needed.

Turning over national BW defence programmes to an international authority would go against this tendency, often referred to as the 'renationalization' of security policy. There is no bloc-to-bloc confrontation any more. As a consequence, the world faces numerous conflicts in the eastern part of Europe, some of which have already resulted in wars or civil wars between small states or ethnic groups. However, after the break-up of both the Warsaw Pact and the Soviet Union there is also a move towards renationalization in the West. NATO still exists, but now that the enemy has gone, its future is in doubt.[16]

In any case, Erhard Geissler's premise, that the role of the United Nations in international relations is becoming more and more important, is questionable. This might be wishful thinking, but it is hard to imagine it becoming a reality. The Persian Gulf War is no case against this argument. In that war, the United Nations had no political control and did not participate in any decision made

[15] Western European Union Council of Ministers, Bonn, 19 June 1992, Petersberg Declaration, p. 7.

[16] Honig, J. W., *NATO: An Institution Under Threat?*, Institute for East–West Security Studies, New York, Occasional Paper Series, no. 22 (Praeger: London, 1991).

during the war such as, for example, the decision concerning the beginning of the ground war.

A national biological defence programme is not essential to military intervention aimed at ending violent conflicts. However, at a minimum, the military leadership and those politically responsible in the various countries will do everything possible to provide their soldiers with optimal protection against even relatively unlikely risks; and this also includes biological defence. As the Persian Gulf War demonstrated, the risk of being attacked by biological warfare agents cannot be ruled out. In the Gulf War it was necessary to vaccinate Coalition soldiers against anthrax and other putative biological warfare agents. Protection provided for soldiers engaged in such missions would also include vaccination against those pathogens which could occur naturally but are more prevalent in times of war.

If access to vaccines, but also to other biological defence measures, were to be under international control, this could circumscribe national freedom of action. Additionally, those states that find themselves in regions with political conflicts that could become military conflicts—again the Middle East comes to mind—would be especially unlikely to limit their national manœuvring room by transferring biological defence to an international authority. It should also be remembered that most states in the world are not democracies. These states generally reject the idea of giving up national control in such sensitive fields as defence policy.

Moreover, the 1992 Chemical Weapons Convention clearly allows national chemical defence programmes. If what is intended is not only to place under international control vaccine programmes but also all biological defence programmes that work with pathogens, then biological defence, including technical biological defence, is no longer possible under national jurisdiction. If, on the other hand, only vaccine production and development, but not the other aspects of biological defence programmes are internationalized, then the question arises as to whether the most important components of biological defence will even be included. As Graham S. Pearson has shown, there are three key elements of a biological defence programme: detection, protection and medical countermeasures.[17] Vaccination is one aspect of medical countermeasures; the development and production of vaccines, however, is by no means the only part of a biological defence programme in which pathogens are needed. In the area of detection and perhaps in that of physical protection they may also be needed.

At any rate the development, for example, of early-warning systems for biological agents on the battlefield requires real pathogens in order to determine whether the new systems will work. This in turn means that in regard to the BWC, the key problem of the verification issue—namely, what amount of which types of pathogens are necessary for peaceful or defensive military uses—still remains unresolved. This does not mean, however, that the problem is inevitably unsolvable. The ongoing talks between governmental experts might approach agreement on what amount of biological agents can be permitted, but again it is hard to see how the VFP programme could lead to the strengthening of the BWC.

[17] See the contribution by Pearson, chapter 14, in this volume.

V. Problems of establishing the VFP programme

It is also questionable whether it is appropriate to establish a 'super authority' to control vaccines and the development of vaccines. The make-up and decision-making power of such an authority is completely unclear to the author of this chapter. Should it be an authority where those states that can offer the know-how, primarily the industrialized countries, have control and where the dependence of the developing countries becomes institutionalized? Or on the contrary, should it be an authority where the developing countries make the demands and the industrial countries place their knowledge at the disposal of all? Would not such an enormous bureaucracy also produce excessive and unnecessary costs?

The financing of a project such as the VFP programme appears questionable—despite Geissler's proposed savings (peace dividend)—when it is recalled that the United Nations is suffering enormous financial problems. Currently, members owe the United Nations $1.85 billion.[18]

The United Nations is growing ever more overburdened. In particular, it is unclear how the numerous peace-keeping operations should be paid for. In the United States, which carries 30 per cent of total UN costs for peace-keeping activities, the opinion is spreading—particularly in Congress—that Germany and Japan should take on a greater share and relieve the United States of part of its burden.[19] In view of the precarious budgetary situation of almost all the industrialized countries, not to speak of the developing countries, there is little reason to believe that the VFP programme would not be affected by such financial constraints.

Additionally, there is the question of how the interests of the national pharmaceutical industries should be taken into account. They produce vaccines for the civilian sector that could, of course, be used at any time by the military. The best example of this is that before Operation Desert Shield/Desert Storm the United States bought vaccines against anthrax and botulism on the open market. Are industries in free-market economies prepared to act under the oversight of an international authority instead of on the basis of supply and demand?

VI. Conclusion

The idea of international co-operation in the area of biological defence is basically sound. More openness is indeed needed, so that the states do not suspect each other of hiding offensive biological programmes behind declared defensive endeavours. However, whether this goal could be achieved by the proposed Vaccines for Peace programme is doubtful.

As long as the BWC remains practically unverifiable and as long as far from every state is a State Party to the Convention, it is especially unlikely that the most powerful countries will be willing to give up national competence in such sensitive areas as biological defence. This is also—and even particularly—valid

[18] 'UNO-Sitzung mit 20 neuen Mitgliedern' [UN meeting with 20 new members], *Süddeutsche Zeitung*, 16 Sep. 1992.

[19] Oberdorfer, D., 'Congress warns Baker over aid for truce forces', *International Herald Tribune*, 5 Mar. 1992.

after the cold war. Smaller wars are not only more probable, they are actually taking place. Those who intervene in such wars, even be it with the goal of bringing such wars to an end, will at least want to immunize their soldiers against diseases that tend to occur under combat conditions. They will hardly want to make themselves dependent on an international authority in order to do this. In view of the lack of interest of the 'key players' in the VFP programme, it is not very likely to be realized.

The realization of the VFP programme, as proposed by Geissler, could even be dangerous in that it would not prevent, but promote proliferation. In any case, the VFP programme would hardly contribute to the intended strengthening of the BWC because it would not motivate those non-signatories to the BWC that are problem cases in terms of proliferation to enter the regime. Even if they were to do so, this would not necessarily mean that these states would abandon programmes they might be conducting in violation of the BWC.

The author of this chapter would recommend that the VFP programme be run as a civilian programme aimed at providing developing countries with needed vaccines for civilian purposes. Apparently, the Biesenthal Consensus[20] already reflects the change of the VFP programme in that direction. The goal of strengthening the BWC should be pursued both by improved and better implemented CBMs and by trying to build up at least a rudimentary verification regime for this Convention.

[20] See annexe C in this volume.

6. Control and co-operation in biological defence research: national programmes and international accountability

NICHOLAS A. SIMS

I. Introduction

The treaty regime flowing from the 1972 Convention on the Prohibition of the Development, Production and Stockpiling of Bacteriological (Biological) and Toxin Weapons and on their Destruction, the Biological Weapons Convention (BWC), is in full evolution. Its Third Review Conference, in 1991, confirmed a widespread perception that the regime not only needed to be strengthened but could and should be without further delay. At last, in the 1990s, it became 'practical politics' to explore the potential always present in the Convention but previously held back by the adverse conditions of the international political environment, notably the mutual suspicion between the Soviet Union and the West. Foundations had already been laid for the reinforcement of the treaty regime by the interpretations of the Convention, and agreements on the implications for States Parties' conduct in ensuring its implementation, which the first two Review Conferences had recorded in their final declarations, in 1980 and (less tentatively) in 1986. Now it was time to build systematically on those foundations. Eventually, this may lead to certain additional obligations, notably in respect of openness to international verification, being negotiated as Protocols to the Convention. However, for the moment at least, and perhaps for rather longer, the strengthening of the treaty regime depends upon States Parties realizing the possibilities latent in the text of the Convention as it stands.

The Vaccines for Peace (VFP) initiative is a welcome part of this process, enabling States Parties to give practical effect to the principle of international co-operation for peaceful purposes, in particular for the prevention of disease, which is affirmed in Article X of the Convention.

II. Return to earlier proposals

Another part of this process is the return to consideration of earlier proposals which envisaged a more open and comprehensive system for dispelling fears that offensive military capabilities for biological and toxin warfare might be developed in national defence establishments. The problem is this: how can research and development (R&D) programmes aimed at protection against biological and toxin weapons (BTWs) which are a fully legitimate and indeed necessary concomitant of BTW disarmament (adding a further disincentive to any potential aggressor which might think of violating the Convention), be distinguished from programmes with offensive intent?

Part of the attraction of the VFP initiative[1] and of the International Program of Development and Use of Vaccines (IPDUV) proposals[2] which preceded it lies in the prospect of military and civil facilities being harnessed together in a common effort to combat disease through the development of more and better vaccines. Vaccine development is an important part of the mission of national defence establishments in so far as it contributes to prophylaxis against attack, through the immunization of troops against certain agents (for example, *Bacillus anthracis*, the causative agent of anthrax). How can general reassurance best be given that such protective programmes mask no offensive intent?

III. International accountability through greater openness

Originally it was envisaged that the Convention would constrain research, through an obligation 'not to conduct, assist or permit research aimed at production of the kind prohibited',[3] but one of several casualties of the 1971 negotiations was any reference whatever to research. The Convention, as negotiated, only subjects development, not research, to the Article I qualifying criteria of 'prophylactic, protective or other peaceful purposes'.[4] Research which did not amount to development was left unconstrained, however offensive its aims and purposes. This has complicated attempts to make the Convention more effective.

In its working paper on microbiological warfare, the United Kingdom had recognized that the constraint on research which, as just quoted, it was then proposing would entail a regime of correspondingly greater openness:

> [The Convention] should also provide for the appropriate civil medical or health authorities to have access to all research work which might give rise to allegations that the obligations imposed by the Convention were not being fulfilled. Such research work should be open to international investigation if so required and should also be open to public scrutiny to the maximum extent compatible with national security and the protection of industrial and commercial processes.[5]

This is just the kind of proposal which deserves reconsideration in the changed world of the 1990s. It may well have been ahead of its time. While it may still be difficult to negotiate an acceptable balance between 'public scrutiny' and 'national security and the protection of industrial and commercial processes', the attempt should now be made both to define a workable balance between those desiderata and to arrange for research in certain categories to be 'open to international investigation'. How to prevent an 'international investigation' leaking information to governments still interested in developing offensive biological and toxin warfare capabilities, in such a way as to diminish the effectiveness of the protective programmes deriving from such research,

[1] Geissler, E., 'Vaccines for Peace: an international program of development and use of vaccines against dual-threat agents', *Politics and the Life Sciences*, vol. 11, no. 2 (Aug. 1992), pp. 231–43.

[2] Proposals circulated at the Third Review Conference (Geneva, Sep. 1991) and subsequent revisions; see also chapter 3 of this volume.

[3] United Kingdom, 'Working paper on microbiological warfare', Eighteen-Nation Disarmament Committee document ENDC/231, 6 Aug. 1968.

[4] Article I of the Convention; see annexe A in this volume.

[5] See United Kingdom (note 3).

would no doubt be high on the agenda of the negotiators. Other obstacles may also be identified, but to note that there are obstacles to be tackled does not invalidate the attempt to see how practical effect could be given to the 1968 proposal.

The aim must be to establish a norm of international accountability to which effect can be given through greater openness.

It is possible that the International Biological Monitoring Agency proposed by Dr Herbert Marcovich in 1990[6] might be adapted to serve as a mechanism for the proposed 'international investigation' of research programmes. Alternatively, the States Parties to the Convention might prefer to create their own Scientific Advisory Panel for this purpose, perhaps basing themselves on earlier proposals of Professor Richard Falk in 1984 that an 'inter-governmental select body of experts . . . be established to investigate the general directions of biological research and to set forth guidelines to sustain the prohibition on military development',[7] or in 1986 that this might be one of the roles of a panel of scientific experts whose principal function would be 'to consider seriously investigation of non-compliance allegations'.[8] The present author recommended in 1991 that the Scientific Advisory Panel, as one of a set of supportive institutions serving the States Parties as a whole, should not be inter-governmental but 'should consist of eminent individuals acting in a personal capacity. It is likely to have plenty of work to do assessing new developments in science and technology, and advising States Parties on their implications for the resilience of the constraints on biological and toxin weapons, and for new pressures and incentives to disregard them'.[9]

In short, international co-operation demands accountability through greater openness in defence research against BTWs. The challenge of the 1990s is to devise appropriate procedures, empower appropriate institutions and negotiate appropriate safeguards against unintentionally assisting potential aggressors to make their biological and toxin warfare capabilities more effective.

IV. International control

Another proposal which may be worthy of reconsideration in the new climate of determination to make the biological disarmament regime work effectively is that of international control over biological defence research. In so far as this implies direction, it goes further than the proposals considered in the preceding section, which had to do rather with accountability through greater openness.

It was on 10 March 1980, at the First Review Conference, that Dr L. D. Thomson, in his opening plenary statement for Australia, addressed the problem of internationalizing biological defence research. The official summary record reads:

[6] Marcovich, H., 'Proposal for an international biological monitoring agency', ed. E. Geissler, *Strengthening the Biological Weapons Convention by Confidence-Building Measures*, SIPRI Chemical & Biological Warfare Studies, no. 10 (Oxford University Press: Oxford, 1990), pp. 198–201.

[7] Falk, R., *Science*, 15 June 1984, cited in Institute for Defense and Disarmament Studies, 'Application of genetic engineering to biological warfare', *Arms Control Reporter* (IDDS: Brookline, Mass.), sheet 701.C.2, July 1984.

[8] Falk, R., 'Strengthening the Biological Weapons Convention of 1972', ed. E. Geissler, SIPRI, *Biological and Toxin Weapons Today* (Oxford University Press: Oxford, 1986), p. 117.

[9] Sims, N. A., *Reinforcing Biological Disarmament: Issues in the 1991 Review*, Faraday Discussion Paper no. 16 (Council for Arms Control: London, 1991), p. 21.

Besides favouring the exchange of information for the prevention of disease, his delegation wondered whether consideration should not be given to the possibility of internationalising research into means of defence against bacteriological weapons. For example, it might be possible to arrange for the exchange of scientists between establishments or to place all research activities under international control. Although there would be practical difficulties in so doing, the Conference could perhaps consider the question.[10]

The version of the middle part provided by the Australian Department of Foreign Affairs and Trade reads slightly more strongly in that it specifies *free* exchange of scientists,[11] which suggests that this mode of internationalizing research would be essentially unrestricted.

At the time Ambassador Thomson's paragraph on internationalizing research struck at least one participant as 'the most intriguing proposal made during the conference on the subject of international cooperation'. The same account of the conference continued: 'Possibly, in a more propitious international climate it might become "practical politics" and at a further review Australia's bold and imaginative proposal might not be given such short shrift as it was in 1980'.[12]

However, this was a time of rapidly worsening East–West relations and Ambassador Thomson's suggestion of international control was not pursued at the First Review Conference or subsequently. It is possible that the suggestion was coolly received because of its implications for national security, or for commercial confidentiality, or simply because it appeared inopportune in the climate of mutual suspicion and accusation which characterized the BTW disarmament regime in the wake of the 1979 'Sverdlovsk incident'[13] and other alleged instances of (mainly) Soviet non-compliance with the Convention.

Because no delegation placed on record its views on the suggestion of international control, it is impossible to do more than speculate on the reasons for its non-acceptance. It may be significant that the Australian delegation itself made no further reference to the proposal, even in its committee interventions or in informal working papers, although on other issues in that Review Conference it was one of the most active delegations. The only conclusion which can be drawn is that it was a very tentative suggestion, perhaps in the nature of a *ballon d'essai*, and not one to which Australia was strongly attached.

Instead, Australia in common with other States Parties pursued the confidence-building measure (CBM) route favoured in Ambassador Thomson's reference to 'arranging for a free exchange of scientists between establishments'.[14] This was seen as a more feasible approach. It did not address the issue of international control but it did look to a future of greater transparency, in which international exchanges would generate a confidence-building effect and render protective programmes less susceptible to suspicion and misinterpretation. In this spirit Australia promoted the adoption of CBMs at the Second

[10] BWC/CONF.I/SR.8, paragraph 31.

[11] 'One possible solution would be for BW defence research to be international, either by arranging for a free exchange of scientists between establishments or by placing all research under international control.' Text supplied by the Australian Department of Foreign Affairs and Trade, Chemical and Biological Disarmament Section of Arms Control Branch, 5 Mar. 1993.

[12] Sims, N. A., *The Diplomacy of Biological Disarmament: Vicissitudes of a Treaty in Force, 1975–85* (Macmillan: London; St Martin's Press: New York, 1988), p. 146.

[13] See Geissler, chapter 3, section VIII, in this volume.

[14] See note 11.

Review Conference in 1986 and their enhancement and expansion at the Third Review Conference in 1991.

Much has changed since 1980, and it is timely to ask whether, and if so how, substance might be given in the 1990s to the idea of 'placing all research under international control'.

To go the whole way would necessitate willingness on the part of national defence establishments to accept direction from an international agency, to which moreover they would have had to entrust information on all their R&D programmes in sufficient detail to give meaning to the concept of international control. This is not immediately a plausible prospect. National defence establishments are likely to resist both the divulging of sensitive information (noted above as an obstacle to implementation of the 1968 proposal) and the acceptance of external direction. Yet even if this prerequisite condition is unlikely to be fulfilled, it may still be possible to move some way towards international control. The immediate way forward may lie in: (*a*) the development of transparency mechanisms, which help to dispel suspicions surrounding the anti-BTW defence research programmes of governments, and (*b*) a recognition of the need to assure a continuous demonstration of compliance, combined with (*c*) the VFP initiative as a framework for co-operation between national defence establishments and the civil pharmaceutical research sector (academic and commercial) in carefully selected areas.

In the longer term, however, a fourth approach should be explored: the extension to a wider spread of States Parties of information-sharing arrangements which have developed among certain governments. Canada, the United Kingdom and the United States have long enjoyed privileged access to one another's R&D achievements in defence against BTWs (as also against chemical weapons). This information-sharing arrangement has, since 1965, extended to Australia, although Australia has never actively participated in the collaborative research on biological defence allowed under this quadripartite Technical Cooperation Programme. Knowledge is power, and also currency; governments will not easily give away expensively won information without the near-certainty of fair exchange or compensation in some other form. They will be particularly wary of giving away any information which might point to possible gaps in their protective spectrum. It is, therefore, only as mutual confidence grows that governments will be ready to share much information, and only when governments perceive themselves to belong to a 'security community' (a more nebulous, but also more durable, relationship than that of alliance) that they will be ready to share the kind of particularly sensitive information which may reveal vulnerabilities.

This is likely to be a gradual process. Defence scientists who feel a special responsibility for ensuring the survival of their country's troops in the event of BTW attack will naturally be very cautious in case the sharing of information might, however inadvertently, help an eventual aggressor. The position is well expressed by Dr Graham S. Pearson in his contribution to this volume:

> The aim of biological defence is to ensure that the armed forces can maintain their operational effectiveness despite being attacked by biological weapons. In other words, military personnel need to survive and to be able to use their weapon systems and platforms. Effective biological defence contributes to the web of deterrence which reduces

the utility of biological warfare to a potential aggressor. However, as in all defence, a defence that is freely available to the potential aggressor to examine and evaluate is no defence as he will seek to and be able to circumvent that defence. The objective of an effective defence is to increase the uncertainty of the aggressor as to whether his biological warfare capability will be effective in achieving his military objective as well as to what response the use of BW will provoke. The goal is for the potential violator to judge that his acquisition of biological weapons would be militarily ineffective because of BW defence capabilities, prohibitively expensive because of export controls and arms control measures and liable to detection through verification or monitoring arrangements, and that the consequences would be politically unacceptable.[15]

V. Transparency mechanisms

Canada introduced the concept of transparency mechanisms, under that name, at the Third Review Conference in 1991. The purpose of such mechanisms was to provide reassurance by subjecting a government's anti-CBW programmes to independent scientific scrutiny. In the case of Canada, on the recommendation of the 1988 Barton Report, this function was being performed by a Biological and Chemical Defence Review Committee consisting of three eminent scientists. Its first annual report was made public in August 1991.[16]

If possible, transparency mechanisms should have a dual audience. Then reassurance is transmitted outwards, to other governments, and inwards, to parliament and people. The governments of other States Parties need to be reassured that the programme is purely protective and has no offensive intent which might threaten their security. Parliament and people need that reassurance, too: they want to know that their government is acting fully in compliance with its treaty obligations. However, they will also want to be reassured that the protective programme is generating effective protection for their troops and giving value for money. There may also be concerns to be allayed regarding research ethics, health, safety and environmental protection.

It is always open to governments to create transparency mechanisms independently of their treaty obligations, simply as a matter of prudent policy. However, they may well see advantage in combining the use of transparency mechanisms with the discharge of treaty obligations and providing a single report every year (supplemented as necessary in the course of the year) which goes to other governments and to parliament and people with the added value of comment appended by the Review Committee, or whatever the group of independent scientists appointed to scrutinize the programme is called.

Under the BWC there is no direct obligation to report on protective programmes. In practice information is exchanged under CBM 'A',[17] as enhanced at the Third Review Conference, and under the new CBM 'F'[18] as regards past activity. As more States Parties start to honour the politically binding commit-

[15] Pearson, G. S., 'Vaccines for biological defence: defence considerations', chapter 14 in this volume.

[16] Canada, 'Transparency mechanisms for the Canadian chemical and biological defence program', BWC/CONF.III/10, 11 Sep. 1991.

[17] Confidence-building measure 'A', Part 1. Exchange of data on research centres and laboratories, Part 2. Exchange of information on national biological defence research and development programmes.

[18] Confidence-building measure 'F', Declaration of past activities in offensive and/or defensive biological research and development programmes.

ment to engage in annual data exchanges under the CBMs, more information may be expected to come into the public domain by this means.

There is a way in which reporting on protective programmes could be more expressly defined as an obligation under the BWC, derived from its Article V. It would be desirable for the Fourth Review Conference to make an explicit declaration that the existence of R&D programmes which are intended as protective but may (however mistakenly) be regarded as offensive or potentially offensive in intent constitutes a 'problem which may arise in relation to the objective of, or in the application of the provisions of the Convention' and is accordingly subject to the Article V obligation 'to consult one another and to cooperate in solving' any such problems. Prompt and full exchange of data could then become the recognized 'best practice' by which States Parties gave continuous effect to that part of their Article V problem-solving obligation.

Because the same government establishments are usually responsible for R&D programmes against both BW and CW agents, transparency mechanisms may most conveniently be applied to both. Although the content of such programmes differs in some respects as between anti-CW and anti-BTW protection (most obviously in the relevance of prophylaxis and the technology of detection and identification of agents), the need for reassurance both nationally and internationally is common to both kinds of programme. Hence the desirability of a common standard of transparency, equally applicable to both.

The 1993 Chemical Weapons Convention (CWC), on an initiative of Australia[19] which eventually found its way into Article X without opposition, refers directly to 'the transparency of national programmes related to protective purposes' and lays down an annual reporting requirement (see below). Although its scope is, evidently, limited to chemical weapons, this requirement could have important implications for reassurance on biological defence research, too.

Eventually, if agreement is reached on expanding the ambit of the Organization for the Prohibition of Chemical Weapons (OPCW) to embrace biological defence research as well, an equivalent provision could be added as an amendment to the BWC. That, however, is a distant and controversial prospect. The OPCW does not come into existence until 1995 at the earliest and it will have its work cut out to implement the CWC through its early years in force. Conversely, the biological disarmament regime has its own distinctive features (including a quite different history with regard to verification) and its own institutional requirements, which may or may not converge on those of the CWC.

What seems more likely in the short run is an informal spillover from the CWC requirement. What is legally mandatory in respect of chemical disarmament may be seen as good practice in respect of biological disarmament, developing all the more easily because of organizational arrangements for defence research within government establishments.

Article X of the CWC is concerned with Assistance and Protection Against Chemical Weapons. The relevant paragraphs are 2 and 4:

[19] Australia initially proposed what is now CWC Article X.4 as Article VI.9 in its Model Draft Convention; see Conference on Disarmament document CD/1143, 12 Mar. 1992, p. 15.

2. Nothing in this Convention shall be interpreted as impeding the right of any State Party to conduct research into, develop, produce, acquire, transfer or use means of protection against chemical weapons, for purposes not prohibited under this Convention.

4. For the purposes of increasing the transparency of national programmes related to protective purposes, each State Party shall provide annually to the Technical Secretariat [of the OPCW] information on its programme, in accordance with procedures to be considered and approved by the Conference pursuant to Article VIII, paragraph 21 (i).

The subparagraph specified is that which empowers the Conference of States Parties, the highest organ of the OPCW, when it comes into being upon the CWC's entry into force, to 'consider and approve at its first session any draft agreements, provisions and guidelines developed by the Preparatory Commission'.

Narrowly construed, Article X.4 could be interpreted as requiring governments only to communicate in confidence with the Technical Secretariat. It is to be hoped, on the contrary, that the procedures to be elaborated by the Preparatory Commission will ensure that the annual reports are circulated to all States Parties and are also made public. This greater openness with regard to chemical defence research could, and should, spill over into the biological defence research sector.

It would then be open to governments to channel their annual reports through Biological and Chemical Defence Review Committees or other transparency mechanisms: to use them, in short, not merely to reassure other States Parties through the OPCW but at the same time to reassure parliament and people through the chosen mechanism.

The inclusion of a ban on TW agents in both the BWC and CWC means that at least the element of protection against toxin warfare in anti-BTW programmes should be reported under CWC Article X.4. This is a further reason to take advantage of the frequent organizational unity (or at the very least proximity) of chemical defence and biological defence. Reporting may not be quite so explicitly required by the BWC, but it is a good way of strengthening confidence in States Parties' compliance with it. If governments are reporting annually on protective programmes against toxin warfare, as they are obliged to do under CWC Article X.4, why go to the trouble of withholding equivalent information regarding their protective programmes against biological warfare, especially when the very act of withholding such information is liable to misinterpretation?

VI. Demonstrating compliance

So long as national defence establishments maintain anti-BTW programmes which are not subject to international control of one kind or another, they should recognize that it is incumbent upon them to demonstrate the innocuous character of the R&D activities for which they are responsible.

Transparency mechanisms may help to increase confidence in the veracity of national defence establishments' declarations that prophylaxis, protection and other peaceful purposes account for the entirety of their programmes. Exchanges of scientists, visits and other manifestations of openness at the international level may also help. As familiarity with the CBM requirements[20] laid down by the Third Review Conference develops, so States Parties may find themselves asked for further information to clarify their declared data, including data provided under CBM 'A'.

The limits of parliamentary accountability will vary from one country to another, and the extent of international accountability is ill-defined. What is certain, however, is that both kinds of accountability will have to be taken increasingly into consideration. A government must not only satisfy itself that its defence scientists are fully under its control and innocent of any offensive intent; it must be ready to satisfy parliament and people, and other governments, that its confidence is well-founded.

All these possibilities raise the question of how compliance can best be demonstrated. What features are there, in a legitimate R&D programme, which reliably indicate its legitimacy?

Tackling the question the other way round, what was it about the purported biological defence research undertaken at Salman Pak in Iraq which convinced UNSCOM inspectors of its offensive intent when they inspected the site in August 1991 and subsequently? Concerns over Biopreparat in Leningrad (now St Petersburg) and other R&D facilities in the former Soviet Union, concerns which have since 1992 been jointly addressed by the Russian, British and US governments, may also have yielded significant indicators. The absence of certain indicators may render implausible the performance of legitimate research functions; the presence of others may point to the likelihood of research in the facility in question being directed towards preparation of an offensive biological warfare programme. To the extent possible, such indicators should be made public. It would then be easier for legitimate defence establishments to demonstrate the innocuous character of their anti-BTW research profile and thereby dispel genuine suspicions and mischief-making allegations alike.

Even with such indicators made public, however, certain problems of ambiguity and disbelief are likely to persist, even if on a smaller scale. The approach just outlined cannot, therefore, be relied upon to provide a complete solution. It is worth repeating that the legitimacy of vaccine and other research programmes in biological defence will continue to depend critically on the perceived good faith of those conducting and those controlling the programmes, and on the transparency of the institutional and procedural safeguards installed in order to prevent anyone who may nourish offensive intentions from diverting the research effort at any level. In so far as safeguards set in place by national governments alone will not always satisfy the sceptics (who can now point to Boris Yeltsin's admitted ignorance of what was happening in Sverdlovsk in 1979 during his tenure as Party Secretary there) some kind of international accountability would seem to be essential, however difficult it may be to give practical effect to this principle.

[20] Annex to the Final Declaration of the Third Review Conference, BWC/CONF.III/23, Geneva, 1992, pp. 27–49.

VII. Civil–military co-operation

Within the framework of the VFP initiative there may be scope for civil–military co-operation. Much depends upon the ability to identify the vaccines for which there is the greatest need.

It may be that the vaccines most urgently needed to protect vulnerable populations against diseases endemic in poor countries are not the vaccines most urgently needed to protect troops against the agents with which, should an enemy resort to biological warfare, they are thought likely to be attacked. In that event, civil–military co-operation will take the form of complementarity, perhaps involving advances in the general technology of vaccine production and development rather than identical vaccines. Or it may be that a certain vaccine appears to demand priority attention for both civil and military protection purposes, since troops also need to be vaccinated against diseases endemic in any theatre of operations to which they may be sent: the very same diseases against which the local population needs protection. In that case the challenge will be to find both nationally and internationally acceptable safeguards over R&D and production of the vaccine in question.

As noted in 1991,

> It would be idle to pretend that states will find it easy to take all the necessary decisions. There is a delicate balance of risks and a long tradition of secrecy which together incline governments to regard both their BW threat assessments and their consequential anti-BW countermeasures as national assets to be closely guarded. However, if full reciprocity were assured, there need logically be no diminution in security. The difficulty lies in effecting the transition from here to there.

The dilemma facing governments is this:

> Will the gains for international confidence outweigh the losses to national security? It may be shortsighted of governments to pose the issue in such terms, but it would be unrealistic to suppose that they will not. The challenge is for them to find ways of making the transition to openness, in which governments worldwide share the 'state-of-the-art' in anti-BW prophylaxis and protection as a universal safeguard against terrorist groups or maverick states, and to retain undiminished security throughout that transition.[21]

Against this background, it is understandable that governments remain reticent about their national intelligence estimates and assessments of the 'agents of choice' against which they deem their armed forces to be in greatest need of protection. They fear that if they made such assessments public and revealed the full extent of their prophylactic and other precautions they would draw undesirable attention to the gaps in their protective spectrum, and would thereby render their troops more vulnerable to an attack which used unexpected agents to exploit those very gaps.

This understandable reticence does not in any way diminish the obligation on those responsible for biological defence programmes to find ways of assuring the continuous demonstration of compliance; but in the matter of prophylaxis by vaccines it undoubtedly sets limits to the scope for civil–military co-operation. Yet national defence establishments can perceive, as clearly as any-

[21] Sims (note 9), pp. 13–14.

one else, the global predicament of applied immunology, which can be simply stated: commercial vaccine production is skewed by the profit-seeking strategies of the major pharmaceutical companies away from the development of effective vaccines for immunization against many of the diseases (other than AIDS) endemic in poor countries.

Intervention along the lines of the VFP initiative is indicated, if this distortion caused by market forces is ever to be rectified. In principle, too, such intervention should contribute to discouraging resort to biological warfare. The higher the level of immunity from endemic diseases in the general population, the harder it will be to disguise any attack as being of natural origin (something which has often complicated investigation of allegations involving diseases endemic to the region in question) and the stronger, in consequence, will be the incentive to remain in full compliance with the obligations of the Convention, because any effective warfare agent would have to be exotic and hence more readily detectable.

Careful selection of areas for civil–military co-operation will be required. This is yet a further reason for the States Parties to the BWC to endow their treaty regime with supportive institutions in which they can confer at diplomatic or scientific levels, as required, in the long intervals between Review Conferences. The *Ad Hoc* Group of Governmental Experts to Identify and Examine Potential Verification Measures (VEREX) which was set up by the Third Review Conference was a start, but it had a very narrow, precisely negotiated, mandate[22] and only a two-year (1992–93) existence. Until the States Parties correct the mistake they made in 1991, when the Third Review Conference lamentably failed to create an intersessional committee of oversight (under that name or any other) or even a dedicated secretariat unit to serve the implementation of the Convention,[23] they are scarcely equipped to take collective action in support of the Vaccines for Peace initiative or other proposals for greater international co-operation.

22 Part of the Article Five section of the Final Declaration of the Third Review Conference, BWC/CONF.III/23, Geneva, 1992, pp. 17–18.

23 Sims, N. A. 'Achievements and failures at the Third Review Conference', *Chemical Weapons Convention Bulletin,* no. 14 (Dec. 1991), pp. 4–5.

7. Verification of the BWC

TIBOR TÓTH,* ERHARD GEISSLER and THOMAS STOCK

I. Introduction

The Convention on the Prohibition of the Development, Production and Stockpiling of Bacteriological (Biological) and Toxin Weapons and on their Destruction (BWC) was opened for signature in April 1972, more then 20 years ago.[1] As of 31 December 1993, 130 countries had become States Parties to the Convention.[2] The BWC was the first convention to prohibit an entire class of weapons. Nevertheless, at the time that it was agreed it made no provision for monitoring compliance or verification.

The Chemical Weapons Convention (CWC) was successfully concluded in 1992 and will presumably enter into force in 1995.[3] By the end of 1993, it had been signed by 154 states.

One of the most heavily criticized and debated elements of the BWC is the lack of a reliable, effective verification mechanism. The 1991 Persian Gulf War reminded many people very clearly of the impact chemical weapon (CW) and biological weapon (BW) proliferation can have, despite the fact there was no actual use of such weapons.[4] Delegations at the Third Review Conference of the BWC in 1991 devoted a major part of their time to discussion of finding a remedy to this deplorable situation. No one was surprised, however, when it became apparent that the issue of verification was a very delicate one, both in the political and the technical sense. The United Nations Special Commission on Iraq (UNSCOM),[5] which was established in the aftermath of the Persian Gulf War, has proved the ability of the United Nations to carry out intrusive on-site verification and monitoring activities, disposal of weapons of mass destruction and long-term monitoring of compliance obligations, albeit under special conditions.

Two main schools of thought have emerged in relation to verification. One takes the approach that verification measures under the BWC must be introduced regardless of whether they will be effective or possible to implement. The second approach is one which says that, of course, there is a need to intro-

[1] The text of the BWC is reproduced in annexe A in this volume.

[2] Ferm, R., 'Major multilateral arms control agreements', SIPRI, *SIPRI Yearbook 1993: World Armaments and Disarmament* (Oxford University Press: Oxford, 1993), p. 763.

[3] Conference on Disarmament document CD/1173, 3 Sep. 1992; Robinson, J. P. P, Stock, T. and Sutherland, R. G., 'The Chemical Weapons Convention: the success of chemical disarmament negotiations', *SIPRI Yearbook 1993* (note 2), pp. 715–34; for the text of the CWC, see *SIPRI Yearbook 1993* (note 2), pp. 735–56.

[4] In 1993 numerous articles and investigations reported illnesses suffered by Gulf War veterans. One possible explanation of this so-called Gulf War Syndrome was the accidental release of chemical agents during the war. See Staff Report to U.S. Senator Donald W. Riegle, Jr, *Gulf War Syndrome: the Case for Multiple Origin Mixed Chemical/Biotoxin Warfare Related Disorders*, US Senate, 9 Sep. 1993.

[5] See Ekéus, R., 'The United Nations Special Commission on Iraq', SIPRI, *SIPRI Yearbook 1992: World Armaments and Disarmament* (Oxford University Press: Oxford, 1992), pp. 509–30; Ekéus, R., 'The United Nations Special Commission on Iraq: activities in 1992', *SIPRI Yearbook 1993* (note 2), pp. 691–703.

* Ambassador Tóth co-authored sections I–III.

duce verification measures, but first there must be an evaluation of all of the scientific and technical arguments associated with such measures. In any case, verification under the BWC must serve to deter a possible violator from seeking to acquire biological weapons and provide a degree of assurance that any such violation is likely to be detected by these verification measures. In addition, an independent international authority must have the power to evaluate verification results and to draw conclusions about compliance or non-compliance. Conducting such verification on an international level will require both resources and personnel.

A Review Conference of only three weeks duration was not able to iron out and co-ordinate all of the various verification proposals which have been made,[6] thus a decision was taken to use a previously successful mechanism and to establish a technical working group to examine potential verification measures. This was done based on the experience of the *Ad Hoc* Group of Governmental Experts set up by the Second Review Conference of the BWC, which worked out the first set of confidence-building measures (CBMs).[7] This mechanism was further strengthened in 1991 and could form one of the basic building blocks of a future verification system.

The 1991 Third Review Conference established an *Ad Hoc* Group of Governmental Experts to Identify and Examine Potential Verification Measures from a Scientific and Technical Standpoint (VEREX). After thorough discussion, the group was given a clearly defined mandate for its work.[8] Nevertheless the official name of the *Ad Hoc* Group does not indicate clearly what is to be verified; in fact it is compliance with the BWC. The mandate of the *Ad Hoc* Group is to identify measures which could determine whether a State Party to the BWC is engaged in prohibited activities either with regard to agents, or to weapons and means of delivery.

Perhaps the most important words in both the official name of the *Ad Hoc* Group and its mandate are 'verification measures'. There are six main criteria for the evaluation of these measures: (*a*) their information-providing ability, (*b*) their ability to differentiate between prohibited and permitted activities, (*c*) their ability to resolve ambiguities about compliance, (*d*) their technical, financial, legal and other implications, (*e*) their impact on scientific activities, and (*f*) their relation to the requirements for confidentiality. The *Ad Hoc* Group was asked to complete its work before the end of 1993 and to present a consensus report to all States Parties,[9] which described the work of the *Ad Hoc* Group and the views expressed during its sessions.

The *Ad Hoc* Group held four sessions: VEREX I (identification of measures) on 30 March–10 April 1992, VEREX II (examination of measures) on 23 November–4 December 1992, VEREX III (evaluation of measures) on

[6] See Atlas, R. M. and Goldberg, M., 'Biological warfare: examining verification strategies', *ASM News*, vol. 59, no. 8 (1993), pp. 393–96; Rosenberg, B. H., 'Progress toward verification of the Biological Weapons Convention', VERTIC *Verification Report 1993: Peacekeeping, Arms Control and the Environment* (Brassey's: London, 1993), pp. 189–96.

[7] *Ad Hoc* Meeting of Scientific and Technical Experts from States Parties to the Convention on the Prohibition of the Development, Production and Stockpiling of Bacteriological (Biological) and Toxin Weapons and on their Destruction, BWC/CONF.II/EX/2, 21 Apr. 1987.

[8] Third Review Conference of the Parties to the Convention on the Prohibition of the Development, Production and Stockpiling of Bacteriological (Biological) and Toxin Weapons and on their Destruction, Geneva, 9–27 September 1991, *Final Document*, BWC/CONF.III/23, part II, pp. 16–17.

[9] *Ad Hoc* Group of Governmental Experts to Identify and Examine Potential Verification Measures from a Scientific and Technical Standpoint, *Report*, BWC/CONF.III/VEREX/9, Geneva, 1993.

24 May–4 June 1993 and VEREX IV (preparation of a consensus report) on 13–24 September 1993. As many as 53 States Parties participated in the sessions as did an observer representing the World Health Organization (WHO). An additional observer representing the United Nations Industrial Development Organization (UNIDO) took part in VEREX I.

The basic task of the first session of the *Ad Hoc* Group (VEREX I) was to identify and compile a list of potential verification measures which could determine whether a State Party is engaged in prohibited activities. Though different stages of the work might not be clearly identifiable, logic dictates that this phase of identification and compilation was followed by more detailed description and analysis (VEREX II). The third phase was the evaluation of the measures (VEREX III), and the last—and most difficult—part was the preparation of the report. The success of the group was achieved by its concentration on technical rather than political aspects; the following is a short assessment of the achievements of the group.

II. Identification of potential verification measures: VEREX I

In the first session, VEREX I, the *Ad Hoc* Group tried to apply the 'measure-oriented' approach. Thus, the basis for identification and compilation was not the list of prohibited activities, but rather the specific nature of the measures themselves. Within the two major categories, namely off-site and on-site, the different measures were clustered into subcategories such as information monitoring, data exchange, remote sensing and inspections for the off-site category; and exchange visits, inspections, and continuous monitoring for the on-site category. It was at the level of these subcategories that the possibly differing requirements of different types of prohibitions were taken into account. The identified measures were further categorized according to their relevance to the phases of development, acquisition or production, and stockpiling.

Within these subcategories a total of 21 measures was identified for further examination (see table 7.1): (*a*) surveillance of publications, (*b*) surveillance of legislation, (*c*) data on transfers and transfer requests and on production, (*d*) multilateral information sharing, (*e*) declarations, (*f*) notifications, (*g*) surveillance by satellite, (*h*) surveillance by aircraft, (*i*) ground-based surveillance, (*j*) sampling and identification off-site, (*k*) observation, (*l*) auditing off-site, (*m*) international arrangements, (*n*) interviewing, (*o*) visual inspection, (*p*) identification of key equipment, (*q*) auditing on-site, (*r*) sampling and identification on-site, (*s*) medical examination, (*t*) continuous monitoring by instruments, and (*u*) continuous monitoring by personnel.[10]

In the subcategory 'information monitoring' the *Ad Hoc* Group listed the following concrete measures: surveillance of publications, surveillance of legislation, data on transfers and transfer requests and on production, multilateral information sharing and exchange visits. Certainly these measures are still too broad, which means their actual application will require addressing numerous practical details. A recurring theme was the establishment of data banks openly

[10] *Ad Hoc* Group of Governmental Experts to Identify and Examine Potential Verification Measures from a Scientific and Technical Standpoint, 'Summary of the work of the *Ad Hoc* Group for the period 30 March to 10 April 1992', BWC/CONF.III/VEREX/2, 13 Apr. 1992.

Table 7.1. Potential verification measures

Off-site measures
Information monitoring
Surveillance of publications
Surveillance of legislation
Data on transfers and transfer requests and on production
Multilateral information sharing
Exchange visits
Data exchange
Declarations (including notifications, data on transfers and transfer requests and on production)
Remote sensing
Surveillance by satellite
Surveillance by aircraft
Ground-based surveillance
Inspections
Sampling and identification
Observation
Auditing
On-site measures
Exchange visits
International arrangements
Inspections
Interviewing
Visual inspections (including observation and surveillance by aircraft)
Identification of key equipment
Auditing
Sampling and identification
Medical examination
Continuous monitoring
By instruments (including ground-based surveillance)
By personnel

Source: *Ad Hoc* Group of Governmental Experts to Identify and Examine Potential Verification Measures from a Scientific and Technical Standpoint, *Report*, BWC/CONF.III/VEREX/9, Geneva, 1993, pp. 132–33.

accessible to all States Parties. Many delegates stressed the importance of the availability of relevant information not only in the area of civilian but also military activities. It was also obvious that the close monitoring of transfers and transfer requests offers significant potential to strengthen the capability to uncover prohibited activities.

The subcategory 'data exchange' comprises declarations and notifications. Declarations could encompass description of a wide range of activities, programmes and facilities, while notifications could relate to changes in declared activities or specific events such as disease outbreaks, military exercises and the like. It is important to keep in mind that large parts of these two subcategories—information monitoring and data exchange—are already covered to some extent by the confidence-building reporting system.[11] Any future verification mechanism will rely on the experience gained from this system.

[11] Geissler, E. (ed.), *Strengthening the Biological Weapons Convention by Confidence-Building Measures*, SIPRI Chemical & Biological Warfare Studies, no. 10 (Oxford University Press: Oxford, 1990); Geissler, E., 'Contribution of confidence-building measures to greater transparency in activities

A rather interesting and novel subcategory is 'remote sensing', which includes three measures in particular: surveillance by satellite, surveillance by aircraft and ground-based surveillance. Satellite surveillance has a long history in arms control and disarmament, although so far it has only served as a national technical means to verify bilateral agreements between the two major nuclear powers. Surveillance by aircraft made its way into arms control recently with the finalizing of the 1992 Treaty on Open Skies in Vienna.[12] Surveillance by aircraft was first considered a CBM, but even before completion of the Treaty on Open Skies, the negotiators of the 1990 Treaty on Conventional Armed Forces in Europe (CFE)[13] considered such surveillance an effective means of verification. Nevertheless, it would be a qualitative change in the history of both methods if they were to be applied in a truly multilateral framework. Ground-based surveillance, in the context of the BWC, implies the possibility of instrumental monitoring, visual surveillance of facilities and their shipping activities, regular checks of the environment and other methods.

The fourth subcategory of off-site measures is inspections. The word 'inspection' is usually connected with on-site activities, but during the discussions at the first session, delegations were able to set up quite a remarkable list of inspection-like procedures that could be used without actually going to the 'site' concerned. The three measures identified in this subcategory were sampling and identification, observation and auditing. Sampling and identification in this regard relate to the possible analysis of air, water, soil, sewage and appropriate biological specimens from animals and plants from the environment of a given facility. Observation mainly involves surveillance of different outdoor activities, while auditing concerns the examination of records, safety and training manuals, financial and commercial documents, and could even include the questioning of local residents.[14]

It is obvious that this fourth subcategory, the last of the off-site measures, is closely related to on-site measures. It would be difficult to conduct a detailed review of documents, for example, from a long distance. Still, these measures were considered as belonging to the off-site measures.

The basket of 'on-site measures' consists of three subcategories, namely exchange visits, inspections and continuous monitoring. With regard to exchange visits, the delegations underlined the importance of international arrangements. The need for such arrangements is clear if the parallel requirements of long-term visits are considered on the one hand, and the commercial and confidentiality implications on the other.

Not surprisingly, the subcategory 'on-site inspections' presents the greatest number of practical procedures and activities. They range from interviewing staff and authorities to visual inspection of facilities and equipment, from identification of key equipment to auditing procedures. Perhaps the most interesting and challenging aspect is sampling and identification. It is a delicate issue not only from the scientific but also from the political point of view. It must not be

directly related to the Biological Weapons Convention', ed. S. J. Lundin, *Views on Possible Verification Measures for the Biological Weapons Convention*, SIPRI Chemical & Biological Warfare Studies, no. 12 (Oxford University Press: Oxford, 1991), pp. 10–25; Stock, T., 'Chemical and biological weapons: developments and proliferation', *SIPRI Yearbook 1993* (note 2), pp. 286–87.

[12] For the text of the treaty, see *SIPRI Yearbook 1993* (note 2), pp. 653–71.

[13] For the text of the treaty see SIPRI, *SIPRI Yearbook 1991: World Armaments and Disarmament* (Oxford University Press: Oxford, 1991), pp. 461–74.

[14] See note 10.

forgotten that the circle of prohibited activities is, at least in some cases, very close to that of permitted ones. Unfortunately for verification efforts, the very nature of biological activities and living material excludes the possibility of copying the quite clear-cut approach used in the case of chemical weapons. While there is no peaceful use for chemicals like sarin or VX, dual-threat agents (DTAs) can be used both for healing people and for killing them. Consideration was given to the possibility of conducting medical examinations on the staff of the given facility and trying to draw the appropriate conclusions from their medical and immunological condition.

The last subcategory is 'continuous monitoring', which can be conducted either by instruments or by personnel. This kind of verification is without doubt the most intrusive, and as such it will probably be the subject of not only scientific but political debate.

III. Evaluation of possible verification measures: VEREX II–IV

At the following two VEREX meetings[15] the advantages and disadvantages of possible application of the 21 verification measures identified above were re-evaluated in terms of the kind of quantitative and qualitative information which a particular measure will provide, how it will answer questions about compliance and how it will be possible to differentiate between legitimate and illegitimate activities, taking into account the state of the art in the various areas of science and technology.

The evaluation of each potential verification measure was based on the following criteria: (*a*) strengths and weaknesses based on, but not limited to, the amount and quality of information it provides and fails to provide; (*b*) ability to differentiate between prohibited and permitted activities; (*c*) ability to resolve ambiguities about compliance; (*d*) technological material, manpower and equipment requirements; (*e*) financial, legal, safety and organizational implications; and (*f*) the impact on scientific research, scientific co-operation, industrial development and other permitted activities, and their implications for the confidentiality of commercial proprietary information.

Evaluation of the potential verification measures revealed that, from a technical and scientific standpoint, no single measure is able to distinguish conclusively between activities permitted or prohibited by the BWC. At VEREX III the experts therefore evaluated these measures in combination and came to the realization that a combination of several measures results in synergistic values as compared to their value singly (see table 7.2).

The group also considered the question of types and quantities of microbial and other biological agents and toxins when it became apparent during the meetings that identification of potential verification measures presupposes the availability of lists of agents. In addition, the group discussed the experiences gained by trial inspections carried out by Canada, the Netherlands and the UK,

[15] *Ad Hoc* Group of Governmental Experts to Identify and Examine Potential Verification Measures from a Scientific and Technical Standpoint, 'Summary of the work of the *Ad Hoc* Group for the period 23 November to 4 December 1992', BWC/CONF.III/VEREX/4, 8 Dec. 1992; *Ad Hoc* Group of Governmental Experts to Identify and Examine Potential Verification Measures from a Scientific and Technical Standpoint, 'Summary of the work of the *Ad Hoc* Group for the period 24 May to 4 June 1993', BWC/CONF.III/VEREX/6, 8 June 1993.

Table 7.2. Illustrative examples of combinations of potential verification measures

Combination A
Declarations + multilateral information sharing + satellite surveillance + visual inspection

Combination B
Information monitoring (surveillance of publications + surveillance of legislation + data on transfers, transfer requests and production + multilateral information sharing + exchange visits)

Combination C
One-site inspection (interviewing + visual inspections, identification of key equipment + auditing + sampling and identification)

Combination D
Declarations + multilateral information sharing + on-site visual inspection

Combination E
Declarations + information monitoring

Source: *Ad Hoc* Group of Governmental Experts to Identify and Examine Potential Verification Measures from a Scientific and Technical Standpoint, *Report*, BWC/CONF.III/VEREX/9, Geneva, 1993, pp. 5, 273.

and considered a Swiss study on Q-fever, a disease caused by a DTA, which showed that the inspection scheme used in that study could identify a violation of the BWC with a high degree of reliability.

During VEREX III a statement was made by the non-aligned and other developing countries participating in the meeting requesting the identification of potential verification measures 'which . . . should be the least intrusive as possible, while still reliable and capable of deterring any States Parties from engaging in or being involved with activities which run counter to the object and purpose of the Convention'.[16] The non-aligned and other developing countries referred in this connection to 'their legitimate interests in the field of biotechnological development for peaceful purposes'. Accordingly, the *Ad Hoc* Group examined potential verification measures not only in terms of their impact on scientific research, industrial development and other activities permitted by the Convention, but also with regard to Article X of the BWC which calls for peaceful co-operation in microbiology (and biotechnology). The *Ad Hoc* Group stressed that the provisions of the Convention should not be used to impose restrictions and/or limitations on the exchange of equipment, materials and scientific and technological information for peaceful purposes.

During its final session, VEREX IV, the *Ad Hoc* Group prepared a final consensus report which

> concluded that potential verification measures as identified and evaluated could be useful to varying degrees in enhancing confidence, through increased transparency, that States Parties were fulfilling their obligations under the BWC. While it was agreed that reliance could not be placed on any single measure to differentiate conclusively between prohibited and permitted activity and to resolve ambiguities about compliance, it was also agreed that the measures could provide information of varying utility in strengthening the BWC.[17]

[16] See BWC/CONF.III/VEREX/6 (note 15), pp. 173–74.
[17] See BWC/CONF.III/VEREX/9 (note 9), p. 9.

The *Ad Hoc* Group came to the conclusion that 'some measures in combination could provide enhanced capabilities by increasing, for example, the focus and improving the quality of information, thereby improving the possibility of differentiating between prohibited and permitted activities and of resolving ambiguities about compliance'.[18]

Although the *Ad Hoc* Group recognized that a number of further scientific and technical questions remain to be addressed—such as the identity of agents, types and quantities—it came to the conclusion that, from the scientific and technical standpoint, 'some of the potential verification measures (identified) would contribute to strengthening the effectiveness and improve the implementation of the Convention, also recognizing that appropriate and effective verification could reinforce the Convention'.[19]

In accordance with the decision of the Third Review Conference the consensus report was transmitted to the States Parties to the BWC by the chairman of the *Ad Hoc* Group. In December 1993 the United Nations General Assembly adopted without vote a resolution commending the VEREX report.[20] It was hoped that after considering the report, a majority of States Parties would ask the Depositary Governments to convene a conference to examine the report and to decide on further action with regard to verification of the BWC.

The decision was taken to convene a special conference in 1994. By December 1993, 53 nations had requested or expressed interest in such a conference.[21] By mid-February 1994, the number had increased to 67 countries thereby initiating convening of a conference (requests were needed from 65 countries to initiate a conference). Such a conference could make use of the experience of the CWC negotiations in considering the feasibility of BWC verification.

IV. Lessons from the CWC negotiations

The Chemical Weapons Convention will presumably enter into force in 1995, and there is already evidence that some lessons have been learned from the CWC negotiations. However, possible future verification measures for the BWC must be considered in a different light because the CWC: (*a*) is already negotiated and agreed; (*b*) contains a definition of prohibited activities under Article I; (*c*) has a national implementation provision; (*d*) includes verification measures such as on-site inspections and monitoring; (*e*) to solve ambiguities concerning non-compliance, permits on-challenge inspections; and (*f*) includes an obligation to co-operate and assist.

The political climate has changed since the CWC negotiations were concluded, and States Parties seem to have become less willing to accept international on-site inspection and monitoring. The following general conclusions can be drawn about a possible future verification regime under the BWC, based on the experience of the CWC negotiating process:

1. If international verification is to be effective, it must be linked to an organization or agency which will oversee such activities.

18 See BWC/CONF.III/VEREX/9 (note 9), p. 9.

19 See BWC/CONF.III/VEREX/9 (note 9), p. 9.

20 Institute for Defense and Disarmament Studies, '16 December 1993', *Arms Control Reporter* (IDDS: Brookline, Mass.), sheet 701.B.121, Jan. 1994.

21 '13 December 1993', *Arms Control Reporter,* sheet 701.B.120, Jan. 1994.

2. There is a need to clearly define the subject of verification.

3. In light of the concluded CWC, the prerequisite for verification is the clear distinction between prohibited and non-prohibited activities, based on definitions and criteria.

4. Mere monitoring of activities will not solve problems of distrust or concerns about non-compliance.

5. The prerequisite for verification activities is the availability of data which States Parties must provide in national declarations.

6. If a verification mechanism has to be built into a multilateral treaty which includes disarmament requirements while also allowing other non-prohibited activities, there must be procedures which will allow the resolving of concerns about non-compliance, and the re-establishment of confidence when questions about ambiguities have been resolved.

7. Verification must be based on a routine inspection process which is transparent for States Parties, which includes clear procedures for handling incidents of alleged use and which addresses security concerns.

8. Verification under the BWC must rely on data provided by States Parties. These data have to be defined by definitions which are not overly complicated and which are acceptable to all parties. From the political point of view, the provision for data declaration will allow the active involvement of each State Party in at least some aspects of verification.

9. If verification measures are accepted, a certain deterrence effect has to be incorporated—in other words, there must be a high likelihood that non-compliance will be detected.

10. New agents cannot be incorporated easily into routine verification schemes. The CWC takes the approach that there is a need to define a 'general purpose criteria' under which new agents can be defined as falling under the scope of the Convention. A mechanism should be built into the BWC to cope with such new agents.

11. As in the CWC, a mechanism must be provided to clarify concern about non-compliance with the BWC that is under the leadership of an international authority. Such a mechanism, like challenge inspection, must be seen as a tool which has a deterrence function and which allows for the re-establishing of compliance.

Another aspect of the CWC negotiations deserves mention. Verification has a tendency to conflict with industry interests. Unique evidence exists to support this point from the novel approach of the CWC negotiations, where industry representatives were invited to meet with negotiators for consultations on the design of the future verification machinery. Such meetings are particularly helpful in dealing with certain types of requested information which industry considers commercially sensitive, such as specific data on production volumes or capacity utilization. Industry should be involved now in the discussion of possible verification measures under the BWC. However, a BWC verification regime may interfere with industry to a lesser extent than in the case of the chemical industry since the relevant companies have limited interest in DTAs.[22]

It is clear that if the BWC is amended by the addition of verification measures there will need to be a follow-up mechanism either to record compliance

[22] See Geissler, chapter 3, section III, in this volume.

or to respond to incidents of verified non-compliance. Verification is not only the registering of compliance or non-compliance by a State Party, it is also the initiating of a process to resolve disputes and tension between nations in order to re-establish compliance—far more important in the long run. Verification is only one instrument in a comprehensive compliance policy. Its credibility is based on the political will to act if non-compliance is detected.

Now that the CWC has been agreed and is open for signature and UNSCOM has demonstrated that a strong compliance-monitoring system can be implemented, there is a 'window of opportunity'[23] for improving the BWC by means of a specifically designed verification regime.

[23] Pearson, G. S., 'Biological weapons: the British view', ed. B. Roberts, *Biological Weapons; Weapons of the Future?*, Significant Issues Series, vol. 15, no. 1 (Center for Strategic and International Studies: Washington, DC, 1993), pp. 7–18.

8. The conversion of biological warfare research and development facilities to peaceful uses

MILTON LEITENBERG

I. Introduction

To the very great surprise of international observers of arms control, Russian President Boris Yeltsin referred to 'a lag in implementing' the 1972 Biological Weapons Convention (BWC) by the former Soviet Union,[1] in a speech on 29 January 1992.[2] Thus began a series of disclosures regarding the biological weapon (BW) research and development (R&D) programme of the former USSR—and, in fact, of Russia as well—that continued until mid-September 1992. Despite a history of allegations in the Western press dating back to 1975 that the USSR had maintained a covert BW R&D effort, it had never been possible to substantiate any of the specific charges in an authoritative way, and there was substantial scepticism regarding their accuracy. Now, as one disclosure followed another from Russian authorities in 1992, they were a continual surprise.

Two days after his initial speech, on the eve of a trip to the United States, President Yeltsin granted a television interview to the US television network ABC and its interviewer, Barbara Walters. Mrs Walters asked Yeltsin whether 'right now', Russia was 'still making chemical and biological weapons'. The Russian President refused to answer. When pressed, he would only say, '[I]n the next few months we're going to take steps to discontinue this kind of activity in accordance with international agreements on chemical and biological weapons'. He promised to have more to say on the matter in his private meetings with President George Bush.[3]

Similarly, on his return to Russia, Yeltsin was paraphrased in the press as having said that the 'Union leadership' had 'deceived the Americans, particularly on the issue of chemical and bacteriological weapons'.[4] In 1987, Soviet President Mikhail Gorbachev had reported that the Soviet Union had ceased producing *chemical* weapons, and the USSR and the USA formally agreed to cease such production in 1990. This left biological weapons as the overwhelming likelihood for the substance of President Yeltsin's remark, which was borne out by yet another interview Yeltsin gave in Russia in April 1992.

When the three of us were alone—Bush, his interpreter and I . . . I said that I could not yet give firm guarantees of honest cooperation. Probably this is not the thing done among politicians but I said, 'We are still swindling you, Mr Bush. We promised to scrap bacteriological weapons. But some of our experts did everything possible to keep

[1] The USSR had signed the BWC in 1972 and ratified it in 1975.

[2] Statement on Disarmament by Russian Federation President Boris Nikolayevich Yeltsin on 29 Jan. 1992, Moscow Teleradiakompaniya Ostankino Television, First Program Network, 29 Jan. 1992, Text.

[3] ABC News, '20/20', 31 Jan. 1992.

[4] See Devroy, A. and Smith, R. J., 'U.S., Russia pledge new partnership', *Washington Post*, 2 Feb. 1992; and *Nezavisimaya Gazeta*, 5 Feb. 1992, trans. in Foreign Broadcast Information Service, *Daily Report–Central Eurasia* (*FBIS-SOV*), FBIS-SOV-92-031, 14 Feb. 1992, p. 26.

the truth from me. It was not easy, but I outsmarted them. I caught them red-handed. I found two test sites . . .'[5]

In Washington on the day following the meeting of Presidents Yeltsin and Bush, Lieutenant General Dmitri Volkogonov, one of Yeltsin's top military advisers, also spoke to the press. According to the *Washington Post*: 'Volkogonov also said Yeltsin had pledged for the first time to halt Russian research into biological weapons, an area where he suggested past military efforts had crossed the line set out by international treaties. He said Yeltsin disclosed that, "a number of centers dealing with this issue have been closed", and said that, "from 1992 [forward], there will be no [military] budget allocations coming to that program"'.[6]

On 28 February 1992 the Russian press reported that a Committee on Convention Problems relating to chemical and biological weapons had been set up under a decree by President Yeltsin. The committee's tasks are: to resolve problems related to the Chemical Weapons Convention (CWC) and the BWC, to implement international and internal monitoring [Russian: kontrol], to prevent their development [Russian: razrabotka], production and stockpiling, and also to organize the elimination of stocks of chemical weapons (CW). General Anatoly Kuntsevich, formerly Deputy Head of Soviet Chemical Troops and the Soviet military representative at the CW arms control negotiations, was appointed committee chairman.[7] On 27 May 1992 another interview with President Yeltsin was published in the USSR which made explicit that BW R&D had continued in the USSR until *after* the 28 February decree. When asked when he became aware 'of the development of biological weapons in Sverdlovsk', and what his response to it had been, Yeltsin replied:

> when I learned that such development was underway, I visited Andropov . . . when an outbreak of anthrax occurred. . . . Andropov called Ustinov and ordered the liquidation of these production facilities completely. I believed it had been done this way. However, it turned out that the laboratories had simply been moved to another oblast, and the development of this weapon continued. And I told about this to Bush, Major and Mitterrand, i.e. this program is going on . . . I signed a decree to establish a special committee and banning the program. Only following this, experts flew there and put an end to the development.[8]

Finally, on 11 April 1992, President Yeltsin signed a decree committing Russia, as successor to the Soviet Union, to the 1972 BWC.[9] The signing followed Russian Government assurances that it intended to strictly abide by the limitations on biological warfare R&D stipulated by the BWC. The assurance was prompted at least in part by conditions legislated by the US Congress on the expenditure of $400 million in US aid to dismantle nuclear and other weapons of mass destruction in the former USSR. The condition stipulated that President Bush certify that the USSR (and therefore subsequently Russia as the inheritor of the agreements) was committed to moving toward compliance with all arms control agreements. As late as 30 March 1992, in submitting its latest report to

[5] Zakharov, M., 'A visit to the President', *Izvestia*, 23 Apr. 1992, in FBIS-SOV-92-079, 23 April 1992, pp. 26–29.
[6] See Devroy and Smith, (note 4).
[7] *Rossiyskaya Gazeta*, Moscow, 28 Feb. 1992, quoted in BBC-SWB, SU/1317 C3/1, 29 Feb. 1992.
[8] President Yeltsin's interview in *Komsomol'skaya Pravda*, 27 May 1992.
[9] 'Yeltsin commits to germ warfare ban', *Washington Post*, 17 Apr. 1992.

Congress on *Soviet Non-compliance with Arms Control Agreements*, the Administration had stated that the 'Soviet Union continues to be in violation of the 1972 Biological and Toxin Weapons Convention'.[10] Other pressures may also have contributed to forcing President Yeltsin's disclosures: the public testimony of senior KGB and military officials in Moscow in November and December 1991 regarding the cause of the 1979 outbreak of anthrax in Sverdlovsk,[11] and the defection to the West in 1989 of the director of one of the USSR's BW-related R&D laboratories, which is discussed in more detail below. The greatest surprises were still to come.

On 31 August 1992, 'senior US officials' disclosed to the press that: 'The United States and Britain are worried that the Russian Government may not have fulfilled a six-month-old promise to shut down the Soviet Union's extensive programme for making illicit germ weapons'.[12] General Kuntsevich had prepared a report for President Yeltsin which 'revealed that the military had illicitly developed aerial bombs and rocket warheads capable of carrying deadly anthrax, tularaemia, and Q fever biological warfare agents'. The report had not been released, but General Kuntsevich informed *The Washington Post* 'that the illicit weapons effort was maintained at least through 1990 after being steadily scaled back during the six years of Gorbachev's presidency'. In September 1992 General Kuntsevich stated in a Russian interview that:

> Indeed these clear violations on the convention were only admitted after the totalitarian regime collapsed and duplicity in politics was abandoned . . . . The remnants of the offensive programs in the area of biological weapons were still around as recently as 1991. It was only in 1992 that Russia absolutely stopped this work.
>
> . . .
>
> We did not have stockpiles of biological weapons. The point is that they cannot be kept for a long time. Therefore, the question of their destruction does not come up.
>
> . . .
>
> Within the Russian Defence Ministry's structure the relevant directorate has been abolished and a directorate for radiological, chemical, and biological protection has been set up.[13]

President Yeltsin's April 1992 decree ordering such work halted and its funding withdrawn was ostensibly in response to General Kuntsevich's report. US intelligence sources were in agreement that the programme had been scaled back, but could not determine if it had been eliminated. US officials were also claiming that the USSR had 'stockpiled substantial germ weapons'. General Kuntsevich, however, 'denied that such stockpiles existed and said that most development work was halted when weapons reached the prototype stage'. There were still difficulties, however, in the documentary submission that the Russian Government was to have made to the United Nations by 15 April 1992

[10] *Soviet Non-compliance with Arms Control Agreement,* 30 Mar. 1992 (White House, Office of the Press Secretary: Washington, DC, 9 Apr. 1992).

[11] Leitenberg, M., 'A return to Sverdlovsk: allegations of Soviet activities related to biological weapons', *Arms Control*, vol. 12, no. 2 (Sep. 1991), pp. 161–90, see especially p. 166; Leitenberg, M., 'Anthrax in Sverdlovsk: new pieces to the puzzle', *Arms Control Today*, vol. 22, no. 3 (Apr. 1992), pp. 10–13; Smith, R. J., 'Yeltsin blames '79 anthrax on germ warfare efforts', *Washington Post*, 16 June 1992.

[12] Smith, R. J., 'Russia fails to detail germ arms', *Washington Post*, 31 Aug. 1992; see also 'Cheating on biological weapons' (editorial), *Washington Post*, 11 Sep. 1992.

[13] Interview with General Kuntsevich, *Rossiyskiye Vesti*, 22 Sep. 1992, in FBIS-SOV-92-186, 24 Sep. 1992.

regarding its BW R&D facilities. US officials were charging that provisional drafts which the Russian Government had provided contained less information than had already been supplied by the USSR in 1988. What all this strongly implied was that the Yeltsin Government and Russian civilian political leadership may not yet have had total control, access or knowledge of the BW facilities and programme that it had inherited. The Russian Defence Ministry's credibility was still nil. The Defence Ministry's Directorate for Bacteriological, Radiation and Chemical Defence told the Russian newspaper *Izvestia* that charges of an active Soviet germ warfare programme were all lies, and that 'all work on biological weapons stopped in 1975'.[14] It can also be noted that despite the explicit admissions of Convention violation by President Yeltsin and General Kuntsevich, the directors of individual laboratories continue to profess the total innocence of their respective institutions.

The 31 August disclosures went further. The Russian defector was Vladimir Pasechnik, and he had been the Director of the Leningrad All-Union Scientific Institute for Especially Pure Preparations.[15] He named his own institution and three others that belonged to a conglomerate named Biopreparat as being part of a covert Soviet biological warfare programme aside from that funded and managed directly by the Defence Ministry. President Bush and British Prime Minister Margaret Thatcher had taken these charges up directly with President Gorbachev. In response President Gorbachev acceded to the visit of a US and British inspection team, which reportedly visited the four institutions in two weeks early in 1991.[16] At least some of these facilities have since also been visited by representatives of US and other Western pharmaceutical firms interested in forming joint ventures.[17] More recent and more detailed disclosures concerning Biopreparat—its size, purpose and operations—appeared in January and February 1993, and are described in subsequent portions of this chapter.

Finally, on 15 September 1992, following negotiations in Moscow, the UK, the USA and Russia signed a joint statement on the status of the Russian BW R&D programme. At a press conference, the Russian negotiator Deputy Foreign Minister Grigory Berdennikov stated that: 'The Soviet Union was violating this [BW] Convention and was running a program in the sphere of offensive biological research and development, which has been declared unlawful by the convention. . . . These activities were in progress from 1946 until March of 1992'.[18] Perhaps the most significant provision of the statement was one which 'Confirmed the termination of offensive research, *the dismantlement of experimental technological lines for the production of biological agents*, and the closure of the biological weapons testing facility'[19] (emphasis added). Although

[14] Gordon, M. R., 'U.S. asking Russia to show it has ended germ weapons program', *New York Times*, 1 Sep. 1992. The name of the 'new' directorate appears in varying versions in English translation with the word 'protection' appearing at times in place of 'defence'. More significant is that it appears to be only a change of name, retaining its existing staff, etc. It is headed by General Valentin Yevstigneyev.

[15] Umnov, V., 'Investigation: the danger of biological warfare remains', *Komsomol'skaya Pravda*, 19 Sep. 1992 (trans. by Joint Publications Research Service, *JPRS Reports*).

[16] See Smith (note 12). The information was contradicted in a subsequent report in 1993 which stated that only one site (the Leningrad laboratory) was visited, that the visit did not occur until November 1992, and that it took 'nearly a year' for the next two sites at Berdsk and Pokrov to be visited. Gordon, M. R., 'Moscow making little progress in disposal of chemical weapons', *New York Times*, 1 Dec. 1993.

[17] See also Netesov, chapter 12, in this volume.

[18] Dahlburg, J. T., 'Russia admits violating biological warfare pact', *Los Angeles Times*, 15 Sep. 1992.

[19] *Joint Statement on Biological Weapons By the Governments of The United Kingdom, The United States, and The Russian Federation*, 15 Sep. 1992, 4 pp., mimeo.

there was no mention of 'stockpiles', the 'experimental technological lines for the production of biological agents' seems a transparent although mildly diplomatic admission of production, without identifying if and when the lines had been in operation and what quantities had been produced in the 'experimental' programme. The agreement also provided for inspection visits at any time to 'any *non*-military biological site' and 'visits to any *military* biological facility, on a reciprocal basis . . . on the basis of agreed principles'. Although not specified in the statement, Russian officials stated that the number of personnel working in military biological programmes would be cut in half, and funding would be reduced by 30 per cent.[20] This partial reduction was demonstrably less of a curtailment than the zero budget allocation and the 'halt [in] Russian research into biological weapons' that General Volkogonov and President Yeltsin had promised in February 1992, but the reconcilement is perhaps that the remaining programmes were now to be wholly 'defensive' in nature.

On 19 January 1993, the US Government released its arms control treaty compliance report for the previous year. It stated:

> The United States has determined that the Russian offensive biological warfare program, inherited from the Soviet Union, violated the Biological Weapons Convention through at least March 1992. The Soviet offensive BW program was massive, and included production, weaponization, and stockpiling. The status of the program since that time remains unclear. Despite the inadequate BWC declaration, and continued leadership by 'old hands' of BW arms control negotiations and the BW defensive program, there has also been a marked increase in cooperation from President Yeltsin and other members of the Russian leadership to attempt to resolve compliance issues. We are now engaged in an effort to work with the Russian leadership to help terminate the illegal program and to pursue a number of measures to build confidence in Russian compliance with the BWC:
>
> . . .
>
> The modernization of biological agent capability and its toxin research and production in the territory of the former Soviet Union remains a concern.[21]

As previously indicated, these events, transpiring between late January and mid-September 1992, were a series of surprises. There are few instances in the thirty-plus years of post-World War II international arms control agreements in which any state has admitted to an overt violation of an arms control treaty which it signed and ratified. In addition, they directly posed the issue of the conversion of the USSR's BW R&D facilities. As is seen below, the size of the USSR's BW programme appears to have been at least an order of magnitude larger that those of the USA and the UK, which were converted, respectively, between 1970 and 1972 (the USA) and in 1979 (the UK). The question of defence industry conversion in general has been an active issue in Soviet and Commonwealth of Independent States (CIS) affairs since the time of President Gorbachev's address to the United Nations in December 1989. It is extremely rare, however, that anyone examines the conversion of *military R&D* institu-

[20] See Dahlburg, (note 18), and Gordon, M. R., 'Russia and West reach accord on monitoring germ weapon ban', *New York Times,* 15 Sep. 1992; Smith R. J., 'Russia agrees to inspection of its biological research facilities', *Washington Post,* 15 Sep. 1992.

[21] *Text of a Letter from the President to the Speaker of the House of Representatives and the President of the Senate,* Pursuant to Public Law 99-145; 22 U.S.C. 2592a as amended, and section 52 of the Arms Control and Disarmament Act (White House, Office of the Press Secretary: Washington, DC, 19 Jan. 1993).

tions along with defence production enterprises. The situation presented by the Russian—or the CIS—BW R&D laboratories provides an excellent opportunity to do exactly that. Finally, there is the equally rare precedent in which the USA totally converted its own biological warfare R&D facilities in the 1970s, and this experience can be examined as a guide to what might be feasible for Russia and the present-day CIS. Therefore before looking at the Russian BW R&D facilities and the conversion possibilities for them, a review of the mid-1970s US experience is perhaps in order.

II. The conversion of the US biological warfare facilities

The control of BW provides a very rare case of the recorded conversion of military R&D facilities. This instance is all the more interesting because the nation concerned was producing biological weapons. The USA closed and converted its two main BW R&D and production facilities, Fort Detrick and Pine Bluff Arsenal, subsequent to the renunciation of the US military biological warfare capability.

Britain also converted its single biological warfare R&D facility, but its size was much smaller and it had not been doing offensive work for many years. After the end of World War II Britain's biological warfare laboratory was renamed the Microbiological Research Department. In 1957 it terminated work on the development of offensive BW programmes and the facility was again renamed as the Microbiological Research Establishment (MRE). In 1979, after the BWC had come into force, the MRE was transferred from the Ministry of Defence to the Department of Health, and became the Centre for Applied Microbiology and Research within the Public Health Laboratory Service. At the same time Britain's Chemical Defence Establishment (CDE) assumed responsibility for work on biological defence as well by setting up a new Defence Microbiology Division, and eventually the entire facility at Porton Down was renamed the Chemical & Biological Defence Establishment (CBDE).[22]

In the United States the process began in March 1969 when the US National Security Council began a major review of US policy concerning biological warfare. The government agencies participating in the review were the Department of State, Department of Defense (DOD), Arms Control and Disarmament Agency (ACDA) and the Office of Science and Technology. Comments were also received from the scientific community and evaluated by the President's Science Advisory Committee. Pending the outcome of the study, the Department of the Army ceased all production of toxins and biological agents and the filling of dissemination devices with these agents on 15 August 1969. On 25 November 1969 the President issued an announcement of US policy regarding biological warfare which included the following:

1. The USA would renounce the use of lethal biological agents and weapons and other methods of biological warfare.

[22] Carter, G. B., '75th anniversary: the chemical and biological defence establishment (CBDE), Porton Down, 1916–1991', *ASA Newsletter,* no. 4 (Aug. 1991); Carter, G. B., 'The Microbiological Research Establishment and its precursors at Porton Down, 1940–1979', *ASA Newsletter*, no. 6 (Dec. 1991); Carter, G. B., 'The Microbiological Research Department and Establishment, 1946–1979', *ASA Newsletter,* no. 1 (Feb. 1992).

2. The USA would confine its biological research to defensive measures such as immunization and safety measures.

3. The DOD would prepare recommendations for the disposal of existing stocks of bacteriological weapons.[23]

On 14 February 1970, a White House announcement extended the policy to military programmes involving toxins, whether produced by biological means or chemical synthesis, and directed the destruction of toxin weapons and stocks which were not required for defensive research programmes.

There were two primary results of these policy decisions: first, 'demilitarization', the name given to the programme to destroy existing BW stockpiles, and second, the conversion of BW R&D and production facilities. In addition, the US Congress passed legislation which mandated the preparation of a public semi-annual and later annual report to the Congress by the DOD on funds obligated in chemical warfare and biological research programmes. Subsequently, when annual Arms Control Impact Statements were initiated by the US Government in the late 1970s, these routinely included an analysis on chemical warfare.

Before turning to an examination of the conversion experience, it is useful to provide a brief description of the 'demilitarization' programme and the subsequent public reporting of information on R&D activities in the chemical and biological area.

Plans for the destruction of BW stockpiles were approved by December 1970.[24] Stocks were located and would be destroyed at four separate sites. The destruction plans were reviewed by officials from several different federal and state agencies, including the US Department of Health, Education and Welfare (HEW) and the Department of Agriculture. Observers from both of these agencies were also appointed to monitor the entire programme. The agent destruction was carried out with substantial publicity which included press briefings, information releases and public tours.

On 1 May 1972 the former Pine Bluff Arsenal was turned over to the Food and Drug Administration (FDA) of the Department of HEW as a new National Center for Toxicological Research (NCTR).[25] The entire destruction programme was carried out on the schedule outlined in table 8.1.

For some years prior to 1973, the DOD supplied Congress with a semi-annual report on its chemical and biological warfare research, development, training and evaluation (RDT&E) programme. Beginning with the report transmitted in November 1973, classified information was removed from the report so that it could be released publicly.[26] This would presumably enable any interested foreign nation to satisfy itself that the United States was adhering to the restrictions that had been established on its biological warfare R&D programme.

[23] *Statements by the President* (White House, Office of the Press Secretary: Washington, DC, 25 Nov. 1969), 2 pp., mimeo.

[24] *Pentagon Press Briefing on the Biological Demilitarization Program*, 21 pp., mimeo.; US Department of Defense, 'Demilitarization of biological agents and weapons', *Press Release*, no. 1025-70 (18 Dec. 1970), 1 p.

[25] 'Demilitarization' (annex L), *US Army Activity in the US Biological Warfare Program*, vol. 2 (US Army: Washington, DC, 24 Feb. 1977), pp. L-1–L-11.

[26] 'Department of Defense Semi-Annual Report on Chemical and Biological Warfare Programs', *Congressional Record,* Senate, 2 Nov. 1973, pp. S-19818–S-19830.

Table 8.1. Destruction of US biological warfare agents

Facility	Stored agents	Destruction completed during
Directorate of Biological Operations, Pine Bluff Arsenal	Antipersonnel	10 May 1971–1 May 1972
Beale Air Force Base	Anticrop	By 10 Mar. 1972
Rocky Mountain Arsenal	Anticrop	By 15 Feb. 1973
Fort Detrick	Anticrop	17 Jan.–18 May 1972

Source: 'Demilitarization' (annex L), *US Army Activity in the US Biological Warfare Program*, vol. 2 (US Army: Washington, DC, 24 Feb. 1977), pp. L-1–L-11.

Subsequent reports were published in the *Congressional Record*, at first bi-annually, and after a congressional modification in the reporting requirements, annually.[27] A further mechanism which enhanced the transparency of the US chemical and biological R&D programmes were the *Arms Control Impact Statements* submitted to Congress beginning in 1978.[28]

The two major facilities affected by the US decision of November 1969 were the Army's Biological Defense Research Center at Fort Detrick, and the Division of Biological Operations, the production facility at Pine Bluff Arsenal. The disposition of the biological complex at Pine Bluff (which was physically distinct from a CW production area that was also in operation at the arsenal) turned out to be the simpler of the two.

It consisted of 33 buildings, in operation since around 1953, at which about 300 people were reportedly involved in as many as 40 R&D programmes.[29] The solution of engineering problems associated with the safety and control of the production processes necessary to culture and store infectious micro-organisms and toxins had resulted in very specialized facilities. Nevertheless on 12 January 1971, very soon after the announcement of the approved plans to destroy the biological stockpiles at Pine Bluff, the Commissioner of the FDA wrote to the Secretary of the Army proposing that the FDA take over the installation and establish a National Center for Food and Drug Safety at the site. Pine Bluff Arsenal had by then already been visited by FDA personnel, who found that it could be adapted to the needs of their agency. The new centre would 'examine the biological effects of a number of chemical substances which are found in man's surroundings, such as pesticides, food additives, and therapeutic

[27] *Congressional Record,* Senate, 11 Mar. 1974, pp. S-3334–S-3348; *Congressional Record,* Senate, 12 Sep. 1974, pp. S-16508–S16521; *Congressional Record,* Senate, 17 Mar. 1975, pp. S-3999–S-16349; *Congressional Record,* Senate, 19 Sep. 1975, pp. S-16348–S-16357; *Congressional Record,* Senate, 11 Feb. 1977, pp. S-2709–S-2723; *Congressional Record,* Senate, 17 Mar. 1978, pp. S-4025–S-4040; *Congressional Record,* Senate, 19 July 1979, pp. S-9921–S-9939.

[28] For example, US Congress, Joint Committee Print, *Fiscal Year 1980: Arms Control Impact Statements*, 'Chemical warfare', 96th Congress, 1st Session (US Government Printing Office: Washington, DC, Mar. 1979), pp. 218–83; US Congress, Joint Committee Print, *Fiscal Year 1981: Arms Control Impact Statements*, 'Chemical warfare', 96th Congress, 2nd Session (US Government Printing Office: Washington, DC, May 1980), pp. 306–38; *Fiscal Year 1982: Arms Control Impact Statements*, 'Chemical warfare', 97th Congress, 1st Session (US Government Printing Office: Washington, DC, Feb. 1981), pp. 34717–52.

[29] *Problems Associated with Converting Defense Research Facilities to Meet Different Needs: The Case of Fort Detrick,* Report to the Congress, by the Comptroller General of the United States, B-160140 (US Government Printing Office: Washington, DC, 16 Feb. 1972), pp. 9–10. An unpublished study was prepared for a UN Secretary-General's working group on military R&D in 1983–84; see Longwell, V., *Fort Detrick: From Biological Warfare to Cancer Research,* mimeo., undated. It was not used in preparing this paper.

drugs. Pine Bluff Arsenal would become a major research centre for the purpose of studying the significance to man of toxicological data obtained from animal testing'. The main effort would be a very large-scale animal screening programme. FDA officials expressed their intention of employing all of Pine Bluff's professional personnel and most, if not all, of the other personnel. The new centre was named the National Center for Toxicological Research and conversion was completed in an opening ceremony in the spring of 1972.

Determining what new research would be undertaken at Pine Bluff Arsenal was free of the decision-making elements that introduced complications at Fort Detrick. Aside from the main effort in animal testing, which seemed clearly established as the primary programme, a study paper proposed a large group of research projects that might be undertaken in the future. These fell into two groupings. One group was clearly based on new priorities and needs, and concerned pollution and pesticide problems, recycling and food production. These included: (*a*) selective biological destruction of undesirable plants; (*b*) viral control of algae; (*c*) disposal of toxic wastes by micro-organisms; (*d*) destruction of pesticides by micro-organisms; (*e*) control of oil spills with micro-organisms; (*f*) utilization of waste material; (*g*) production of single-cell protein food supplements, amino acids and growth factors; and (*h*) production of cellulose and other enzymes.[30]

A second group of research topics, however, was either much more closely related to and/or made more particular use of Pine Bluff's existing specialized facilities: (*a*) microbial insecticides, (*b*) viral and rickettsial vaccine production, (*c*) production of bacterial and fungal vaccines and toxoids, (*d*) aerosol immunization, (*e*) development of decontamination systems, (*f*) aerosol applications of air pollution control, and (*g*) development of rapid, automated bioanalysis techniques.

Hedén has pointed out that these topics 'belong to the areas . . . where the reciprocity of international cooperation and fellowship programs might serve a verification purpose', as it is this group that comes closest to classical biological warfare research. He indicated that 'it would be unwise to initiate one of the projects: "production of toxins, specific bacterial pathogens, viruses and rickettsiae", before such international cooperation had started'.[31]

It is not clear to what degree, if at all, any of these proposed projects were subsequently carried out at the new NCTR.[32] The important context is the intent to convert facilities in which military R&D has been carried out, after weapon development of that type is renounced. If existing biological warfare facilities are converted, it is clearly beneficial from the disarmament and arms control standpoint the more 'distance' there is in the projects chosen for the converted facility from those that might have biological warfare relevance as well. Thus *from this standpoint* research in production of cattle feed from paper waste, or of fertilizer, cattle feed or single-cell protein from mixed waste—all processes in which there already existed research in 1972—would clearly have been pre-

[30] *Concepts for Future Utilization of the NCTR Facilities*, 1 June 1972.

[31] Hedén, C. G., 'Global monitoring of the environment, a factor in the control of CBW-research', Seminar on Chemical and Biological Disarmament, Helsinki, Finland, 20–30 Sep. 1972, pp. 13–14. See also Hedén, C. G., 'The opportunity for a redeployment of military microbiology', Seminar on Microbiological Control of Insects, Helsinki, Finland, 8–9 June 1977, mimeo.

[32] Schmeck, Jr, H. M., 'Deadly arsenal turned into a health research center', *New York Times*, 23 Feb. 1975.

ferable to projects in biological methods of pest control or in aerobiological aspects of disease spread or control, and even more so to viral and rickettsial production, however useful knowledge or products in the latter areas might be. It would simply allay suspicion of intent. This would be so despite the fact that research in biological methods of pest control might already be under way in the laboratories of an agriculture ministry in the same country, and that such research would continue. It would equally be so even if a military agency possessed the ability to monitor and attempted to adapt such research results in the absence of any other analogous research of its own. This example in fact points to the explicit formal relationships that underlie judgements of intent in areas of prospective weapon development.[33]

At the time of the US decision in November 1969 to curtail its biological warfare R&D programme there were roughly 1800 professional, technical and support personnel employed at Fort Detrick.[34] It was a very much larger facility than Pine Bluff Arsenal, with 460 individual structures and a value of $190 million. The Army estimated that the number of people required and the basic operating costs of the Fort Detrick facilities—300 people and $6 million annually—were alone equal to the totals involved in the transfer of Pine Bluff to the FDA. An additional complication was that the Army had originally hoped to retain all of Fort Detrick's research personnel—which turned out not to be feasible—and that while several different federal agencies expressed interest in the laboratories none of them seemed willing to allot the funds required for the conversion out of their existing budgets.[35] The final resolution was that some portions of the military programme were moved from Fort Detrick, some remained, and several new research institutions arrived with the result that after 1972 some half dozen federal programmes shared the facilities:

1. 240 civilian and 190 military personnel were relocated to the Dugway Proving Grounds in Utah. This represented 19 to 24 per cent of the research personnel of the original installation.[36]

2. The Analytical Science Office and the Biological Defense Material Division studying physical defences against BW, representing some 40 research personnel, were transferred from Fort Detrick to Edgewood Arsenal, Maryland.

3. Civilian personnel, equipment and facilities of the Plant Sciences Directorate of Fort Detrick were transferred to the US Department of Agriculture in April 1971 to continue the work on defence technology against crop disease, in accordance with a recommendation made by the President's Science Advisory Committee. This involved 20 researchers.

[33] These interrelationships were investigated in a larger study by the author, *Research and Development in Chemical and Biological Warfare: An Examination of the Possibility of Distinguishing Between Civil and Military, Offensive and Defensive R & D.* This study was prepared for the Ministry for Foreign Affairs, Sweden, in 1983, and an earlier examination of some of the same issues was presented by the author in a paper to the International Congress of Microbiology, Mexico City, 1970.

[34] *Problems Associated with Converting Defense Research Facilities to Meet Different Needs: The Case of Fort Detrick* (note 29), pp. 16, 27. The exact number given in the GAO report to Congress is 1 792. Other numbers have appeared in the literature: 1 595 civilians and 650 military, for a total of 2 245 in Goldhaber, S. Z., 'CBW: interagency conflicts stall administration action', *Science*, vol. 169, no. 3944 (31 July 1970), pp. 454–56; and 1 685 civilian plus 160 military, for a total of 1 845 in Boffey, P. A., 'Fort Detrick: a top laboratory is threatened with extinction', *Science*, vol. 171 (22 Jan. 1971), pp. 262–64.

[35] See Boffey (note 34).

[36] See Goldhaber (note 34).

4. Research in the field of medical defences against biological agents was transferred to the US Army Medical Research Institute of Infectious Diseases (USAMRIID) which remained at Fort Detrick. In 1977 it had 461 employees.

5. The US Navy also continued to maintain a small medical research detachment at Fort Detrick.

6. The President's decision in October 1971 to establish a branch of the National Cancer Institute, part of the National Institutes of Health (NIH), Department of HEW, at Fort Detrick reflected purely domestic political considerations rather than scientific priority.[37] Once the decision had been made on the major area of new work to be done at Fort Detrick, it was considered desirable for economic reasons to retain as much of the equipment and performance capacities of the former laboratory as possible. Thus the National Cancer Institute concluded that the principal activities for which the facility was suited were: first, the large-scale production and testing of viruses in cancer research, and second, the breeding and location of animals to be used in large-scale screening programmes. The cancer research programme was to be managed by a contractor, and was expected to employ 200 people.

By early 1972 most of the professional staff not absorbed by these various programmes had sought positions elsewhere, and only some 600 support staff remained. As part of the conversion process, it was arranged for two Soviet officials to visit the facilities in August 1972. These were the USSR Minister of Health and the head of a cancer research institute.[38] The visitors portrayed themselves as relatively unenthused by what they were being shown, and could not reply to a question of whether the Soviet equivalent(s) to Fort Detrick were also being converted. The Minister of Health replied that he could only state that his ministry had no such facilities, which was at one and the same time a partial truth and a gross evasion. The USSR's Ministry of Health was responsible for the 'medical' aspects of the R&D that took place in the USSR's biological warfare R&D laboratories. The laboratories themselves were under the authority of a special section of the General Staff of the USSR, but it was none other than the Deputy Minister of Health of the USSR who was the liaison with them.[39] An offer, first made by President Richard Nixon in October 1971, that several laboratories at Fort Detrick be set aside for use by foreign scientists, including scientists from the USSR, was repeated, but there was no response to this. Official representatives of Soviet ministries—including the then Deputy Minister of Health of the USSR—again visited the laboratories in 1988, at the time of their visit to the US National Academy of Sciences to present the Soviet

[37] A Republican, President Nixon, made the decision to pre-empt the calls by a major Democratic opponent, Senator Edward Kennedy, for a national cancer research programme. See Meyer, L., 'U.S. to use Ft. Detrick for research in cancer', *Washington Post*, 15 Oct. 1971; Meyer, L., 'Cancer research lab planned at Ft Detrick', *Washington Post*, 19 Oct. 1971; Semple, R. B., 'Nixon counting on conversion of military facilities', *New York Times*, 19 Oct. 1971; Greenberg, D., 'Washington view: modern cancers', *New Scientist*, vol. 54, no. 796 (18 May 1972), p. 393; 'NCI announces award for Fort Detrick', *Science*, vol. 176, no. 4042 (30 June 1972), p. 1402; Schmeck, Jr, H. M., 'Litton will run cancer unit lab', *New York Times*, 25 July 1972.

[38] Wade, N., 'Russians reserve doubts: is Fort Detrick really de-tricked?', *Science*, vol. 177, no. 4048 (11 Aug. 1972), p. 500; Auerbach, S., 'Russians see once-secret germ lab', (from the *Washington Post*), *International Herald Tribune*, 5–6 Aug. 1972; 'Fort Detrick converting to major medical research center', *Army Research and Development News Magazine*, vol. 14, no. 4 (July/Aug. 1973), pp. 16–19.

[39] See Leitenberg (note 11).

version of what happened during the epidemic of anthrax in the Soviet city of Sverdlovsk in April to June 1979.[40]

In February 1970, early in the conversion process, a senior US Government official apparently implied that all future defensive biological warfare research would be carried out on an unclassified basis, and was quoted as saying 'there will be no need for secret research in this field under this program'.[41] That this was obviously not the case was quickly realized, and either the original reports were incorrect or any such intention was revoked. Classified biological warfare research was still going to be carried out, which rapidly led to criticism that the Army had not reduced or altered the types of research it was doing after the President's renunciation of biological warfare and the announced closing of Fort Detrick.[42] Testimony to Congress, however, indicated the degree of change that had taken place in funding levels.

Immediately following the President's policy announcement of 25 November 1969, all offensive biological research and development was terminated. The defensive effort has also been reduced as the following figures show (in millions of dollars):

Fiscal year	1969	1970	1971	1972
Biological offense	3.158	3.964	0	0
Biological defense	18.378	14.376	15.585	13.200
Total	**21.536**	**18.340**	**15.585**	**13.200**

The portion of the program comprising the technological base is unclassified and will remain at Fort Detrick. This will require approximately 160 civilian personnel. The Army considers defensive work in biological alarms and physical defense, and vulnerability analysis to be classified since knowledge of alarm characteristics or U.S. vulnerability to attack would be an invaluable asset to a potential enemy. Consequently, 52 civilian spaces will be transferred to Edgewood Arsenal for the alarm and physical defense work, and 9 civilian spaces will be transferred to Dugway Proving Ground for the vulnerability analysis work.[43]

From the point of view of arms control, the combination of the conversion of the BW production facilities *as well as* the cessation of the 'offensive' R&D programme is almost the best thing that could possibly have happened. Perhaps the very best would have been if it could have taken place even without the stated maintenance of 'defensive' research. In the mid-1980s (under the Reagan Administration), US defensive BW research was sharply expanded and sub-

[40] See Leitenberg, 'A return to Sverdlovsk: allegations of Soviet activities related to biological weapons' (note 11), p. 187.

[41] See Goldhaber (note 34). The official who made the remarks was President Nixon's National Security Advisor, Henry Kissinger.

[42] US Department of Defense Statement, 'U.S. curtailing chemical biological weapons research', 6 Dec. 1971, *Press Release*, no. 350, 8 Dec. 1971; 'Fort Detrick's future disputed', *Baltimore Sun*, 20 June 1970; Smith, R. M., 'U.S. slow to dismantle germ-war arsenal despite Nixon stand', *New York Times*, 10 Nov. 1970; Getler, M., 'U.S. issues plan to destroy biological warfare stocks', *International Herald Tribune*, 19–20 Dec. 1970; Schmidt, D. A., 'Senator asserts army plans to expand biowar research', *International Herald Tribune*, 25 Jan. 1971; Lewis, F., 'Full speed ahead on chemical and biological weapons', *Washington Post*, 6 Dec. 1971.

[43] Authorization For Military Procurement, Research and Development, Construction and Real Estate Acquisition for the Safeguard ABM and Reserve Strengths, Fiscal Year 1972, 'Research and development', Hearings before the Committee on Armed Services, US Senate, 92nd Congress, 1st Session (US Government Printing Office: Washington, DC, Feb.–May 1971), Part 3 of 5 parts, p. 2605. Under the Reagan Administration in the 1980s, US expenditure for all chemical and biological weapons R&D increased by an order of magnitude, including that for defensive BW R&D. See also footnote 44, below.

stantive questions were raised as to whether particular research projects were of an 'offensive' or a 'defensive' nature.[44] It may also be considered advantageous that the 'defensive' biological warfare R&D was not transferred to an existing civil installation, since in that case all the problems of distinguishing between 'military' and 'civilian' research would descend in turn on the civilian institution. On the other hand there would presumably be much less suspicion of 'offensive' research being carried out under a 'defensive' guise in such circumstances. In other cases in which limitations on military R&D are conceivable, a reduction in production capability might not necessarily be expected. Conversely, in cases in which there were decisions not to produce and deploy a particular system—such as the anti-ballistic missile (ABM) system—continued ABM R&D was frequently supported even by those who strongly opposed the procurement of ABM systems.

III. The biological warfare facilities of the former Soviet Union

The first task would be to establish the magnitude of the former USSR's biological warfare R&D programme:

1. Just how many biological warfare R&D and production facilities did it have?
2. What is the size of those institutions (physical plant)?
3. What are the sizes of the programmes in them?
4. How many people are working in them?

The United States had to convert two facilities; how many must the Russians now convert? Substantially more it would seem, and to a surprising degree. The exact number is still not known.

Until quite recently it was not possible to have any real understanding of the nature of the Soviet programme. Any interested researcher was forced to depend on a handful of scattered reports and press accounts, none of which could be verified or corroborated by Soviet sources. The USSR did have a biological warfare R&D programme in the years prior to and during World War II. It apparently began in the mid-1930s but its details are not publicly known.[45] As

[44] Since this chapter focuses on conversion, the disputes regarding US BW research projects in the 1980s are not discussed here. The reader will find them covered in King, J. and Strauss, H., 'The hazards of defensive biological warfare programs'; Piller, C., and Yamamoto, K. R., 'The US biological defense research program in the 1980's: a critique'; and Wright, S. and Ketcham, S., 'The problem of interpreting the US biological defense research program', all in ed. S. Wright, *Preventing a Biological Arms Race* (MIT Press: Cambridge, Mass., 1990); *Biological Warfare: Role of Salk Institute in Army's Research Program*, Report to the Chairman, Committee on Governmental Affairs, US Senate, GAO/NSIAD-92-33 (US General Accounting Office: Washington, DC, Dec. 1991); Norman, C., 'Army shifts on Dugway lab', *Science*, vol. 241, no. 4874 (30 Sep. 1988), p. 1749; Norman, C. 'Biological defense defended', *Science*, vol. 240, no. 4855 (20 May 1988), p. 1749, Smith, R. J., 'Under pressure, army scales back plan for germ warfare lab', *Washington Post*, 30 Sep. 1988; ter Haar, B., *The Future of Biological Weapons* (particularly chapter 2), The Washington Papers, no. 151 (CSIS and Praeger: Westport. Conn., 1991); Dickson, D., 'Gene splicing dominates review of weapons pact', *Science*, vol. 234 (10 Oct. 1986), pp. 143–45; Callaham, M. B. and Tsipis, K. M., *Report on a Meeting to Discuss the Applicability of the Biological Weapons Convention to Recombinant DNA Work*, Program in Science and Technology for International Security, Report no. 2 (Massachusetts Institute of Technology, Cambridge, Mass., Aug. 1978); Wright, S., 'Biowar treaty in danger', *Bulletin of the Atomic Scientists*, vol. 47, no. 7 (Sep. 1991), pp. 36–40.

[45] The only known source regarding the USSR's BW R&D programme between the mid-1930s and 1945 is the Hirsch report, based on German interrogations of captured Soviet scientists, and prepared after the end of World War II. It alleges a range of agents, weapon types, natural vectors, experiments and testing sites, and laboratories or sites of their location (Chkalov, Perm, Gorodomlia Island in Seliger Lake

already noted, Deputy Foreign Minister Berdennikov's statement on 15 September 1992 referred to the post-World War II programme existing 'from 1946'. A 1992 Soviet publication states, in relation to the Vozrozhdeniye Island BW test site in the Aral Sea, 'The order to create a secret subunit on Vozrozhdeniye Island was signed in 1952. The work, however, began two years later'.[46] (As noted, however, this test site apparently had existed since 1936.)

Between 1975 and 1977, just after the BWC came into force, the first press accounts appeared in the United States suggesting that the USSR was building or had recently built three to six facilities 'that may be capable of producing biological warfare weapons'. The first report mentioned three sites: at Zagorsk (80 km north of Moscow), Omutninsk and Sverdlovsk.[47] The second report added three more sites: at Berdsk, Pokrov and Aksu (160 km south-west of Omsk).[48] It was explicit that the sources of the information were members of the Government and US intelligence reports. The judgements were apparently based on satellite photography evidence. The crucial indicators were 'very high incinerator stacks and large cold storage bunkers', and one US intelligence report stated that the plant designs 'indicate they were built for biological warfare capability'. However, the ambiguity was substantial: 'Some intelligence reports describe the plants as suspected biological warfare production and storage facilities. Other sources say the plants may be making biological-associated products for agricultural purposes but could be adapted easily to turn out warfare materials'.[49]

Responsible US congressional officials were sceptical; the Chairman of the Subcommittee on International Security and Scientific Affairs of the Committee on International Relations wrote in a personal communication:

> As you know, the issue has been raised in the past, at which time I conferred with appropriate officials in various government agencies, including the U.S. Arms Control and Disarmament Agency. On the basis of my discussion with those officials, I do not believe those reports have any basis in fact.[50] . . . I have noted that these stories periodically appear in the press. One can only speculate that they are leaked by sources intent on creating a base of apprehension on which they might hope to establish support for a renewed BW program in the United States.[51]

near Ostashkov, a series of frequently renamed institutes in the 1930s belonging to the Red Army, and the 'Velikanovskiy Institute'—or V/2-1094—which also established and was responsible for the Vozrozhdeniye Island test site in the Aral Sea used for BW testing starting in the summer of 1936). Oleg Penkovsky referred to Kaluga being a site of BW R&D, and US intelligence in the mid-1960s named Saratov as such a site as well. In *Manipulated Science: The Crisis of Science in the Soviet Union* (Doubleday: New York, 1979), Mark Popovsky claims that Professor Velikanov's institute existed from 'the late twenties onward'. He also claims that a secret bacteriological laboratory existed in Suzdal between 1930 and 1937.

46 Kozlov, S., 'Secret Vozrozhdeniye Island BW lab abandoned', *Nezavisimaya Gazeta*, 23 June 1992; in JPRS-TND-92-022, 10 July 1992, pp. 25–26. Detailed maps showing the island and its relation to Aralsk appeared in *National Geographic,* vol. 177, no. 2 (Feb. 1992), pp. 74, 75, 80.

47 Beecher, W., 'Soviets feared violating germ weapon ban', *Boston Globe,* 28 Sep. 1975.

48 'Russia: 6 "germ" plants?', AP dispatch, in Scripps-Howard newspapers, 15 June 1976; see also Wade, N., 'Biological warfare: suspicions of Soviet activity', *Science*, vol. 172, no. 4234 (2 Apr. 1976), pp. 38–40; Toth, R. C., 'Russ believed plunging into gene study: new labs could lead to development of biological weapons', *Los Angeles Times,* 20 Feb. 1977.

49 'Russia: 6 "germ" plants?' (note 48).

50 Personal communication, Representative C. J. Zablocki, 1 July 1976. (This author had made an attempt at the time to resolve the allegations.)

51 Personal communication, Representative C. J. Zablocki, 21 July 1976.

In mid-1976 the US ACDA reportedly urged, unsuccessfully, a comprehensive National Security Council study of the satellite intelligence.[52] It is interesting in retrospect to match the sites referred to, and in the subsequent US intelligence disclosures in 1984, with the information which began to be supplied by Soviet sources between 1987 and 1992.

In 1984, eight years later, the United States again repeated these charges, identifying these and several additional sites, but this time in publicly released official US Government reports. The first occasion was in a report by the President to Congress in January 1984,[53] but the most detailed was in the widely distributed report, *Soviet Military Power, 1984*. It referred to 'at least seven biological warfare centers in the USSR that have the highest security and are under the strictest military control', and added the explicit charge that the 'Soviet Union has an active R&D program to investigate and evaluate the utility of biological weapons and their impact on the combat environment . . . [which] violates the Biological and Toxin Weapons Convention of 1972'.[54] The Sverdlovsk site was described as a 'BW research production and storage facility'. Articles which subsequently appeared in the US press referring to 'US intelligence reports' named 'major BW-related research and production installations' as 'identified' at Sverdlovsk and Zagorsk, and six others 'suspected' at Omutninsk, Aksu, Pokrov, Berdsk, Penza and Kurgan, and 'a storage depot' at 'Malta'.[55] In 1986 a public US Defense Intelligence Agency (DIA) report on the USSR's biological warfare programme stated:

> We have also identified a number of installations capable of producing disease agents and toxins on a large-scale and placing them in munitions and delivery/dissemination systems. These installations have been established by the Ministry of Defense and are under its control. One such facility is in the city of Sverdlovsk and has a long history of biological warfare R&D and production with emphasis on the causative agent of anthrax. In addition to anthrax, we believe the Soviets have developed tularemia, plague, and cholera for BW purposes, as well as botulinum toxin, enterotoxin, and mycotoxins.[56]

In 1984[57] and 1986[58] several articles based on interviews with *émigré* Soviet microbiologists were published which charged that the USSR had inaugurated a programme of research utilizing genetic engineering for the purposes of design-

[52] Robinson, J. P., 'The Soviet Union and the Biological Weapons Convention, and a guide to sources on the Sverdlovsk incident', *Arms Control* vol. 3, no. 3 (1982), p. 54.

[53] 'Soviet non-compliance with arms control agreements', *Fact Sheet*, issued in conjunction with a classified National Security Council report to Congress on that subject, 23 Jan. 1984. In a statement to the Informal Heads of Delegation Meeting of the CSCE in Madrid on 16 Feb. 1982, US Ambassador Max Kampelman stated that the USSR had five 'production plants . . . devoted to the production of biological agents'.

[54] US Department of Defense, *Soviet Military Power 1984* (US Department of Defense: Washington, DC, 10 Apr. 1984), p. 73. This summary is based on Robinson, J. P. P., 'Chemical and biological warfare: developments in 1984', *World Armaments and Disarmament: SIPRI Yearbook 1985* (Taylor & Francis: London, 1985), pp. 178–79.

[55] Anderson, J. and Van Atta, D., 'How Russia fights with poison and germs', *Reader's Digest*, Sep. 1984, pp. 54–58; Anderson, J. and Van Atta, D., 'Sanitation institute a Soviet front', *Washington Post*, 3 Aug. 1989.

[56] US Defense Intelligence Agency, *Soviet Biological Warfare Threat*, DST-1610F-057-86 (DIA: Washington, DC, 1986), pp. 1–2.

[57] Kucewicz, W., published seven articles in the *Wall Street Journal* between 23 April and 21 May 1984. The substantive information in them is, however, quite limited and of very variable reliability.

[58] Finder, J., 'Biological warfare, genetic engineering, and the treaty that failed', *Washington Quarterly*, vol. 9, no. 2 (spring 1986), pp. 5–14.

ing biological weapons. This was the state of knowledge until the USSR began to release information during President Gorbachev's tenure.

As a result of agreements reached at the Third Review Conference of the BWC in 1986, the USSR agreed to an exchange of information dealing with certain categories of its microbiological research institutions. On 13 October 1987 the USSR provided the first such exchange of information which was subsequently to be deposited annually. It reported five laboratories under Ministry of Defence control: (*a*) Leningrad (now St Petersburg); (*b*) Kirov; (*c*) Sverdlovsk (now Ekaterinburg); (*d*) Zagorsk (subsequently also referred to under its pre-1917 name, Sergiyev-Posad), Moscow oblast; and (*e*) Aralsk, Kzyl-Ordinsky oblast.[59] The Leningrad site was under the jurisdiction of the USSR Ministry of Defence Scientific Research Institute for Military Medicine, the remaining four were under the USSR Ministry of Defence Scientific Research Institute for Microbiology. The documentation also listed 14 civilian laboratories, for a total of 19 sites, including those in Ukraine and what was then Byelorussia.

There are strong reasons to believe however that the 1987 documentation is incomplete:

1. When secret portions of the Sverdlovsk facility were moved in the mid-1980s, after years of clean-up and decontamination, they were reportedly moved to 'a location near Irkutsk',[60] (and portions possibly also to an area 'near Moscow'). The 1987 Soviet documentation listed a Ministry of Health facility called the Irkutsk Anti-Plague Scientific Research Institute of Siberia and the Far East.

2. A 4 February 1992 *Pravda* article discusses another institute 'established two decades previously at Obolensk, near Moscow to work on . . . biomedical means of protection against BW'.[61] Obolensk was not mentioned in the 1987 Soviet documentation, neither among the military *nor* the civilian institutions, but appeared in the 1989 submission as the All-Union Scientific Institute of Applied Microbiology under the jurisdiction of the USSR Ministry of the Medical and Microbiological Industry.[62] It clearly met the criteria which should have mandated its inclusion in 1987.

3. A subsequent Russian press item which also mentioned Obolensk goes on to infer that a large number of additional institutions were established or diverted into the Soviet biological warfare R&D programme *after* the signing of the BWC.

The convention had already been signed when a bacteriological center was opened in Obolensk, near Moscow and a virology center in Koltsovo near Novosibirsk.[63] Insti-

[59] 'Exchange of data on research centers and laboratories: information presented by the USSR [to the UN Department of Disarmament]', 13 Oct. 1987, mimeo.; see also Geissler, E. (ed.), *Strengthening the Biological Weapons Convention by Confidence-Building Measures*, SIPRI Chemical & Biological Warfare Studies, no. 10 (Oxford University Press: Oxford, 1990).

[60] See Leitenberg (note 11).

[61] Kaisyn, V., 'Visiting a caged beast', *Pravda*, 4 Feb. 1992; in JPRS-TAC-92-008, 9 March 1992, pp. 47–48; see also Litovkin, V., 'Yeltsin bans work on bacteriological weapons. This means: work was under way, and we were deceived', *Izvestia*, 27 Apr. 1992, in FBIS-SOV-92-084, 30 Apr. 1992, p. 7.

[62] 'Information submitted by the USSR [to the UN Department of Disarmament] in fullfillment of agreements reached at the Second [Review Conference of the BWC]', 12 Apr. 1989, mimeo.; see also Geissler (note 59).

[63] 'Koltsovo', the All-Union Research Institute for Molecular Biology, was listed in the original Soviet submission of 1987, again under the jurisdiction of the USSR Ministry of the Medical and Microbiological Industry. The Leningrad facility was not mentioned, however.

tutes were built in Moscow—the Biological Instrument Building Institute and the Biochemical Machine Project. The Institute for Ultrapure Drugs appeared in Leningrad. Industrial test bases were opened.

Entire faculties at a number of higher educational institutions in Moscow were entirely redirected—the Moscow Higher Technical School Imeni Bauman, Moscow State University, the Second Medical Institute . . . .[64]

4. A 3 March 1992 US press report, attributing information to an unreleased February 1992 CIA report, referred to '16 known and suspected biological weapons facilities', including 'special military-secured storage facilities for' BW.[65] This was reported as an increase from 'nine biological weapons facilities' which had been 'identified' by US intelligence in the previous year. The Vozrozhdeniye Island testing area in the Aral Sea, Sverdlovsk and Zagorsk were referred to as 'confirmed sites'.[66]

5. A 17 April 1992 US press report stated that 'US intelligence officials said they have found more than 20 sites in the former Soviet Union for germ-warfare work'.[67] It also claimed that 'Western intelligence' had developed an estimate of the size of Soviet BW stockpiles by stating that the USSR was only reporting '10 per cent' of the amount that Western sources believed Russia had.

6. The Soviet defector, Dr Vladimir Pasechnik, identified four institutes involved with the Biopreparat conglomerate as involved in BW programmes: his own Institute of High Purity Preparations in Leningrad, the two institutes referred to above in Obolensk and Koltsovo,[68] and a fourth institute not previously mentioned. Since the institutions associated with the Biopreparat organization varied over the years, it seems evident that this was the cause of the increase in Western intelligence estimates of from around 10 to 16 or 20 following his defection.[69]

Perhaps the most significant disclosures aside from the official Soviet and Russian documentation released since 1987 appeared in a 19 September 1992 *Komsomol'skaya Pravda* article. It described the origin and bureaucratic role of the Biopreparat organization in the USSR's biological warfare development programme. It was apparently spun off from the Ministry of Medium Machine Building, one of the former USSR's eight defence industrial ministries, and the one responsible for producing nuclear weapons. It acted as an intermediary for funding and for the supply of resources to its affiliated members, and would therefore appear to have been a smaller and highly specialized analogue to the

[64] Umnov, V., 'After 20 years of silence the Soviet microbes are talking', *Komsomol'skaya Pravda*, 30 Apr. 1992, in FBIS-SOV-92-087, 5 May 1992, pp. 4–6.

[65] Gertz, W., '16 biological weapons sites identified in ex-Soviet Union', *Washington Times*, 3 Mar. 1992. The coincidence of the numbers might lead one to think that the '16' or '20' facilities referred to in these US intelligence reports could be those identified by the USSR in October 1987 as *civilian* microbiology research centres, or includes some portion of them. However, there is reason to think that is not the case. One press account explicitly stated that British officials had raised their estimate from 10 to 20 following Dr Pasechnik's disclosures.

[66] See Umnov (note 64). See also FBIS-SOV-92-040, 28 Feb. 1992, pp. 54–55; JPRS-TAC-92-015, 8 May 1992, pp. 27–28; JPRS-TND-92-014, 14 May 1992, pp. 28–29.

[67] 'Yeltsin commits to germ warfare ban', *Washington Post*, 17 Apr. 1992; see also Gertz, W., 'Russia told to unveil all biological arms', *Washington Times*, 24 July 1992.

[68] The All-Union Scientific Institute of Applied Microbiology and the All-Union Research Institute for Molecular Biology.

[69] One press account explicitly stated that British officials had raised their estimate from 10 to 20 following Dr Pasechnik's disclosures.

USSR's Military Industrial Commission (VPK). The important particulars of the article were as follows:[70]

1. It was established by Central Committee directive in 1973, and its first head was General V. I. Ogarkov.
2. 'Technical and scientific documentation was transferred to [it] from the Ministry of Defence'. A directorate of the Defence Ministry (presumably the one that directed the Ministry's own biological warfare R&D institutes) was its 'customer', and it had 'strictly military tasks'.
3. Its staff, in 1991 composed of 150 managers, operated 'independently of the structure to which it technically belonged', and were 'officers on loan, who had gained experience at the biological facilities of the Ministry of Defence'.
4. It was responsible for the construction of the institutes in Obolensk and Koltsovo, but other enterprises as well (two in Vilnius are mentioned) that had nothing to do with the biological warfare programme, and were allegedly a 'cover'. It also acquired several operating plants.
5. A 'mobilization' programme and department was organized within the Biopreparat organization to begin production at short notice. 'The equipment was mothballed in special shops (as a rule operating biochemical production facilities were used). Such shops were idle at the Berdsk and Omutninsk Chemical Plants and the Progress Plant in Stepnogorsk. In addition there was a plant within the organization of the Ministry of Agriculture and two plants within the Ministry of Health'. It is not stated, but the 'short notice' production presumably would have been BW agent and not vaccine. It is very likely that this 'mobilization department . . . [and] . . . equipment' is the same 'experimental technological lines for production of biological agents' referred to in the US, British and Russian statement of 15 September 1992.
6. After Dr Pasechnik's defection 'the special equipment in the mothballed shops . . . was shipped out', some destroyed and some re-stored elsewhere. Allegedly, documentation was also destroyed.

Another summary of the Biopreparat organization appeared in a 1993 *Izvestia* article:

The bitter irony is that work on bacteriological weapons developed especially vigorously precisely after the convention was signed. The accomplishments of biotechnology were the scientific basis for this. In the mid-1970s a highly secret Scientific-Technical Council staffed by the country's leading scientists was established as part of the Main Administration of Microbiological Industry.

The production tasks were imposed upon the large Biopreparat Association, which had shops and plants all over the country. This association was referred to colloquially as 'Ogarkov's system', after the name of the general who served as its first director. The system contained 18 scientific institutes employing 25 000 associates, five plants and a large storage facility in Siberia. Several institutes and plants formerly subordinated to purely peaceable departments such as the Ministry of Agriculture and

[70] See Umnov (note 15). The names assigned to the Biopreparat organization have changed numerous times, in a manner not atypical of certain Soviet organizations: The All-Union Research and Production Association Biopreparat, The Special Directorate of the Main Administration of the Microbiological Industry, The Main Directorate Biopreparat of the USSR Ministry of the Medical Industry, The State Concern Biopreparat. 'On 5 December 1991, it was transferred to the jurisdiction of the Ministry of Health of Russia . . . It is still run by a general. The facility is guarded, just as before, by warrant officers of the internal troops . . .'.

the Ministry of Health also worked for 'Ogarkov's system'. 'Ogarkov's system' did not involve itself in mass production of weapons, but a so-called 'mobilization plan' existed. This plan specified the quantity and the sort of concoctions that were to be produced in response to a particular command.[71]

The significance of these disclosures is that it indicates that the USSR had at least two separate systems for funding and managing biological warfare R&D: the first in the Ministry of Defence, and the second in the Ministry of the Medical and Microbiological Industry, via Biopreparat. (There are in fact three other 'state concerns' that act as intermediaries between government ministries and production facilities in the same way that Biopreparat does and in the same general product area as Biopreparat, one of which even split off from Biopreparat. It is not known, however, if any of these also played some role in BW development.) There were apparently also various degrees of co-operation between the Ministry of Health and the Ministry of Defence. Biopreparat, for example, acted as a channel for funding from the Ministry of Health to some of its affiliated institutes. Other indications of close relations between the Ministries of Health and Defence are the roles played by senior generals, for example, General Y. I. Smirnov, as Minister of Health.

In January and February 1993, two additional disclosures became available concerning Biopreparat. The first appeared in an interview with Dr Pasechnik, made by the BBC and *The Spectator*.[72] It reported that:

Biopreparat had 25 000 employees and a budget of 100 million roubles each year in the 1980s.

Its present head was Yuri Kalinin, another former General of the Soviet Army's Chemical Troops.

It quoted Deputy Foreign Secretary Berdennikov to the effect that the Russian Foreign Ministry did not really know what Biopreparat did: 'When we speak to those people they say "no". So what can we do?' If this truly represents the status of the Russian government knowledge and its ability to govern crucial affairs, it would be an incredibly damaging admission.

A letter from US Secretary of State Eagleburger and UK Foreign Minister Hurd to the Russian government in August 1992 alleged that work was underway 'to allow industrial production of a strain of plague resistant to cold and heat and to 16 antibiotics—for offensive purposes'.

An article by John Barry in *Newsweek* again quoted Deputy Foreign Minister Berdennikov, saying that Biopreparat 'was one of the best guarded secrets in the old Soviet Union'.[73] Apparently a second Biopreparat official, senior to Dr Pasechnik, had also defected more recently and had reported that offensive biological warfare work had continued within the Biopreparat system even after President Yeltsin's decrees in February and April 1992, but the production plants had reportedly been mothballed. The two reports substantially corroborated one another.

[71] Leskov, S., *Izvestia*, 26 June 1993, in JPRS-TND-93-025, 2 Aug. 1993, pp. 13–17.

[72] Urban, M., 'The cold war's deadliest secret', *The Spectator*, 23 Jan. 1993, pp. 9–10.

[73] Barry, J., 'Planning a plague?', *Newsweek*, 1 Feb. 1993, pp. 40–41. The Soviet programme to produce the genetically engineered plague strain, resistant to antibiotics and in dry form, dated from 1984 and was 'a top priority of the five-year plan for Biopreparat during the second half of the 1980s, the heart of the Gorbachev era'.

In an interview with *Pravda* on 15 October 1992, General Kalinin claimed that only 1 per cent of the 'general budget' of Biopreparat was devoted to biological warfare.[74] Without access to the relevant documentation, scepticism is warranted of the claim, unless it is taken to suggest that there may have been an additional 'specific' budget as well as the 'general budget'. Kalinin admitted to Biopreparat's development of a 'mobilization capacity', which he implied was intended only to be activated in wartime, the production of 'gene engineered medicines of viral and bacterial source, and the technology and equipment for their production'. What is of interest is that if General Kalinin's estimate were even approximately correct, it would mean that Biopreparat's facilities and its staff would need virtually *no* 'conversion', since they would presumably already be engaged for the overwhelming part in civilian production.

This situation also complicates the problem of estimating how many Soviet, or currently Russian, research and production institutes were devoted to biological warfare—and hence how many now require conversion programmes. Those not directly managed by the Ministry of Defence may have had other primary responsibilities, and only varying or small portions of their facilities or staff may have been directly engaged in biological warfare R&D. This would appear to be the case, for example, according to evidence presented below, for the large institute at Koltsovo. In addition to the five institutes that the USSR reported in 1987 as under the management of the Ministry of Defence, the Vozrozhdeniye Island test site is certain. (President Yeltsin's April 1992 reference to 'two test sites' has never been further explained). If the Irkutsk, Obolensk and Koltsovo laboratories are then added, this could mean *anywhere from 9 to over 20* biological warfare R&D facilities, all or in part. That would mean that the USSR had between 5 and 10 times as many biological warfare facilities as did the United States. Interestingly, in September 1992 General Valentin Yevstigneyev reported that, in addition to the 70 million rouble expenditure for the USSR's programme in 1991, 'In our country no more than ten establishments are engaged in protective military programs . . . . Just over ten specialists work in the Defence Ministry's directorate'.[75]

It is interesting to note that in 1975, reporting on a visit by a US National Academy of Sciences delegation to the USSR, Dr Alexander Rich remarked that 'One of the things I learned there was that their government Central Committee had made a decision to emphasize the science of molecular biology and to go into that area heavily'.[76] It seems quite plausible that Dr Rich was being given a public portrayal of what was in effect the Soviet Government's decision to sponsor a resurgence of BW R&D—*following* their signing of the BWC—through an extensive programme of research in molecular genetics and the establishment of new institutes for that purpose.

The Scientific Research Institute of Applied Microbiology was set up in the early seventies. The foundations of the first houses in the settlement of Obolensk, which still does not appear on the map of the oblast, were laid simultaneously. The official reason for the start of construction was a CPSU Central Committee and USSR Council of

[74] Kaisyn, V., 'Medicines: shield or weapons', *Pravda*, 15 Oct. 1992.

[75] Golts, A., *Krasnaya Zvezda*, 29 Sep. 1992, in FBIS-SOV-92-194, 6 Oct. 1992, pp. 2–4.

[76] *US–USSR Cooperative Agreements in Science and Technology*, Hearings before the Committee on Science and Technology, US House of Representatives, 94th Congress, 1st Session (US Government Printing Office: Washington, DC, Nov. 1975), pp. 27, 240. (Dr Rich is a noted US molecular geneticist.)

Ministers resolution on boosting the role of genetic engineering and microbiology in the country's national economy but, as is customary in our country, different purposes were concealed beneath the official statement. A very strict secret was made of the fact that the institute was earmarked for the study of the existing biological and bacteriological weapons and the development of reliable vaccines to protect the Army and the civilian population.[77]

It is also interesting to note that in March 1973 a US–Soviet Joint Commission on Science and Technology agreed to develop 'cooperative projects' in six areas of scientific research, one of which was 'microbiological synthesis', more specifically, The US–USSR Joint Working Group on Scientific and Technical Cooperation on the Production of Substances by Microbiological Means.[78] The exchange programme was managed on the US side by the National Science Foundation and the American Society for Microbiology, while the Soviet counterpart was the Ministry (then the 'State Committee') of the Microbiological Industry. Researchers from literally dozens of major Soviet research institutes working in the field of molecular biology participated, and the programme continued through 1982.

IV. Conversion of the former Soviet biological warfare facilities

With some conception of the number of institutes that are involved it is now possible to turn to the question of conversion. In order to assess the possibilities as well as the problems that would be faced in converting each of these facilities it would be well to know, aside from their location: (*a*) the number of research personnel employed at each site; (*b*) the products currently produced, and in what quantities; and (*c*) the kinds of equipment in the facility and their volumetric capacities.

Varying amounts of information became available in 1991 and 1992 regarding four of the Soviet facilities: Obolensk, Kirov, the Vozrozhdeniye Island test site and Koltsovo. The first information to become available was for the Scientific Research Institute of Applied Microbiology at Obolensk. It reportedly consisted of five buildings, one of them eight stories tall, and out of '1200 employees . . . the biggest and best part of the scientific cadres' were assigned to work dealing with BW.[79] The agents causing anthrax, plague and tularaemia were among the organisms reportedly being worked on. The most recent work orders (before September 1991) had dealt with studies of the immune system, and 'to create micro-organisms capable, "according to a set program" of producing substances unknown in nature'. According to the Deputy Director of the Institute, the officials who delivered the state work orders were allegedly unknown to the staff. At the time of the press report (September 1991) it was claimed that 'there [is] already no money to pay the next wages' and there 'is no other employment for [the staff] at present', although this is contradicted by several

[77] Nedogonov, V., 'Directed-energy plague, or what the secret scientific research institute near Moscow did', *Komsomol'skaya Pravda*, 24 Sep. 1991, in FBIS-SOV-91-191, 2 Oct. 1991, pp. 48–50.

[78] *Review of the US–USSR Joint Working Group in Microbiology*, Final Report, Technical Note, SSC-TN-7557-5 (SRI International: Arlington, Va., Sep. 1980).

[79] See Nedogonov (note 77).

other reports quoted below. Obolensk was reported to 'cost the state 150 million roubles', presumably in capital construction costs.[80]

More detailed information on personnel numbers became available in a June 1992 *Izvestia* report on a visit to the institute at Kirov: 'The institute has 36 State Prize winners, five doctors of science, 82 candidates [of science, ed.], and a total of 114 officers who are scientists. . . . Their range of interests includes microbiology, epidemiology, immunology, genetics, aerobiology, biochemistry, biophysics, physical and colloidal chemistry, and biotechnology'.[81]

The wording is somewhat ambiguous, but this appears to mean 237 senior professional personnel. Making the *roughest* extrapolation from these numbers, if the USSR had five biological warfare R&D facilities, there might be 1185 senior scientists involved; if 10 biological warfare R&D facilities, 2370 scientists; if 20 facilities, 4740 scientists. In his September 1992 interview, General Yevstigneyev claimed that only 'Approximately 400 scientists in Russia are engaged in this research'.[82] Much would depend on the number of scientists in an individual institution that were specifically assigned to BW R&D, but given the other figures accumulated in this chapter, the number 400 continues to arouse scepticism. The *Izvestia* report also claimed that one-third of the 'employees' had already left the institute due to reductions in the institute's budget, although full salaries remain in force. It also claimed that there was a 'conversion program', valued at 8 million roubles, but paradoxically, that the institute's 'hands are tied by the ban on their commercial activity'. Significantly, the disciplinary interests listed for the research personnel indicate that they would be able to carry out work on any of the multiple kinds of problems within their individual research disciplines. This report also claimed that the USSR spent 70 million roubles annually for operating the laboratories, although other statements by Soviet officials in April and October 1992 referred to the 70 million figure as the expenditure for 1991 only.

The information on the Vozrozhdeniye Island test site was rather general. It was part of the Aralsk (or Aralsk-5) facility, and was in fact managed by the Ministry of Defence's laboratory in Sergiyev-Posad (formerly Zagorsk). 'A regiment . . . was quartered on the island', and the base had a population of 'over a thousand' (this presumably does not include the regiment).[83]

In contrast, information that became available at the end of 1992 regarding the Institute of Molecular Biology in Koltsovo is extremely detailed.[84] Together with the Institute of Biologically Active Substances at Berdsk, near Novosibirsk, and the Experimental Production Plant also in Koltsovo, it had 182 PhDs and DScs on its staff, out of a total staff which 'exceeds 3000 persons'—by another count, close to 4000 including the Experimental Agricultural Production Enterprise which is a food collective supplying the research institutes with some of the food their employees require, as well as such agricultural products

[80] See Kaisyn (note 61). Kaisyn refers to Obolensk only as a 'nine-story glass building'.

[81] Litovkin, V., 'We have no bacteriological weapons, military bacteriologists maintain', *Izvestia*, 12 June 1992, in JPRS-TND-92-019, 19 June 1992, p. 22.

[82] See Golts (note 75).

[83] See Kozlov (note 46), and Safulin, D., 'Status of biological lab remains unclear', *Nezavisimaya Gazeta*, 1 July 1992, in JPRS-TND-92-026, 31 July 1992, p. 27.

[84] Netesov, chapter 12, in this volume.

as may also be needed in the research and production programme.[85] If it can be assumed that this ratio of scientific personnel to supporting staff was representative of other Soviet BW-related institutions, about 1 to 20, or between 5 and 10 per cent—it would be quite interesting. The support personnel, who would be preparing media and the like should not need any 'conversion'; their tasks would remain the same so long as the institution can continue to function. The range of organisms that Koltsovo has worked with, as well as the range of products that it and the institute at Berdsk produce, is extremely wide by Western standards. In addition, the Koltsovo facility carries out about 30 per cent of the work done in Russia for the Human Genome Project. The Experimental Production Plant is occupied in manufacturing human and veterinary medicines. The capital value of the four combined institutions is 250 million roubles (in 1984 prices). A report late in 1993 indicated that US intelligence agencies believed that the facility at Berdsk had been 'used to develop biological weapons'.[86]

What is currently known about relevant conversion capabilities in the former USSR, or what kinds of alternative work have some of these institutes already themselves suggested or embarked on?

1. The USSR had a very large biotechnology programme. Roger Roffey refers to 'a national committee and a national program for biotechnology [which] encompassed 150 institutes in the former Soviet Union'.[87] A portion of that programme consisted of extremely large factories for the production of single-cell protein that was packaged for use as livestock food, for cattle, hog and chicken feed.

2. The institute at Obolensk, in addition to its work on BW, was occupied in 'the struggle against plant pests and efforts to develop new medicines', and 'At present people [t]here are urgently trying to re-qualify for the production of medical preparations'.[88]

3. For Koltsovo, which admits to having been 'a secret institution' between 1974 and 1990, but claims not to have been 'a BW laboratory', its product line in vaccines, medical diagnostic aids and molecular reagents is so wide as to scarcely need any change other than to increase its production of these commercial products and to develop its own marketing network within the former Soviet Union. The same holds for its current sister institute in Berdsk.

4. In a press conference given in the spring of 1990 by the Sverdlovsk Ministry of Defence BW facility, now renamed the Sector for Military Epidemiology of the Microbiology Research Institute, the spokesman listed the following capabilities of the laboratory that could be applied to civilian problems:

production of nutrients for bacteriological cultures,
chemical analysis,
monitoring of urban and industrial air quality,

[85] A Russian epidemiologist speaking at a US research centre quoted a figure of 20 000 employees in the nine older plague laboratories that had existed in the USSR. Plague incidence in the USSR was no higher than that in the USA, at under 100 cases per year, and at first sight this figure seems implausible.

[86] See Gordon (note 16).

[87] Roffey, R., 'Bioteknisk forskning i Ryssland: målinriktad satsning, ökande konkurrens' [Biotechnical research in Russia: target-oriented venture, increasing competition], *FOA Tidningen*, vol. 30, no. 3 (Nov. 1992), pp. 16–17 (in Swedish).

[88] See Nedogonov (note 77).

assaying and combating damage to metal structures by bacteriological organisms,
detection of harmful substances in the environment, and
other ecological research'.[89]

In June 1992 the Deputy Chief of the Center for Science at the same facility listed a slightly different agenda of projects in the civilian sector that could be performed by their staff:

They are preparing to do the following:
cleanse maternity hospitals of *Staphylococcus,*
disinfect poultry farms and railroad cars, removing every kind of fungus or mould,
destroy chemical weapons and highly toxic waste with their own bacteria,
clean up spills of oil and kerosene with micro-organisms that will reprocess the oil into protein that will go in food for fish, [and]
set up production of the very antibiotics that hospitals are so catastrophically short of.[90]

Two of these proposals made use of the facility's clean-up capacity, turned to commercial use, two had been proposed earlier, and CW detoxification was newly added. In March 1992 it was claimed that work was under way on two of these technologies. Scientists at the Sverdlovsk laboratory had developed a method of eliminating water and soil contamination by fuel oil and other oil products, using micro-organisms that metabolize the fuel oil, and producing a protein product that could be used as a fish food. The process was developed jointly with researchers at the Tyumen Petroleum and Gas Institute.[91] The organisms that degrade petroleum residues have long been known and have been commercialized in the West, and given the degree of oil pollution being reported in the former USSR and in Eastern Europe this should certainly be a viable project. Research was reportedly also under way on the bacterial degradation of the active agents in chemical weapons.

5. Perhaps of greater immediate significance and need, in a country where virtually every single hospital in every city and town claims a near-total absence of antibiotics, there should be little problem in finding immediately useful application for former biological warfare R&D laboratories. There appears to be at least some attempt to move in this direction, but antibiotics production is clearly needed on a massive scale.[92] Any medium or large-scale fermentation

[89] Bogomolov, S., '19th cantonment: a reporter is a rare guest here', *Ural'sky Rabochiy,* 12 Mar. 1990, in JPRS-TAC-91-025, 24 Oct. 1991, pp. 53–56.

[90] Belyaninov, K. *et al.*, 'Anthrax epidemic linked to biological war', *Komsomol'skaya Pravda,* 10 June 1992, in JPRS-TND-92-022, 10 July 1992.

[91] Usacheva, L., 'Nine hours behind the barbed wire: reporting from the 19th military installation', *Poisk,* 7–13 Mar. 1992.

[92] The actual picture seems somewhat confusing. Virtually all foreign observers report a massive deficit in all kinds of pharmaceuticals in the former Soviet Union, with bribes required to obtain medication, or seeking it on the black market, etc. None other than Arkadiy Volskiy, the leader of the USSR's former defence industrialists, included in the four main 'conditions' that he put to President Yeltsin on 28 Oct. 1992 a demand for 'the provision of medicines, of which only 60 per cent of the needed amount was available' (Lloyd, J. and Boultan, L., 'Industrial czar puts Russia's leader on spot', *Financial Times,* 29 Oct. 1992). Most Western observers would consider the figure of 60 per cent a gross overestimate, and most likely a number that was selected at random. On the other hand, the facility at Koltsovo reported in the autumn of 1992 that it was producing antibiotics and that its storage facility was full, but that local communities and hospitals did not have the funds to purchase them. At the same time as the USSR may have simultaneously had both overcapacity and insufficient production of pharmaceutical products and antibiotics for *civilian* use in the past, there were reports for many years that it was buying antibiotics from Cuba, and may have continued to do so in the early 1990s.

capacity could be immediately put to use 'to avoid unemployment . . . the scientists in Obolensk established ten small enterprises for the production of medicines that are in very short supply'.[93]

The same practice has been followed at Koltsovo: the staff has been divided into smaller production units and shareholder companies, and these have funds with which to procure the raw materials needed for production.

The point is that biological conversion does not necessitate major expenditure. Strains, serums, vaccines, and other output developed previously can with comparative ease become the basis of new medical preparations. The money spent on biological weapons research will not have been wasted, it will start to work for people.

Such programs already exist. The Yekaterinburg [Ekaterinburg] Center's buildings and laboratories are being transferred to medicine production. It is already ready to produce medicine. A special program is also being formulated for the institute at Sergiyev-Posad, which develops vaccines that are of great interest to foreign countries. Scientists at the center in Kirov are also working successfully on conversion and are providing their city with great assistance in creating its agro-industrial complex.[94]

In a June 1992 interview General A. T. Kharechko, now the head of the Ekaterinburg laboratory, reported that 'the cantonment is now geared exclusively for medical needs and is going to produce antibiotics and artificial blood substitutes',[95] and in April 1992 the General Staff claimed that 'We have an entirely realistic plan to set up a production facility for antibacteriological agents based on the Yekaterinburg [Ekaterinburg] Center'.[96] The problem is that these various statements are at best imprecise and more frequently contradictory.[97] It is not possible to know what is a 'plan' and what is now 'geared . . . to produce'. As late as October 1993 General Kuntsevich was still using phrasing that appeared to be anticipatory of first 'formulating programs': Now we are formulating programs to retool the relevant scientific centers, former participants in military–biological programs, for general scientific activity to supply our population with effective medicines'.[98] In an earlier statement in September 1992, he had them already so occupied: 'This facility [Ekaterinburg], like similar centers

[93] See Kaisyn (note 61).

[94] See Litovkin (note 61). Regarding the vaccine which the Sergiyev Posad facility hoped to export, the article added the following: 'Our specialists claim that during the Gulf war the Americans were studying the possibility of buying these vaccines because of their great effectiveness', which suggests that the vaccine in question was for anthrax.

[95] Chelikov, V., 'A weapon against their own people', *Moscow News*, no. 23, 7–14 June 1992.

[96] Pashkov, A., 'Military deny involvement in mysterious illness: chief of CIS joint armed forces top secret military laboratories answers journalists questions for the first time', *Izvestia*, 17 Apr. 1992; see also FBIS-SOV-92-082, 28 Apr. 1992, pp. 4–5.

[97] Statements from different Russian sources, military and civilian, as to whether the Vozrozhdeniye Island BW test site was or was not closed, and if so when it had ceased operations, were also widely contradictory during 1991 and 1992. A military official claimed that 'all testing on the island . . . ceased' in June 1991, whereas another report stated that 'in November 1991, at a scientific council in Sergiyev Posad, a decision was made to terminate the experimental work on the island definitively', while other reports had the site 'still operating . . . in January 1992', and on 17 Apr. 1992, the CIS General Staff offices responsible for these installations reported that although the Kazakh Government had taken over responsibility for the island test site, the General Staff had *proposed* 'a more fundamental decision, that this institution be shut down'. There had already been numerous statements that the site had been shut down for some time. In September 1992 General Kuntsevich claimed that 'it has been destroyed' ('Official examines destruction of CBW weapons', *Rossiyskiye Vesti*, 22 Sep. 1992, in FBIS-SOV-92-186, 24 Sep. 1992, pp. 2–5. In August and September 1992 US authorities did state that the BW testing site was closed (see notes 46 and 83).

[98] 'Official surveys CBW destruction process', *Krasnaya Zvezda*, 22 Oct. 1993, in JPRS-TND-93-035, 10 Nov. 1993, pp. 47–49.

in Kirov and Sergiyev-Posad, are now only working on creating means of protection against biological weapons . . . . Apart from the protective means, the facilities are today engaged in developing new highly effective medicines'.[99]

In contrast to all of the above, General Yevstigneyev (in April 1992) claimed that 'the [Ekaterinburg] plant that produced vaccines and diagnostic substances was closed down'.[100] As if to display these contradictions to the maximum, General Kuntsevich stated that 'Having invested our scientists and specialists efforts in this, we are preserving a great intellectual and scientific and technical asset', and only a single sentence later, 'Now that the equipment has been completely dismantled and the resources that previously were used for military purposes have been destroyed . . . .'[101] Few competent observers have been to any of these facilities and there is no real understanding of which of them is doing what, either of previous work or of 'conversion' projects. US and British government officials that have visited some of these facilities have not seen fit to make any public report which would help understand exactly what the institutes are currently doing. Similarly, Western pharmaceutical companies that have visited at least some of the sites since 1990 investigating commercial possibilities, of course, do not make public reports about their visits either.

Biological warfare R&D laboratories that formerly produced vaccines—the Ekaterinburg laboratory was one of these—could also produce vaccines for domestic livestock; cattle, hogs and poultry are all routinely vaccinated against various diseases. Other projects could also be applied to the production of protein feed and fertilizer utilizing bacterial cultures which transform paper waste to cattle feed or to fertilizer. As already indicated, pilot plant installations for these were developed as long ago as the mid-1960s in various US universities. For each of the sites a list of between 5 to 10 alternative research or production priorities should be drawn up. These would fall into two broad categories: (*a*) the production of commodities and services which the institutes by their nature can produce and may already have produced in the preceding years, and which are in the most dire need in Russia and in the other new republics of the former USSR, and (*b*) interdisciplinary problem-oriented research in the fields of public health and ecological and environmental problems.

The entire territory of the former USSR—as well as most of Eastern Europe—suffers from gross pollution in every category: air, water, land and, over large areas, also radiation.[102] Any products these institutions could produce that served environmental protection or recovery would also have immediate application.

V. Prerequisites for conversion

There are several preliminary steps which the Russian authorities and those of any other republic in which any of these facilities exist must take in the process of conversion:

[99] 'Official examines destruction of CBW weapons' (note 97), pp. 2–5.

[100] 'General quizzed on chemical weapons production', *Izvestia*, 17 Apr. 1992, in FBIS-SOV-92-082, 28 Apr. 1992, pp. 4–5.

[101] 'Official examines destruction of CBW weapons' (note 97), pp. 2–5.

[102] Feshbach, M., and Friendly, Jr, A., *Ecocide in the USSR: Health and Nature Under Siege* (Basic Books: Bloomington, Ind., 1992); see also Shapiro, M., 'Ex-Soviet empire the new "sick man of Europe"', *Washington Post*, 3 Oct. 1992.

1. *Absolutely end the offensive BW R&D programme.* This has supposedly been done as of the joint US, British and Russian statement of 15 September 1992, but it is not clear to outside observers exactly what has occurred. The section on the Russian General Staff that formerly controlled the five Ministry of Defence laboratories and the 'offensive' programme was simply renamed and became 'defensive'. It is also not clear whether any or which of the 'number of centers' that General Volkogonov claimed in February 1992 'have been closed' have in fact been closed, and if so, how many and which of them they are. In September 1992 Umnov also reported that 'four divisions of the Central Institute of Microbiology of the Armed Forces of Russia have now been closed'.[103] The announced budget reduction of 30 per cent, however, suggests that they have not actually been 'closed', but only redirected. It is also not clear by when the reduction of personnel by half would be completed.

Perhaps most important of all, there has never been any explanation as to *why*, and *how,* within the Soviet political decision-making structure itself, the violation of the BWC came about. This holds for the period 1972 to 1985 as well as for 1985 to mid-1992, the time of President Gorbachev's tenure and following it.[104] The new agreements on openness and inspections are, of course, extremely important for the future, but there must also be some general confidence based on understanding how the decision to carry out and maintain an explicit violation of the BWC was made and maintained for 20 years, including during a period in which the Soviet General Staff and President Gorbachev were acceding to a wide-ranging group of far more significant strategic arms control agreements, such as the Intermediate-range nuclear forces (INF) Treaty, the US–Soviet Treaty on the Reduction and Limitation of Strategic Offensive Arms and the US–Russian Treaty on Further Reduction and Limitation of Strategic Offensive Arms (referred to as the START Treaty and the START II Treaty), and the Conventional Armed Forces in Europe (CFE) Treaty. That process must be understood in order to be assured that the same situation does not reoccur.

2. *The institutes should by and large be removed from control by the Russian military; they should be placed under civilian control.* 'Experts from the committee for conversion problems consider that these institutes must in time be removed from the tutelage of the military. The highly professional scientific forces created there and their experience are a federal asset and must switch entirely to work in the national economy'.[105]

Obviously Russian military authorities may choose to retain one or two facilities for defensive R&D as permitted by the BWC and as the United States also did, but such facilities should also be open for inspection as Fort Detrick has been since Soviet officials first visited it in 1972. As part of the government-to-government initiatives a Russian team carried out an inspection visit in December 1991 at the Salk Institute's facilities which produce vaccines under contract for the US DOD.[106] Another Russian team of 12 scientists visited three US

[103] See Umnov (note 15).

[104] For a general discussion, see 'The sources of Soviet compliance behavior', chapter 7 in ed. G. Duffy, *Compliance and the Future of Arms Control* (Ballinger: Cambridge, Mass., 1988).

[105] See Litovkin (note 61).

[106] The Russian team of 12–14 inspectors was composed of members of the Ministry of Defence, the Ministry of Foreign Affairs, and scientists from the Russian biotechnology industry. The Russian inspection team was well versed in how to seek for violations. (Personal communication with the author.)

facilities under the terms of the 1992 US–Russian–British agreement in March 1994. They visited the Plum Island animal diseases laboratory and two Pfizer Incorporated pharmaceutical facilities at Vigo, Indiana and Groton, Connecticut.[107]

Civilian control is also crucial to providing full availability of information to the government. The General Staff was clearly responsible for the inadequate information in the drafts of Russia's annual submission to the BWC in the spring of 1992. This raised the question of whether the commission established by President Yeltsin still lacked access to information or had yet developed its own authority and ability to survey and to monitor the activities inside the R&D institutions. At a minimum, declassification and removal from military control should be a pre-condition for any Western financial or technical assistance to these institutions. The International Science and Technology Centers established in Moscow and Kiev by Western donors are intended to fund research projects by former Soviet scientists who were previously engaged in work on biological weapons, as well as those who may have worked on nuclear and chemical weapon and missile delivery systems.[108] On a trip to the United States in October 1992 General Kuntsevich apparently also sought additional US Government help for the conversion of Russian biological warfare facilities. He also established a private non-governmental US–Russian organization to facilitate conversion of Russian BW and CW facilities.[109] Unfortunately, as late as March 1992 the directors of some of the former Soviet BW-related facilities expressed the opinion that they were in no need of 'conversion', that they had nothing to 'convert', and that there was nothing wrong with what they currently were doing, at the very same time as they were describing new programmes of work that they were going to engage in.[110] The members of the Russian Committee for Convention Problems, established in February 1992, could not have agreed with that, and hopefully things have changed since September 1992.

3. *All of the institutes in question should be open to international scientific visitors, and secrecy should be removed from any non-military institute.* The All-Union Institute of Molecular Biology at Koltsovo was a totally secret institute until 1990. It has since been visited by representatives of a sizeable number of Western pharmaceutical corporations, as have other institutes in Russia.[111] However as late as September 1991 the *Pravda* correspondent that was permitted to visit Obolensk could not learn where the facility was, and was taken there in a disguised vehicle.[112]

The above three changes are prerequisites for any real conversion: (*a*) a total end to offensive programmes; (*b*) a complete turnover of the laboratories to civilian control, and no covert programmes withheld from government knowledge;

[107] McQuiston, J. T., 'Russians finish an inspection of Plum Island disease lab', *New York Times*, 2 Mar. 1994.

[108] US Department of State, 'Science and technology centers', *Fact Sheet* (US Department of State: Washington, DC, undated); Dowdy, E. J., 'Technology centers for Russian scientists', *Bulletin of the Atomic Scientists*, vol. 48, no. 8 (Oct. 1992).

[109] International Center for Disarmament and Conversion, *Press Release*, 6 Oct. 1992, 2 pp., mimeo.

[110] 'Conversion? . . . This word somehow doesn't apply very well to us. After all, we never were a VPK [military industrial complex] that worked on war. We always worked on defence'. See Usacheva (note 91).

[111] Some of these are Merck, Sharp and Dohme, Ortho Diagnostics, Johnson & Johnson (of the USA), Merieux (France), Glaxo (UK), Pharmacia LKB Pribori, and Lab Systems (Finland).

[112] See Nedogonov (note 77).

and (*c*) an end to secrecy, and complete access to all the facilities by the international scientific community.

Beyond that, conversion is entirely feasible. There is probably no other area of defence-related R&D or defence industrial production in which conversion should be as easy. Facilities require little or no modification and personnel virtually no retraining. Microbiologists, virologists, molecular geneticists, biochemists do not need to be retrained when they turn to a new research problem or work with a new organism; that is part of what they routinely do throughout their careers. Finally, the national need for the converted personnel and products is supremely manifest in Russia and in all of the former Soviet Union, unquestionably more so than anywhere else in the industrialized world. There is no question that they have other constructive and economically viable alternatives to which to turn.

This chapter has not directly addressed the Vaccines for Peace proposal, an international programme for the development and use of vaccines against dual-threat agents. It is clear that it implicitly suggests other avenues of conversion. Every precept of arms control would suggest that an emphasis on vaccine production for 'dual-use' agents in particular should be avoided at all costs. The production of vaccines for use specifically in developing countries, however, as a part of a programme of national aid to developing countries, is eminently desirable. In that case the disease agents selected against which vaccines should be prepared should follow the priority of diseases which most seriously affect developing nations, as listed in the annual reports of the World Health Organization.[113]

For a decade after 1972 there was the hope that the problem of biological warfare was going to be eradicated. However, the last decade has produced indications that some eight developing nations, in addition to China and Israel, have initiated BW development programmes of varying degrees. It is an extremely discouraging development, and if there is to be any hope of reversing this process as soon as possible, it is crucial that all of the major powers—Russia, obviously, having been the problematic party—be known to be in total and rigorous adherence to the BWC.

[113] These tables are reproduced in Cairncross, S. *et al.* (eds), *The Poor Die Young: Housing and Health in Third World Countries* (Earthscan Publications: London, 1990), pp. xxi, xxii and xxiv.

Part III. Vaccine R&D and production

9. Viral vaccines: their evolution and current trends

FLORIAN HORAUD

I. Introduction

It is difficult to clearly and concisely review the topic of viral vaccines. In the past 15 years viral vaccines have been the subject of many international meetings and scientific papers published in major microbiology and public health journals. Exhaustive presentations of viral vaccines are available in several recent books,[1] in the proceedings of specialized meetings and in journals. This chapter presents a review of some aspects of the experience which has been gained in the manufacture and control of viral vaccines, and the likely direction of future developments.

There are many reasons for the current interest in viral vaccines, but there is no doubt that the key role played by viral vaccines in public health is the major factor. Viral vaccines are the only tools available for the control of many severe human and animal diseases, not only because they are highly efficient, but also because other prophylactic or therapeutic anti-viral products simply do not exist.

II. Empiricism and efficacy

Products derived from human or animal tissues and fluids have been used for medical purposes for many centuries, but it was Edward Jenner in the 18th century who laid the foundation for the modern era of vaccination. A century after Jenner's observation, Louis Pasteur developed a scientific approach to vaccine preparation. Pasteur's great achievement was to develop an anti-rabies vaccine, even though he was completely unaware of the nature of the virus causing the disease. His experiments with chicken cholera and anthrax vaccination and his exceptional intuition were the factors that allowed Pasteur to elaborate the strategy for rabies vaccine preparation. However, Pasteur was extremely lucky in choosing rabies, since the nervous tissues of rabies-infected animals contain a large enough antigenic mass of virus to allow a vaccine to be prepared from it.

After Pasteur, the development of new viral vaccines was hindered by the inability to cultivate viruses on substrates other than the tissues of infected animals. Therefore, the development of a new generation of viral vaccines depended on improvement of the technology used in the preparation of the cell substrates necessary to propagate viruses.

The most remarkable fact emerging from the history of viral vaccines is that their reputed efficacy was the result of an extraordinary effort of empirical experiments and epidemiological observations. All marketed viral vaccines consist of killed or live virus, with the exception of the hepatitis B vaccine. This is the first and currently the only vaccine obtained by recombinant DNA (rDNA)

[1] Woodrow, G. C. and Levine, M. M. (eds), *New Generation Vaccines* (Marcel Dekker: New York, 1990); Plotkin, S. A. and Mortimer, E. A. (eds), *Vaccines* (W. B. Saunders: Philadelphia, 1988).

technology. The development of killed viral vaccines followed generally Pasteur's approach to rabies. However, live vaccines containing viral strains with attenuated virulence[2] were based on Jenner's observation, the capacity of cowpox virus to immunize humans against smallpox, or Max Theiler's work on 17D yellow fever vaccine. In the latter case, unlike Jenner's observation, a human virulent strain of yellow fever became attenuated by serial passages on a non-human host (i.e., monkeys, mice and chick embryos).[3] Even today the reasons for many cases of viral attenuation of live vaccines defy scientific explanation. This situation is well illustrated by the use of vaccinia virus as a vaccine against smallpox. This method, developed by Jenner 200 years ago, has led to the eradication of the human disease.[4] However, in other cases, such as live poliovirus vaccine prepared with Sabin strains, André Lwoff was able to demonstrate that low temperature (under 37°C) is the selective factor for mutants with reduced virulence.[5] This concept was later generalized and used for the selection of attenuated variants to be used in the production of live attenuated vaccine. The efficacy of viral vaccines became evident after World War II when large national and international vaccination campaigns were organized. Since then the efficiency and safety of viral vaccines currently used (see table 9.1) have been proved over many years of world-wide use in large vaccination campaigns, and it is likely that they will remain on the market for a number of years.

III. Safety of viral vaccines: the past

In developing a scientific approach to vaccine preparation, Louis Pasteur took a new approach in which the starting material, identified as a human pathogen, is transformed into a clinically useful drug with a specific prophylactic activity. The aim of this process is to destroy the pathogenic potential of the source material while preserving its capacity to induce an immune response in a host. It is therefore clear that there is an inherent risk associated with using vaccines prepared by this method. The same holds true for live viral vaccines, since the attenuation is potentially reversible and because a failure in good manufacturing practice (GMP) could introduce a wild virulent strain of virus into the vaccine. For all these reasons, the clinical acceptability of viral vaccines is still guided mainly by risk–benefit analysis.

However, despite the successful use of rabies vaccine by Pasteur, vaccines have been implicated in serious accidents from the time of their first use. For instance, before Pasteur's time vaccine lymph that was used for smallpox vaccination was involved in the transmission of other diseases. Because calf lymph for smallpox vaccination did not become available in large enough quantities until the mid-19th century, human lymph, transferred from arm-to-arm, was used as the source material for vaccination. Many transmissible diseases were sporadically disseminated by this procedure, but the most dramatic incident

[2] See Woodrow and Levine (note 1).

[3] Freestone, D. S., 'Yellow fever vaccine', Plotkin and Mortimer (note 1), pp. 387–419.

[4] See Fenner, chapter 18, in this volume.

[5] Lwoff, A., 'The thermosensitive critical events of the viral cycle', *Cold Spring Harbor Symposia on Quantitative Biology,* vol. 27 (1962), pp. 159–74.

Table 9.1. Human viral vaccines currently in use

Killed Vaccines
Influenza
Rabies
Polio
Hepatitis A
Hepatitis B (rDNA subunit vaccine)[a]
Japanese encephalitis
Live Vaccines
Polio[b]
Measles[b]
Rubella
Mumps
Varicella
Yellow fever[a]

[a] Vaccine under consideration for use in the WHO Expanded Programme on Immunization
[b] Vaccine used in the WHO Expanded Programme on Immunization

occurred in Italy in 1861.[6] Approximately 46 children and 20 nurses in Rialta were infected with syphilis originating from the lymph of a donor. During his life Pasteur was criticized because rabies vaccine was at the origin of clinical accidents.[7] The rabies vaccine that Pasteur prepared probably contained residual live virus, but there is no evidence that he was aware of this. In any case, the problem of viral inactivation was too complex to be analysed in the early days of microbiology. Historically, viral vaccines were not the only biologicals at the root of clinical accidents; other immunological products, such as toxoids and sera, have also been responsible for adverse reactions. The excellent book by Graham Wilson gives an extensive and valuable review of such occurrences.[8]

Accidents generated by viral vaccines can result from the complex technology of their preparation, which requires a cell substrate system for virus replication. The historical development of viral vaccines is presented in table 9.2. Advances and the development of a new generation of viral vaccines depended on improvement of the technology used in the preparation of cell substrates available for virus production. When viral vaccine development is compared to the appearance of adverse effects after vaccine administration, it can be seen that each new generation of viral vaccine has been responsible for undesirable consequences.[9] For instance, the history of the development of polio vaccine was marked by a series of tragic experiments that started in 1935 with the attempt by Maurice Brody and John Kolmer to obtain a vaccine from the spinal cord of paralysed monkeys and (hopefully) ended in 1968, when there was a large outbreak of polio in Poland as a probable consequence of limited field trials of a new type 3 attenuated poliovirus.[10]

The adverse effects encountered as a result of the clinical use of viral vaccine

[6] Wilson, G. G., *The Hazards of Immunization* (University of London, Athlone Press: London, 1967).
[7] Lutaud, M., 'Pasteur et la Rage', *Journal de Médecine de Paris*, 1887, pp. 387–404.
[8] See Wilson (note 6).
[9] Horaud, F., 'Viral safety of biologicals', *Developments in Biological Standardization*, vol. 75 (1991), pp. 3–7.
[10] Horaud, F., 'Ethical and safety considerations for the use in clinical trials of new attenuated poliovirus strains', *Developments in Biological Standardization*, vol. 78 (1993), pp. 149–55.

Table 9.2. An historical account of viral vaccine development[a]

Year(s)	Vaccine	Cell substrate
1795	Smallpox (Jenner)	Calf lymph and human lymph (variolization)
1885	Rabies (Pasteur)	Rabbit central nervous system
1937–40	Influenza	Embryonated eggs
	Yellow fever	Embryonated eggs
1950–65	Polio	Tissue culture
	Measles	Tissue culture
	Rubella	Tissue culture
	Mumps	Tissue culture
	Foot-and-mouth disease virus and other veterinary vaccines	Tissue culture
Since 1980	Hepatitis B	Blood derived HBs-Ag
	Hepatitis B	rDNA HBs expressed in animal cell or yeast
	Varicella	Tissue culture
	Hepatitis A	Tissue culture

[a] This table shows that every new generation of viral vaccines was related to an innovation in the technology used in the preparation of cell substrates necessary for viral growth.

can be classified into four types of accident: (*a*) inactivated vaccines in which the virus used as immunogen has been incompletely inactivated and residual active virus induces clinical disease; (*b*) components of the cells used as substrates for virus propagation generate severe allergic reactions; (*c*) cells used as substrates were contaminated with endogenous or adventitious viruses that were released into the product; and (*d*) viruses were introduced into the vaccine by the reagents used during manufacture. These various types of accident induced by viral vaccines are presented in table 9.3.

This classification requires further comment (see table 9.3). The clinical accidents induced by incomplete inactivation of viruses used as immunogens have generally been dramatic because of the large number of subjects having a particularly severe clinical disease.

In many cases, vaccines have been recognized as the source of accidents because of the short lag time between vaccine administration and the onset of the disease. This was, for example, the case for the Fortaleza[11] and Cutter[12] accidents. However, in the outbreaks originating from foot-and-mouth disease vaccination, the correlation was only established once a powerful investigative tool for characterizing viral genomes became available.[13] In many other instances, a contaminant in the vaccine has been identified only many years after its licensing and large-scale use. An example illustrating this situation was the presence of hepatitis B virus (HBV) in the human serum used to stabilize

[11] Para, M., 'An outbreak of post-vaccinal rabies (Rage de Laboratoire) in Fortaleza, Brazil, in 1960: residual fixed virus as the aetiolological agent', *Bulletin of the World Health Organization*, vol. 33 (1965), pp. 177–82.

[12] Nathanson, N. and Langmuir, A. G., 'The Cutter incident: poliomyelitis following formaldehyde-inactivated poliovirus vaccination in the United States during the spring of 1955, I. Background', *American Journal of Hygiene*, vol. 78 (1963), pp. 16–81.

[13] Brown, F., 'An overview of the inactivation of FMDV and the implication when residual virus is present in vaccines', *Developments in Biological Standardization*, vol. 75 (1991), pp. 37–41.

Table 9.3. Examples of accidents induced by viral vaccines

Cause of accident	Examples
Incomplete inactivation or the virus present in the vaccine	Early rabies vaccines Fortaleza rabies incident Cutter incident: residual live virulent virus present in the vaccine Foot-and-mouth disease virus vaccine: limited outbreak was caused by residual active virus
Cell-component factors	Allergic encephalitis induced by myelin present in rabies vaccine produced in the central nervous systems of animals
Viral contamination of cell substrate	Yellow fever vaccine containing avian retroviruses Polio vaccines containing SV40, an oncogenic DNA virus
Contamination of vaccines by viruses present in the reagents	Yellow fever vaccine was contaminated with hepatitis B virus present in the human sera used as a stabilizer

yellow fever vaccine. While human serum was quickly recognized as the source of contamination,[14] the identification of the viral agent present in the serum only became possible recently, once the biology of HBV had been described.[15] Similarly, avian retroviruses from the chick embryos used contaminated yellow fever vaccine, and in 1960[16] it was realized that polio vaccine and other vaccines prepared from primary Rhesus kidney-cell culture and administered in the 1950s contained SV40, a DNA virus of monkeys capable of inducing tumours in hamsters.

IV. Safety and efficacy of viral vaccines: the present

The previous section gave an historical account of the major clinical accidents caused by viral vaccines. Because such accidents have become considerably less frequent in the last two decades, they are now mainly of historical interest. It is therefore worthwhile to try to analyse the reasons underlying the progress in the field of vaccine safety in general and of viral vaccines in particular. Both the pressures caused by legal liability and advances in technology have led to improvement in vaccine safety. Table 9.4 reviews the main factors that have contributed to this.

The acceptability of producing vaccines from tissue culture derived from

[14] Findlay, M. G., MacCallum, O. F. and Murgatreid, F., 'Observation bearing on the aetiology of infective hepatitis (so-called epidemic catarrhal jaundice)', *Transactions of the Royal Society of Tropical Medicine and Hygiene*, vol. 32 (1939), pp. 575–80; 'Report: jaundice following yellow fever vaccination', *Journal of the American Medical Association*, vol. 119 (1942), p. 1110.

[15] Leonard, S. B. *et al.*, 'A serological follow-up of the 1942 epidemic of post-vaccination hepatitis in the United States Army', *New England Journal of Medicine*, vol. 316 (1987), pp. 965–70.

[16] Sweet, B. H. and Hilleman, M. R., 'Detection of a "non-detectable" simian virus (vacuolating agent) present in Rhesus and Cynomolgus monkey-kidney cell culture material: a preliminary report', *Live Poliovirus Vaccines*, 2nd conference (PAHO-WHO: Washington, DC, 1960), pp. 79–89; Sweet, B. H. and Hilleman, M. R., 'The vacuolating virus, SV40', *Proceedings of the Society for Experimental Biology and Medicine*, vol. 109 (1962), pp. 965–68.

Table 9.4. Main factors that contributed to the safety of viral vaccines

Replacement of infected animal tissues as source material by viral suspensions obtained by tissue-culture technique; acceptability of diploid and heteroploid cell lines as systems for cell substrates
Development of cell-bank system allowing a full characterization of contaminants potentially present in cell substrate
Scientific knowledge of virus inactivation mechanism
Purification of inactivated vaccines
New approaches to quality control and introduction of good manufacturing practice (GMP) and good laboratory practice (GLP)
International and national guidelines standardizing the manufacture and control of viral vaccines
Viral-vaccine manufacturing is now a specialized branch of large pharmaceutical companies

diploid and especially heteroploid cell lines was an important breakthrough that contributed significantly to the introduction of modern industrial technology in viral vaccine preparation. This approach made possible the production of large batches of viral vaccines with remarkably reproducible quality for two reasons. First, the cells used in the process are derived from a cell bank, and the substrate is thus always the same. Second, bioreactor methodology was introduced for mass cultivation of animal cells. Used first in the manufacture of foot-and-mouth disease vaccine for veterinary purposes, this new technology was successfully adapted to the production of polio and rabies vaccines.[17] Bioreactor technology allows much better control of contaminants and standardization of the whole process. The existence of cell banks eliminates the risk introduced by the large variability of primary cell-culture substrate prepared from animal organs and allows consistent testing for viral and bacterial contaminants of the source material.

The quality of inactivated viral vaccines was also improved by the control of viral inactivation by chemical agents used to abolish viral infectivity such as formaldehyde or beta-propiolactone. There is no doubt that the purification of inactivated vaccines (influenza, polio and rabies) also contributed to their safety and consistency.

For live vaccines, new developments are needed to better characterize in molecular terms the viral genomes of attenuated strains. For Sabin polio viruses, a number of phenotype and genotype markers are available for determining *in vitro* and *in vivo* their identity and the degree of residual and neurovirulence.[18] This is, however, not the case for measles, mumps and rubella vaccines for which the attenuated character has been established by clinical trials, and for which vaccines are produced on the basis of virus seed lots.

The new technology in vaccine preparation, together with the increase in liability, created a new regulatory philosophy[19] and requirements for purity and quality control of vaccines. In the 1970s and 1980s large pharmaceutical companies came to dominate vaccine manufacture mainly because only large-scale

[17] Montagnon, B. J., 'Polio and rabies vaccines produced in continuous cell lines: a reality for vero cell line', *Development in Biological Standardization*, vol. 70 (1989), pp. 27–47.

[18] Minor, P. D., 'The molecular biology of poliovaccine', *Journal of General Virology*, vol. 73 (1992), pp. 3065–77.

[19] Hopps, H. E., Meyer, B. C. and Parkman, P. D., 'Regulation and testing of vaccines', Plotkin and Mortimer (note 1), pp. 576–86.

industry can afford the investment necessary for vaccine development, the cost of scientifically qualified staff and the price of sophisticated quality-control systems. This was in contrast to traditional vaccine production. Especially in Europe, vaccine production had been carried out in many laboratories that belonged to non-profit or academic institutions and that frequently had no well-defined quality-control systems. In many European countries national control authorities were poor, and liability was not clearly defined in law. The introduction of appropriate approaches to quality control, like GMP and good laboratory practice (GLP), also contributed to raising the levels of consistency and safety of viral vaccines. The implementation of new technological and regulatory approaches in viral vaccine preparation is still a problem in many laboratories in developing countries in which viral vaccines, such as rabies, are manufactured with outdated methodology and equipment.

It is important to call attention to the current situation in the European countries of the former Soviet bloc. This part of the world, with a population of approximately 350 million, uses vaccines that are mainly produced locally in numerous laboratories spread over a vast territory. With few exceptions, the vaccines are made in rudimentary conditions with outdated equipment, far-from-modern approaches to quality control and in the absence of qualified regulatory agencies. Furthermore, most of these countries cannot afford to import vaccines from producers in developed countries because of the shortage of foreign currency. In addition, if the laboratories making vaccines in East European countries suddenly stop their activities, the vaccination programmes will be compromised. Although the lag in the technology and philosophy of vaccine preparation is detrimental to the quality of the products, the existence of vaccine-manufacturing facilities supports qualified microbiologists in this part of Europe. This expertise should be maintained, because it could nevertheless be advantageous to public health microbiology, if suitably utilized. For all these reasons, assistance should be offered to the laboratories preparing viral vaccines in order to set up modern systems for quality control of viral vaccines. If this help is not available, production of viral vaccines will continue to pose a potentially large threat of clinical accidents.

V. Recently licensed vaccines

Only three new vaccines became available on the market and were licensed in the last decade: hepatitis B, varicella and hepatitis A vaccines.

At the end of the 1970s, the first anti-hepatitis B vaccine became available.[20] This vaccine was unique: since HBV cannot be cultivated *in vitro*, the starting material used for its preparation (HBs-Ag) was derived from the blood of patients that suffered from hepatitis B. Donors with large amounts of HBs-Ag in their blood, but negative for the marker of infectious virus, were selected. The HBs-Ag obtained from blood was highly purified and submitted to double inactivation procedures (formaldehyde and heat). The vaccine was produced in Europe, the Far East and the USA and was remarkably safe, despite the fact that its introduction into the market corresponded to the early period of the spread of AIDS and before HIV was identified. The rapid progress in the study of the

[20] Krugman, S., 'Hepatitis B vaccine', Plotkin and Mortimer (note 1), pp. 458–73.

molecular biology of HBV at the beginning of the 1980s opened the way for the development of a vaccine by rDNA technology. The biology of HBV replication is particularly appropriate for the development of a genetically engineered vaccine, since HBs is particulate: particles carrying the full human immunogen can be constructed which are non-infectious because they are free of nucleic acid. Thus the immunogen for the vaccine was prepared by cloning HBV genomic fragments containing the s-Ag gene and expressing them in yeast or animal cells; a biosynthetic HBs particle, physico-chemically identical to the natural 22 nm particle, was obtained.[21] Hepatitis B infection prophylaxis by an effective vaccine is an important landmark in the control of severe diseases representing major public health problems world-wide. For this reason, the inclusion of hepatitis B vaccine in the WHO Expanded Programme on Immunization (EPI) is now under consideration.

A live vaccine against varicella (Oka strain) has been extensively studied and tested, first in Japan,[22] and later in Europe and the USA. This vaccine is licensed in Japan and in several European countries, but there is debate about the category of children for whom this vaccine is beneficial. In Europe it was accepted for immunocompromised children, for example, those suffering from cancer or receiving steroids, but in Japan vaccination was extended to normal children. The remarkable fact in the development of the Oka vaccine strain of varicella zoster virus (VZV) was the classic approach used by the Japanese workers to obtain an attenuated varicella virus. The virus was isolated from a typical case of chickenpox and then passaged serially at 34°C, initially on human embryonic lung, then in guinea-pig embryonic fibroblast and finally on WI38 and MRC5 human diploid cells. The Oka strain seems to be a ts^- mutant that occurred during passages at low temperature and selected when virus was grown in guinea-pig embryonic cells. The varicella vaccine has the side-effects of rash and fever, but is generally well tolerated by normal children. The frequency of these side-effects is higher in leukaemic children, and the occurrence of zoster is correlated mainly to a previous history of rash and fever.

The relative simplicity of the methodology used to isolate an attenuated varicella virus shows clearly that low-temperature viral mutants can be generally considered as attenuated, irrespective of whether the virus is a ribonucleic acid (RNA) or a DNA virus. As is discussed below, the efficacy of live attenuated vaccines depends mainly on the type of infection that the virus induces in humans and the characteristics of the immunological response.

In the 1970s it became evident that there are several forms of hepatitis induced by different viruses. They include a long incubation and frequently chronic disease induced by HBV, and a short incubation orally transmitted syndrome which spontaneously resolves that has been called hepatitis A (HAV). In 1979, the virus was isolated and propagated[23] in tissue culture of foetal rhesus kidney and hepatoma cells. It was identified as a picornavirus (i.e., a small single-stranded, RNA-positive virus). Some features of HAV facilitated and justified the development of a vaccine: the virus does not present antigenic variation; there is no post-infection chronic hepatitis; and antibodies induced in humans

[21] Ellis, R. W., 'Recombinant-derived hepatitis B vaccine', Woodrow and Levine (note 1), pp. 439–47.
[22] Takahashi, M., 'Varicella vaccine', Plotkin and Mortimer (note 1), pp. 526–48.
[23] Provost, P. J. and Hilleman, M. R., 'Propagation of human hepatitis virus in cell culture *in vitro*', *Proceedings of the Society for Experimental Biology and Medicine*, vol. 160 (1978), pp. 213–21.

and infected animals by minute amounts of virus are able to neutralize viral infectivity. The vaccine currently available on the market is a formaldehyde-inactivated vaccine, but work continues to develop a live, attenuated vaccine.[24] Vaccination against hepatitis A is not compulsory, but vaccination is justified in some geographical areas where the disease is endemic, or for immunocompromised individuals who risk severe clinical forms of the disease. It has to be remembered that HAV can provoke a fulminating clinical form of hepatitis estimated between 0.04 per cent and 0.4 per cent.

In concluding this chapter it must be noted that among new, licensed vaccines, only that for hepatitis B has been made using a new rDNA technology, whereas the two other vaccines were developed by the classical approach of viral inactivation or the selection of viral attenuated *ts*$^-$ mutants. Again, HBV has particular features allowing the application of rDNA technology for obtaining a vaccine. Conversely, it is also true that without genetic engineering methodology it was not possible to develop a vaccine for a virus that cannot be grown *in vitro* in a sensitive cell-culture system.

VI. Making vaccines by new technology

The remarkable potential of molecular biology technology has created new challenges for all fields of biomedical research and hence also opened the way to novel approaches to the development of new vaccines. In the 1980s, many enthusiastic attempts to apply the technical achievements of molecular biology to vaccinology resulted in failure. This was especially true for existing vaccines, because the new approaches to subunit vaccines were unable to offer vaccines of better design, and thus a higher immunogenicity, than classical vaccines containing the whole virus. This was, for instance, the case with antigens obtained by producing synthetic peptides or anti-idiotypic antibodies.[25] The replacement of existing live or killed viral vaccines by new ones cannot be excluded, but will undoubtedly be preceded by long and careful studies to demonstrate their superiority. The decision by public health authorities to replace existing vaccines in mass vaccination campaigns with new products will require abundant and consistent laboratory and clinical data.

Despite current disappointment about vaccines obtained by non-conventional methods, it is reasonable to assume that in the future live attenuated vaccines will be developed by constructing viruses carrying defined mutations or gene modifications which control a stable attenuated phenotype.[26] In recent years the genomes of several viruses, including adenovirus, herpes and polio, have been genetically modified by the deletion of particular genes without altering their viability.

For instance, a part of the genome of herpes simplex virus type 1 controlling neurovirulence and the thymidine kinase was deleted. The genes coding for the glycoproteins of type 2 virus and thymidine kinase (the enzyme responsible for sensitivity to acyclovir[27]) were then inserted in the region of internal inverted

[24] Deinhardt, F. and Hilleman, M., 'Hepatitis A vaccine', Plotkin and Mortimer (note 1), pp. 549–57.
[25] Murphy, B. R. and Chanock, R. M., 'Immunization against viruses', eds B. N. Fields *et al.*, *Virology*, 2nd edn, vol. 1 (Raven Press: New York, 1990), pp. 469–502.
[26] See note 25.
[27] See Langen, chapter 15, in this volume.

repeat.[28] The resulting mutant showed a stable attenuated phenotype and is a promising candidate for a live anti-herpes vaccine.

A new era in vaccinology opened with the possibility of altering the genomes of large DNA viruses by inserting heterologous genes. Live recombinant viruses can thus be constructed which act as vectors for other genes.[29] In this new approach the most widely used virus is vaccinia[30] since it allows the insertion of large fragments of foreign genomes. A segment of the viral genome, non-essential to viral replication, is cloned in a plasmid, and a gene encoding an immunogenic protein of another pathogen is introduced into this non-essential gene. The plasmid carrying the recombinant vaccinia gene is then introduced into cells in culture together with a wild vaccinia virus. The progeny of this infection will contain recombinant vaccinia virus capable of expressing the foreign protein. The potential use of this powerful technology in vaccinology is fascinating, and all the more so because of its simplicity. Moreover, the eradication of smallpox by vaccination with vaccinia virus demonstrated indirectly the practical value of vaccines using vaccinia vectors. Recombinant vaccinia viruses have been prepared to express many viral immunogens, including those from hepatitis B, HIV and respiratory syncytial virus. In the near future, vaccinia recombinant virus will undoubtedly be a valuable tool in veterinary medicine, since several different immunogens derived from animal pathogens can be carried by a single recombinant viral particle.

VII. Desirable viral vaccines

A number of viral infections are diseases having a particular geographical distribution. This category includes infections caused by dengue, Japanese encephalitis, Lassa and tick-borne encephalitis viruses. Active immunization against diseases induced by these viruses is limited to those individuals exposed to risk of infection. For some of these diseases, killed vaccines are available, while vaccines are in development for dengue, haemorrhagic fever and Lassa virus. The manufacture of killed vaccines for these diseases poses serious problems of safety, because it requires handling large amounts of virulent virus. Therefore the development of live attenuated vaccines able to protect individuals against these severe diseases would be valuable.

Licensed vaccines cover a family of major human diseases that have some common traits. For instance, the mechanism of their transmission involves contact with free virus and, in practically all cases, there is a viremic phase of infection. For this reason the neutralizing antibodies can play an important role in immunity, and their presence in the blood can prevent the occurrence of the clinical disease. Therefore the efficacy of these vaccines is based mainly on stimulating the B lymphocyte system and in some cases also cytotoxic T cells.

There are other diseases of importance to public health for which vaccines are not yet available. For instance, a rotavirus live vaccine protecting children against viral diarrhoea is in development, but in other cases the nature of viral

[28] Whitley, R. J. and Meignier, B., 'Vaccines against herpes simplex infections', Woodrow and Levine (note 1), pp. 825–54.

[29] Flexner, C. and Moss, B., 'Vaccinia as a live vector carrying cloned foreign genes', Woodrow and Levine (note 1), pp. 189–206.

[30] See note 29.

infection of humans is such that vaccination may be ineffective. This is the case with AIDS which is by far a priority.[31] The obstacles to developing a vaccine against AIDS have recently been reviewed,[32] and the difficulty resides essentially in the extraordinary attributes of HIV. Briefly, HIV is transmitted by free virus but also by infected cells which escape attack by neutralizing antibodies. The cDNA transcript of the viral RNA genome is integrated into the host cell genome, and it is practically impossible to excise it from the integration site. The virus is also sequestered in the central nervous system (CNS) where it is inaccessible to the immunological defence system. There is a remarkable natural antigenic variation of the glycoprotein gp120, and finally, the propagation of the disease induces gradual destruction of the immunological system of the host. Despite the fact that efforts continue to be made to find a vaccine, the majority of scientists are sceptical about the possibility of developing an efficient vaccine against AIDS in the near future. Sooner or later the solution will be found—if a solution exists—based on the biology of HIV and the continuing investigations of HIV infection of humans.

Vaccines are also needed for other infections like hepatitis C, which is caused by a virus only recently characterized by molecular biology and which is an important public health problem.[33] For hepatitis C, the key would be a recombinant virus carrying an immunogenic viral protein. However, such a protein remains to be identified and characterized.

[31] Tacket, C. O., 'An overview of approaches to vaccination against AIDS', Woodrow and Levine (note 1), pp. 741–53.

[32] Hilleman, M. R., 'Impediments, imponderables and alternatives in the attempt to develop an effective vaccine against AIDS', *Vaccine*, vol. 10 (1992), pp. 1053–58.

[33] Plagemann, P. G. W. 'Hepatitis C virus: brief review', *Archives of Virology*, vol. 120 (1991), pp. 165–80.

10. Human viral vaccines

NIZAR AJJAN, PIERRE SALIOU and LOUIS VALETTE

I. Introduction

The introduction of vaccines against a variety of different viral diseases has led to some of the major advances in modern medicine, for instance, the world-wide eradication of smallpox with no cases reported in the past 15 years. Poliomyelitis has also become a rare disease in developed countries, and many childhood diseases such as measles, mumps and rubella are now much less prevalent in the industrialized countries but are still world-wide the cause of over two million deaths a year.

Antiviral vaccination was first recorded scientifically by Edward Jenner in England in 1796.[1] One hundred years later, Louis Pasteur administered the first rabies vaccine to Joseph Meister, thus putting vaccination on a sound footing.[2]

The years between 1892 and 1927 saw the development of several bacterial vaccines, and as early as 1932 attempts were made to develop antiviral vaccines. A vaccine against yellow fever was studied but was rapidly abandoned owing to major central nervous system reactions. Eventually, a yellow fever vaccine based on the 17D Rockefeller strain was developed and proved to be effective and only very slightly reactogenic. This vaccine is now heat stable and like many others may be stored at +4°C.

Several vaccines were developed but were later found to be ineffective, for instance, an influenza vaccine developed by Jonas Salk[3] and a mumps vaccine developed by John F. Enders.[4] They have since been abandoned. The true era of viral vaccines began in 1949 with the development by John Franklin Enders of tissue-culturing techniques for growing viruses.[5] This discovery made possible the cultivation of viruses on a large scale and the production of either live or inactivated viral vaccines.

There are currently nine viral diseases for which vaccines are available and commonly or routinely used: hepatitis A, hepatitis B, influenza, measles, mumps, poliomyelitis, rabies, rubella and yellow fever. In some countries where the incidence of diseases is high, vaccines are also used against dengue, Japanese B encephalitis and tick-borne encephalitis. In addition, vaccines are available against cytomegalovirus and varicella but are only used in specialized circumstances. Several other vaccines are in the experimental or developmental

[1] Jenner, E., *Inquiry into the Causes and Effects of the Variolae Vaccina* (Bibliothèque Britannique: Geneva, 1798), pp. 258–399.

[2] Pasteur, L., 'Méthode pour prévenir la rage après morsure', *Comptes Rendus, Academie des Sciences*, vol. 101 (1885), pp. 765–74.

[3] Salk, J., 'Reactions to concentrated influenza vaccines', *Journal of Immunology*, vol. 58 (1948), pp. 369–95.

[4] Enders, J. F., 'Techniques of laboratory diagnosis tests for susceptibility and experiments on specific prophylaxis', *Journal of Pediatrics*, vol. 29 (1946), pp. 129–42.

[5] Enders, J. F., Weller, T. H. and Robbins, F. C., 'Cultivation of the Lansing strain of poliomyelitis virus in cultures of various human embryonic tissues', *Science*, vol. 109 (1949), pp. 85–87.

stage; these include vaccines against various herpes virus diseases, rotavirus and respiratory syncytial virus.[6]

II. Measles vaccine

Measles remains a serious public health problem in many parts of the world, especially in developing countries. It is estimated that 67 million cases of measles occur every year in the developing world, causing over 2 million deaths. Complications, including blindness, diarrhoea, ear infections, encephalitis and pneumonia, occur in approximately 30 per cent of all cases.

Several different strains of virus are presently available for the manufacture of vaccines.[7] The majority of them are derived from the Edmonston A or B strain which is cultivated in chick embryos. The most commonly used vaccine to date is the so-called Schwarz vaccine.

Measles vaccine is indicated for persons who are susceptible to measles, regardless of age, unless otherwise contraindicated. The vaccine should be given at 9 months of age for children in developing countries and between 12 and 15 months for those in industrialized countries. There is no necessity for a booster dose if the vaccine is given on or after the first birthday.

Vaccination with measles produces a mild, non-communicable infection, and antibodies develop in at least 95 per cent of children when vaccinated at the age of 15 months. Studies extending over 23 years indicate that the titres of vaccine-induced antibodies are lower than those following natural disease but still confer protection which appears to be durable.

Contraindications to the use of measles vaccine are pregnancy, because of the theoretical risk of infecting the foetus, and children who have a febrile illness.

The United States vaccination programme has resulted in a marked decline in the cases of measles. Before the vaccination programme came into effect approximately half a million cases were seen every year in the United States. This has now declined to about 10 000 cases annually.

III. Rubella vaccine

The primary goal of vaccination against rubella is to prevent the disease occurring during pregnancy with consequent danger to the unborn child.

The currently available live rubella virus vaccine contains the RA 27/3 strain of rubella virus grown in human diploid cells.[8] Following vaccination, a protective level of antibodies is seen in more than 98 per cent of cases. The available data indicate that one dose confers long-term, probably lifelong, immunity. The vaccine is administered by subcutaneous or intramuscular injection either alone or in combination with mumps and measles vaccines.

[6] Additional information is presented in: Ajjan, N., *La Vaccination* (Institut Mérieux: Lyon, 1986); Grant, J., *La Situation des enfants dans le monde* (UNICEF: New York, 1992); Lerner, R. A., Chanok, R. M. and Brown, F., *Vaccine 85* (Cold Spring Harbor Laboratory: Cold Spring Harbor, N.Y., 1985); Plotkin, S. A. and Mortimer, E. A., *Vaccines* (W. B. Saunders: Philadelphia, 1988); Talwar, G. P., *Progress in Vaccinology* (Springer-Verlag: Berlin, 1989); Woodrow, G. C. and Levine, M. M., *New Generation Vaccines* (Marcel Dekker: New York, 1990).

[7] Enders, J. F., Katz, S. L., Milovanovic, M. V. and Halloway, A., 'Studies on an attenuated measles-virus vaccine I', *New England Journal of Medicine*, vol. 263 (1960), pp. 153–59.

[8] Plotkin, S. A., Farquhar, J. D., Katz, M. and Buser, F., 'Attenuation of AR 27/3 rubella virus in WI 38 human diploid cells', *American Journal of Diseases of Children*, vol. 118 (1969), pp. 178–85.

Women of child-bearing age should only be vaccinated if there is no risk of becoming pregnant during the following two months. The vaccination should not be given during pregnancy, to patients with immunodeficient disorders or to patients who have recently been given preparations of immunoglobulins.

The US vaccination programme has resulted in a marked decline in reported rubella cases with a 99 per cent decrease from 1969 in the reported rates of congenital rubella syndrome (CRS). In 1985, two children were born with CRS in the United States. However, no cases have since been reported.

IV. Mumps vaccine

Approximately 30 per cent of susceptible individuals exposed to mumps never develop clinical disease but only an asymptomatic infection which is followed by lasting immunity. Mumps is usually regarded as a relatively mild disease characterized only by swelling of the salivary glands. However, orchitis does occur in about 20 per cent of patients who become infected after puberty, and deafness and meningo-encephalitis are common complications of the disease.

Two vaccines are available, one based on the Jerryl Lynn strain and the other on the Urabe strain.[9] Both vaccines are produced in chick embryo cell cultures. Experience with these two vaccines shows that they are both immunogenic and induce protective immunity in at least 95 per cent of recipients.

Local and systemic reactions are rare, the most common being fever in 5–15 per cent of cases and parotitis in approximately 1 of 1000 cases. Rare instances of sterile aseptic meningitis have also been recorded with the Urabe strain.

Mumps vaccine should be given routinely to children after the age of 12 months and is usually combined with rubella and measles vaccines. The contraindications to giving mumps vaccine are the same as those noted above for measles vaccine.

V. Poliomyelitis vaccine

Poliomyelitis is the cause of serious public health and socio-economic problems, particularly in developing countries, because of the permanent disabilities that the disease causes. The disease has been virtually eradicated from the developed countries of the world, and even from the developing countries of the Americas, by extensive use of either inactivated or live attenuated vaccines. In contrast, in many developing countries the disease remains a major cause of mortality and permanent disability.

Reports of the disease are mostly based on the subsequent observation of lameness which is one of the long-term effects of poliomyelitis infection. This, however, represents only 15 per cent of the actual cases of the disease which are estimated at approximately 220 000 new cases per year. Reports by the WHO from 118 countries in 1981–84 show persistently high prevalence of poliomyelitis in those countries where vaccine coverage remains low. Reported cases dropped from 52 000 to 36 000 in 1983, and then to 24 000 cases in 1984.

[9] Buynak, E. B. and Hilleman, M. R., 'Live attenuated mumps virus vaccine', *Proceedings of the Society for Experimental Biology and Medicine*, vol. 123 (1966), pp. 768–75.

Surveys show that the disease generally affects children under the age of five or six years. Following this, cases of poliomyelitis are extremely rare, and almost all children possess antibodies for one or several types of the poliovirus. The incidence of the paralytic form of the disease varies from country to country and shows an annual incidence ranging from 5 to 50 cases per 100 000 individuals.

Two types of trivalent vaccine are available: the oral polio vaccine (OPV) and the inactivated polio vaccine (IPV) which is given by injection.[10]

The choice between the live and the killed vaccine has frequently led to fierce debate and continues to do so. Live polio vaccine has been used extensively in the USA which has led to massive reduction in the occurrence of the disease. However, IPVs have been used in the Scandinavian countries, and both vaccines have been employed in France and other European countries. This practice has led to the almost total eradication of poliomyelitis in these regions.

The WHO Expanded Programme on Immunization (EPI) recommends the use of OPV at birth and then at the ages of 10 and 14 weeks. In all, a total of 14 doses of OPV may have to be used in order to confer lasting immunity.

The use of OPV has recently been called into question for two reasons.

1. Neurological complications following vaccination have been seen in the industrialized countries which have been evaluated at a rate of 1 case per 8 million doses as compared to 1 case in 5 million doses among household and community contacts. Between 1973 and 1984, 138 cases of paralytic poliomyelitis were reported; 105 of these cases (76 per cent) were vaccine associated, 35 cases occurred in vaccinees, 50 cases in contacts of OPV recipients and 14 cases in immune deficient individuals. (No serious side-effects have been reported from the currently available IPV.)
2. It is ineffective from a serological and epidemiological point of view.

Several factors seem to be responsible for the relative failure of OPV:

1. The first is the presence of maternal antibodies during the first month of life. According to various surveys, older infants respond better to vaccination than do the very young.
2. Another factor is breast-feeding since colostrum contains large quantities of poliomyelitis antibodies.
3. A third reason is the possible interference by intercurrent intestinal enterovirus infections, making the use of oral vaccines relatively ineffective.
4. Finally, the relative heat stability of the vaccine is such that in many tropical countries failure may be caused by improper storage of the oral vaccine, with subsequent inactivation by heat. In recent years, however, the heat stability of the vaccine has been considerably improved.

The inactivated polio vaccine can now be produced in vero cell cultures and the development of microcarrier techniques has also contributed to its mass production.

[10] Sabin, A. B., 'Oral poliovirus vaccine: history of its development and use and current challenge to eliminate poliomyelitis from the world', *Journal of Infectious Diseases*, vol. 151 (1985), pp. 1151–55; Salk, J. and Salk, D., 'Control of influenza and poliomyelitis with killed virus vaccine', *Science*, vol. 195 (1977), pp. 834–47.

Clinical studies of poliomyelitis vaccine produced in vero cells were begun in France in 1982. Since then, several world-wide investigations have dealt with this vaccine, administered separately or in combination with diphtheria, pertussis and tetanus (DPT) vaccine, in comparison to the oral vaccine. Comparative trials between IPV and OPV show the superiority of IPV, following two injections, compared to OPV, after three or more doses.

VI. Influenza vaccine

Influenza is a serious public health problem, and the annual epidemics lead to large numbers of infections with consequent public health socio-economic problems and also, particularly in high-risk groups, very large numbers of deaths.[11] The high-risk groups for influenza are the very young, the very old and those with chronic conditions such as upper respiratory diseases, cardiovascular diseases, renal diseases and immunodeficiency diseases.

The problem associated with influenza is the extreme variability of the virus which requires a new vaccine to be produced and administered almost every year. Influenza vaccine is an inactivated virus containing representatives of the three main virus strains: two type A and one type B, which need to be altered almost every year because of virus variability.

Influenza vaccine should be given every year before the flu season begins. Unfortunately, the world-wide coverage even in high-risk groups is unsatisfactory.

VII. Hepatitis vaccine

Viral hepatitis is a major cause of public health problems in all parts of the world.[12] Several different types of infections are recognized as being caused by different viral agents: hepatitis A, hepatitis B, hepatitis C, delta hepatitis and hepatitis E. No vaccine exists for the last three of these, but vaccines against hepatitis A and hepatitis B are in widespread use.

Hepatitis B virus (HBV) is a major cause of acute hepatitis and in a proportion of cases, probably around 10 per cent, leads to chronic disease. A late manifestation of chronic hepatitis may be either cirrhosis or in rare cases, again approximately 10 per cent, the development of hepatocellular carcinoma. Persistent infection is common, and it is estimated there are approximately 200 million carriers of the virus world-wide.

Infection can be transmitted from a mother to her child both prenatally and perinatally with a very high incidence of infection. It is thus necessary to immunize children born of a mother carrying or infected with HBV. Immunization should also be considered for people in certain countries where the prevalence of hepatitis B infection is high. In these areas, 10–20 per cent of the population may be carriers, and primary liver cancer is common. These are predominantly tropical areas and unindustrialized countries.

[11] Kilbourne, E. D., *Influenza* (Plenum: New York, 1987).

[12] Kurstak, E., *Viral Hepatitis* (Springer-Verlag: New York, Vienna, 1993); Maupas, P., Goudeau, A. and Coursaget, P., 'Immunization against hepatitis B in man', *The Lancet*, vol. 1 (1976), pp. 1367–70; Zuckerman, A. J., *Viral Hepatitis and Liver Disease* (Alan R. Liss: New York, 1988).

Since 1980 two plasma-derived hepatitis B vaccines have been available, and since 1986 vaccines have been produced by recombinant DNA technology in Chinese hamster ovary cells and in yeast.[13] There has been some concern about the transmission of other viral diseases using plasma-derived vaccines so that these recombinant vaccines now offer a safe and practical alternative.

Hepatitis B vaccine is recommended as pre-exposure prophylaxis for persons at high risk. These individuals include: health care workers, patients on hemodialysis for chronic renal disease, homosexuals, prostitutes, recipients of certain blood products, household members and sexual contacts of hepatitis B carriers, and international travellers going to areas of HBV endemicity. Vaccination is also recommended for individuals who have been exposed following a needle stick, for instance, or children born to mothers carrying the virus, in combination with hepatitis B immunoglobulin.

Some countries, such as Italy, now recommend universal vaccination of infants with hepatitis B vaccine, and the vaccine can be combined with other immunizations as is being done in some areas in the WHO EPI.

Hepatitis A is a viral disease transmitted either directly by sexual contact or as a result of faecal contamination of food and is extremely common in some areas of the world, particularly tropical areas. It causes serious morbidity but very little mortality or long-term effects.

Hepatitis A vaccination is recommended for individuals travelling to endemic areas and for those at high risk for other reasons. The vaccine is highly effective, conferring protective immunity in more than 90 per cent of individuals following one injection. Side-effects have been extremely rare.

VIII. Rabies vaccine

Rabies occurs world-wide. In some areas, such as the UK and the USA, because of intensive control programmes, the disease is rare, whereas in other areas such as India, Thailand, Turkey and Asia in general, it continues to be common. Rabies is commonly transmitted to man by domestic or wild animals, the most common source of infection being dogs, followed by cats, farm animals and wild animals such as foxes, squirrels, and the like. The occurrence of the disease in man can be reduced by either pre- or post-exposure vaccination.

The evolution of the vaccine from its original source in animal organs to cell cultures has now led to the ability to produce a glycoprotein vaccine as a result of recombinant DNA technology.[14] This vaccine is now extremely immunogenic and very safe and can be used before exposure to the infection.

In general, before this improvement in technology occurred, rabies vaccine was used as post-exposure treatment in contrast to all other vaccines in production. There are currently four main rabies vaccines in use: one produced in suckling mouse brains, another produced in duck embryos, a third produced in goat, sheep and rabbit brains (the Semple-Fermi vaccine), and finally the cell-

[13] See note 12.

[14] Wiktor, T. J., Sokol, F., Kuwert, E. and Koprowski, H., 'Immunogenicity of concentrated and purified rabies vaccine of tissue culture origin', *Proceedings of the Society for Experimental Biology and Medicine*, vol. 131 (1969), pp. 799–805; Plotkin, S. A., 'Rabies vaccine prepared in human cell cultures: progress and perspectives', *Reviews of Infectious Diseases*, vol. 2 (1980), pp. 433–47.

culture rabies vaccines made in human diploid cells (HDCV), in purified vero cells (PVRV) and in purified chick embryo cells (PCEC).

IX. Haemorrhagic fever vaccines

Various haemorrhagic fever viruses, which are dual-threat agents, produce similar severe clinical diseases with different aetiologies and epidemiological characteristics in different parts of the world.

Vaccines against a number of mosquito- and tick-borne flaviviruses, causing diseases such as Japanese encephalitis, tick-borne encephalitis and yellow fever, are widely used in several regions of the world where these diseases constitute a major public health problem.

Yellow fever

Vaccine for yellow fever can give lasting protection of at least 10 years, and probably lifelong, after one injection.[15] Immunization against yellow fever is recommended in several areas in the world and is highly recommended for travellers going to these areas. The vaccine is a live attenuated vaccine which is now much more stable than it used to be owing to improved technology.

Japanese encephalitis

Japanese encephalitis is a serious public health problem in South-East Asia. A vaccine containing inactivated vaccine has been available since 1973 and is now produced in infected mouse brains and subsequently purified. Inoculation with this vaccine confers protection in at least 80 per cent of individuals. A live vaccine is now under production in Chinese hamster ovary cells.

X. Herpes virus vaccines

The DNA herpes virus group includes herpes simplex virus (HSV), types I and II, cytomegalovirus, varicella zoster virus and Epstein-Barr virus.

Herpes simplex

Very little progress has been made in controlling herpes infections. No anti-HSV vaccine is currently available. Research is directed towards the development of such a vaccine by genetic engineering. The main problem (and this is true for other herpes viruses as well) is to produce a vaccine which is completely free of the potential for ocogenicity and which is capable of eliminating the persistence of latent virus.

[15] Durieux, C., 'Preparation of yellow fever vaccine at the Institut Pasteur Dakar', *Yellow Fever Vaccination*, WHO Monograph no. 30 (WHO Monograph Services: Geneva, 1956).

Cytomegalovirus

A live attenuated vaccine developed by Stanley A. Plotkin using the Towne strain cultivated in human diploid cells is available for use in individuals in special high-risk groups.[16] This vaccine has shown 95 to 100 per cent seroconversion without major side-effects and is used for the protection of individuals undergoing organ transplantation, who are at very high risk of subsequent development of cytomegalovirus infection with serious consequences.

Varicella

Varicella or chickenpox, which is usually a benign disease, becomes extremely severe or fatal in immunosuppressed individuals or the elderly, in whom the disease may manifest itself as herpes zoster.

In 1974, Michiaki Takahashi *et al.* published the first experiments showing immunization against varicella using a live vaccine prepared from the Oka strain of virus grown in human diploid cells.[17] The results of extensive clinical trials using the Oka strain of live varicella vaccine in Japan over the past 10 years, and more recently in Europe and the United States, show that children with malignant disease can be safely immunized and effectively protected providing that the following conditions are observed:

1. The children should be in remission from the malignant disease.
2. Cell-mediated immunity should be normal.
3. Chemotherapy for the malignant disease should be suspended for a week before and a week after immunization.

The vaccine has been shown to be safe and immunogenic in both normal and immunocompromised children with seroconversion seen in 95–100 per cent. Following vaccination, fever and a slight transient rash were observed in 1 per cent of the normal children and in 16 per cent of leukaemic children. The varicella-like illness was very mild with minimum symptoms.

It has been reported that post-immunization immunity lasts for 2–5 years and may be boosted by silent subclinical infection. A booster dose is indicated for children suffering from malignant disease.

The main question concerning varicella immunization is whether or not it is truly indicated, particularly in normal children. At present, this is not seen as advisable. Vaccination is recommended for children with malignancies or with the immunodeficiency syndrome, for normal seronegative adults in contact with at-risk children and for health care workers.

Epstein-Barr virus

The Epstein-Barr virus is the cause of Burkitt's lymphoma, infectious mononucleosis and nasopharyngeal carcinoma and is possibly involved in the aetiology of Hodgkin's disease and B-cell lymphomas seen in immunocompromised hosts such as those suffering from HIV infection.

[16] Plotkin, S. A., Friedman, H. M., Fleisher, G. R. and Dafoe, D. C., 'Towne vaccine induced prevention of cytomegalovirus disease after renal transplants', *The Lancet*, vol. 1 (1984), pp. 528–30.

[17] Takahashi, M., Otsuka, T., Okumo, Y. and Asano, Y., 'Live vaccine used to prevent the spread of varicella in children in hospitals', *The Lancet*, vol. 2 (1974), pp. 1288–90.

The search for an effective vaccine against this virus has continued for almost 20 years and is currently nearing success with at least one putative vaccine due to go into early clinical trials in the near future.

XI. Rotavirus vaccine

In developing countries, rotavirus infection is probably responsible for approximately 6 per cent of all diarrhoeal disease and 20 per cent of all deaths related to diarrhoeal disease in children under five years of age. The goal of immunization against rotavirus will be to vaccinate all children, particularly in developing countries, as soon as possible after birth and certainly before six months of age.

A live attenuated bovine rotavirus vaccine has been shown in several trials to induce cross-protection against human rotavirus infection.[18] Eighty-four per cent of previously seronegative children have shown antibody responses when the vaccine is administered between 6 and 12 months of age, but only 35–50 per cent in new-born infants following administration of a single oral dose.

XII. Discussion

There are several aspects of the production of viral vaccines which need to be considered. The first is the difficulty of industrial-scale production both from the point of view of ensuring safety and economy, major concerns of manufacturers of biological products. How, for instance, can each person at risk in every country of the world economically be supplied with the necessary vaccines? Owing to safety concerns, the use of primary animal cells is no longer advised. Only cell lines in culture are used, and the production of systems such as vero cells has allowed industrial-scale production of viruses against poliomyelitis and rabies.

One fermenter with a capacity of 1000 litres has the same surface as 300 000 culture bottles. On this scale, the cost of production becomes acceptable for a general immunization programme.

The same industrial and economic considerations apply to the freeze-drying process. Apparatus is now available to freeze-dry in a single stage 300 000 vials of measles vaccine. Modern technology using isolation and high-security laboratory techniques has also allowed environmental and product security with protection both for the product and the environment.

XIII. Conclusion

The basic requirements for effective immunization of large populations worldwide against infectious diseases which formerly caused serious public health and socio-economic problems are in place. When the science of vaccination began in the 18th and 19th centuries, vaccination was a hazardous procedure. It has now become a safe and effective way of protecting the world's population.

[18] Maldonado, Y., Hestvik, L., Wilson, M. and Townsend, T., 'Safety and immunogenicity of bovine rotavirus vaccine RIT 4237 in 3-month-old infants', *Journal of Pediatrics*, vol. 109 (1986), pp. 931–35.

11. Viral vaccine research, development and production in the former Soviet Union: a brief review of the situation

SERGEY G. DROZDOV

I. Introduction

The vaccines routinely used for the prevention of viral diseases on the territory of the former Soviet Union include: rabies (inactivated), tick-borne encephalitis (TBE, inactivated), poliomyelitis (live, Sabin), influenza (both live and inactivated), measles (live, L-16) and yellow fever (live, attenuated). Several other vaccines have been developed almost to the stage at which they could be used; these are hepatitis A (inactivated), Japanese encephalitis (inactivated) and mumps (live, attenuated). Two more vaccines have been under development for a long time: hepatitis B and live, attenuated TBE encephalitis vaccine.

The facilities and scientific centres for the development, improvement and production of vaccines are mostly located in Russia. Thus the Institute of Poliomyelitis and Viral Encephalitides in Moscow covers poliomyelitis, TBE, rabies and yellow fever vaccines. The Institute of Vaccines and Sera, Tomsk, works with TBE. The Institute of Vaccines and Sera, Ufa, works with rabies. The Institute of Viral Preparations, Moscow, covers measles vaccine. In St Petersburg the Institute of Influenza, Institute of Vaccines and Sera and the Institute of Experimental Medicine handle influenza and measles vaccines. Several facilities belonging to 'Microbioprom' have been working on influenza vaccines. Outside Russia, in Ukraine, the Odessa Plant for Bacteriological Preparations and the Kharkov Plant for Medical Preparations produce rabies vaccine.

Most of these institutes and factories combine scientific and production facilities, uniting scientists and producers in the field of viral vaccine development. The needs for and trends in viral vaccine development are well illustrated by the situation regarding some traditional and newly developed vaccines at the Institute of Poliomyelitis and Viral Encephalitides.

II. Poliovirus vaccine

Although the attenuated Sabin strains have proved to be an efficient and safe source for oral poliomyelitis vaccines, they nevertheless have definite drawbacks. Among these are inter-strain interference, which dictates the need for multiple vaccinations in order to achieve immunity to all three serotypes, and a tendency for the strains to revert to virulence, which could, at least in part, be responsible for cases of vaccine-associated paralytic disease. This last property is mainly associated with type 3, and for years attempts have been made to find a substitute strain with more stable characteristics.

One of the ways to solve this problem was pursued by Dr V. Agol and his group at the Institute of Poliomyelitis and Viral Encephalitides in Moscow. They describe as their goal the designing of three poliovirus strains (types 1, 2 and 3) whose genomes would share most segments except the antigen (serotype) specific, capsid protein coding regions. Non-reversion to neurovirulence could probably be achieved either by accumulating as many known attenuation mutations as possible in the shared portion of the genome, or by the creation of new attenuating mutations which do not show reversion. The specific aim of the study is to define such irreversible attenuating mutations and to design a common module for their introduction into each of the three Sabin strains in order to improve their stability and diminish mutual interference. It is known that the level of poliovirus neurovirulence is controlled, in part, by a specific locus of the untranslated region (5-UTR) of the genome. Therefore a large collection of mutant polioviruses of serotype 1, selected or constructed in Dr Agol's laboratory, and having significant alterations within this region, is the main subject of the study. The assay will be done partly in monkeys but mostly in mice, using transgenic mice susceptible to poliovirus, or by engineering viruses having, in addition to the 5-UTR mutation, a determinant in the VP1 capsid protein conferring on the virus the ability to infect mice. The structure of the appropriate region of the genome of viruses isolated from the brain of the infected mice will be investigated to evaluate the stability of the mutations. Depending on the results of these studies, new mutations will be introduced into the viral genome by site-directed mutagenesis.

Eventually genomic module(s) will be selected having an optimal combination of attenuation and genetic stability. The strains containing these modules will be candidate vaccine strains. In this way an improved live poliovirus vaccine could be constructed that would be thermostable and non-cross-interfering.

III. Tick-borne encephalitis vaccine

The first preparation of TBE vaccine was developed in the former USSR by A. Smorodintsev, N. Kagan and E. Levkovitch (1939) using white mouse brain containing a high concentration of virus inactivated by formaldehyde.

In 1963–64 this preparation was replaced by an inactivated chick embryo cell culture vaccine developed at the Institute of Poliomyelitis and Viral Encephalitides by M. Chumakov and co-workers. However, the protective activity of this vaccine was relatively low. In 1974 at the same institute, L. Elbert, V. Grachev and co-workers set out to purify and concentrate this preparation. The concentration technology based on ultra-centrifugation was patented in 1977 just before an analogous method developed by Immuno of Austria.

In 1978–79 studies were begun on a new technology based on ultra-filtration and chromatography. Virus grown in cell culture and inactivated by formaldehyde is concentrated by ultra-filtration (using Pellicon or 'nucleo-filters') followed by purification on chromatography columns with a special type of macroporous glass. This technology allowed reliable production of relatively inexpensive and antigenically highly active vaccine.

In 1988–89 the consensus reached on the use of viral vaccines produced in heteroploid continuous cell lines in humans opened up new possibilities for improving and standardizing the inactivated TBE vaccine. For this purpose, the Institute of Poliomyelitis and Viral Encephalitides carried out studies with cell line 4647, a Vero-like continuous cell line originated at the institute from adult green monkey kidneys by L. Mironova and co-workers. Virus grown in this continuous cell line was treated by the ultra-centrifugation and chromatographic purification technology to produce the vaccine. Special procedures were needed to separate the raw material from cellular DNA.

During recent years M. Chumakov and co-workers have developed an even newer technology based on the transformation of acute infection of tissue culture cells into subchronic form, permitting collection of several lots of virus suspension from the same lot of tissue culture.

However, there is an alternative approach to TBE vaccine. Since the mid-1960s in the former USSR the scientific and practical bases have been laid for the use of live, attenuated TBE virus for vaccine production. In brief, TP-21 Langat virus, a virus belonging to the same serological subgroup as TBE, was first studied for this purpose by A. Smnorodintsev and V. Ilyenko. Then the naturally attenuated Elantsev strain of TBE, isolated from a human in western Siberia, was studied as a candidate vaccine strain by A. Dubov and colleagues, with the permission of the Ministry of Health. In the course of those studies it was found that one in 10 000 vaccinated persons developed the clinical disease, so the studies were stopped.

Recently I. Kamalov (Institute Pasteur, St Petersburg) has been studying attenuated variants of Langat TP-21 virus in order to select candidate vaccine strains. This programme has been adopted in principle by the Russian Committee on Sanitary-Epidemiological Surveillance.

IV. Hepatitis vaccines

Inactivated whole-virus vaccine

Hepatitis A is a world-wide disease. Regions with a stable high level of morbidity have been shown to exist in many countries, including in certain parts of the former USSR where the annual incidence rate reaches from 400 to 600 cases per 100 000 people.

From studies of the epidemiology and pathogenesis of hepatitis A virus, it has been concluded that an adequate vaccine can protect susceptible individuals against infection and effectively control the spread of the disease at a population level. Between 1986 and 1991 M. Balayan and co-workers at the Institute of Poliomyelitis and Viral Encephalitides developed an inactivated whole-virion hepatitis vaccine produced in tissue culture. This vaccine was produced on a semi-industrial (laboratory) scale as follows. Hepatitis A virus was grown in 4647 cells, licensed for the production of inactivated vaccines for human use. Mature virus particles were harvested from both cells and supernatant, and purified by column chromatography on porous silica beads. After inactivation with 1 : 3000 formaldehyde, aluminium hydroxide was added as an adjuvant and the vaccine was ampouled and stored.

Procedures for safety testing, following international requirements, have been developed. These include tests for hepatitis A virus identity, for residual substrate protein and DNA, sterility (for bacteria, viruses and mycoplasma) and an immunogenicity assay in laboratory animals. Protective potency is assayed in susceptible tamarin monkeys. This assay is essential at the development stage, but can be omitted from the large-scale manufacturing process.

Experimental lots of the vaccine have been tested in human volunteers. It was found to be adequately immunogenic and well tolerated by the vaccinees. The virus has now been licensed by the National Control Authorities for large-scale production, and the production technology, seed viruses and cell banks have been transmitted to a commercial manufacturer.

Genetically engineered vaccine

M. Balayan and co-workers, who developed the inactivated vaccine described above, have collaborated with E. Sverdlov (Institute of Bio-organic Chemistry) and O. Andjaparidze and V. Chernos (Institute of Viral Preparations) in studying recombinant and synthetic hepatitis A viral proteins capable of inducing protection against the infection. A preparation consisting of recombinant vaccinia and hepatitis A viral genes has been produced carrying full-length viral RNA which can be expressed in a permissive cell system (primate primary or continuous cell lines) in the form of hepatitis-A-like particles lacking the RNA.

This recombinant vaccine has been administered intradermally to susceptible monkeys, and it produces an intense specific antibody response and solid protection to challenge inoculation with infectious virus. Various vaccination schedules have been tested in 16 monkeys, using recombinant vaccinia/hepatitis B vaccine as a control.

Hepatitis A vaccine was also prepared from the empty particles produced in cell cultures inoculated with the vaccinia/hepatitis A virus vector, and separated from vaccinia virions by rate/zonal centrifugation. The yield of hepatitis A virus in this system was significantly higher than that obtained after inoculation of the cells with virus alone, but the empty particles appear to be unstable. However, it is expected that their stability can be improved by the insertion of RNA fragments or defective (non-infectious) hepatitis A viral RNA.

V. Conclusion

The work described above shows that in the former USSR the group of traditional and recently developed institutions is still functional in the fields of viral vaccine research, development and production. A considerable number of highly qualified scientists and producers are involved; various scientific approaches to vaccine development and production are being used, and significant progress is being achieved in several directions. However, closer involvement of former Soviet scientists and producers in the international community is desirable to increase the possibility of contributing to current activities in protecting human beings from viral infectious diseases.

The Vaccines for Peace programme could receive considerable support and development by involving participants from Russia and the newly independent states in the field of viral vaccines. This would also help the programme towards its goal of utilizing the scientific potential of these states and assist in converting a group of scientists and science institutions from the military field to that of the protection of human beings.

12. The Scientific and Production Association Vector: the current situation

SERGEY V. NETESOV

I. Introduction

The Scientific and Production Association (Nauchno-Proizvodstvennoye Obyedinenie, NPO) Vector was created in 1986 by merging four institutions located near Novosibirsk, Siberia—the Institute of Molecular Biology (VNII MB) in Koltsovo; the Institute of Biologically Active Substances (NIKTI BAV) at Berdsk; the Experimental Production Plant (NOPB) in Koltsovo; and the Experimental Agricultural Production Enterprise (OPSP) in Morosovo, Iskitim District, about 25 km from Koltsovo.

The total value of the main production funds of NPO Vector exceeds 250 million roubles (1984 prices); the total building area is about 200 000 square metres, and the staff numbers 3000, including more than 120 PhD and DSc graduates.

The Institute of Molecular Biology and subsequently NPO Vector were organized for basic and applied research and development (R&D) and production of anti-viral vaccines, diagnostic kits and medicinal drugs for health care of the general public and the Soviet Army.

The head organization of NPO Vector is the Institute of Molecular Biology, which was founded in 1974 by a Special Decision of the Soviet Government. This decision was closely connected with the development of molecular biology and genetic engineering, both of which had been practically forbidden in the Soviet Union for a very long period. The decision opened the door to developing molecular biology research in many institutions of the former Soviet Union.

The main achievements of the Institute of Molecular Biology during the last 10 years have been in the sequencing of viral genomes, the identification of the determinants of antiviral immunity, the construction of recombinant vaccinia strains and the development and production of viral diagnostic kits (see tables 12.1–12.3). The recombinant hepatitis B vaccine was successfully tested in human volunteers in 1991, and field tests are now in progress.

II. Basic research

All basic research is performed at the Institute of Molecular Biology. The primary focus of the basic research carried out is shown in table 12.2.

The sequencing of the variola virus genome is conducted in the framework of a national programme which is co-ordinated with international programmes (such as the World Health Organization).

Table 12.1. Main achievements of the Institute of Molecular Biology

Nucleotide sequencing
Full sequencing of the following viral genomes:
Hepatitis A (a few strains)
Tick-borne encephalitis (TBE)
Marburg
Ebola
Foot-and-mouth disease (a few strains)
Eastern equine encephalitis
Venezuelan equine encephalomyelitis (VEE), (a few strains)
Influenza (a few strains)
HIV-1 (several isolates)
Variola (smallpox)
Construction of a full-length copy of the VEE virus genome and formation of infectious virus from this copy and investigation of the influence of the different substitutions in this copy on attenuation of this virus
Vaccines
Construction of recombinant vaccinia strains producing specific immune response against:
Hepatitis B
TBE
VEE
Pilot production being developed of vaccines for:
Measles
Hepatitis A
Diagnostic kits
Immunoenzyme assay (ELISA) kits for the following:
HBs antigen (hepatitis B)
Antibody to HBs antigen
HIV-1, HIV-2
Hepatitis A (virus specific IgM antibodies)
Delta hepatitis (total and IgM antibody)
TBE (total and IgM antibody)
Cytomegalovirus (total and IgM antibody) and many others

III. Applied research

The development and production of diagnostic test reagents and medicinal drugs at the Institute of Molecular Biology are shown in table 12.3.

The main focus of the work of the Institute of Biologically Active Substances has been on the development of the technology for obtaining and producing a wide range of enzymes, nucleic acids, gene-engineering and other reagents, antibiotics and interferon (see table 12.4).

The Institute of Molecular Biology and the Institute of Biologically Active Substances are active participants in the following Russian Government R&D programmes: the Human Genome Programme, the Gene and Cell Engineering Programme, the Protein Engineering Programme, the Viral Infections Programme, the Gene-directed Biologically Active Substances Programme and the State Programme on Combating AIDS.

The main activity of the Experimental Production Plant is manufacturing medical and veterinary preparations. These are listed in table 12.5.

Table 12.2. Basic research at the Institute of Molecular Biology

Viruses
Variability at the biological and molecular levels
Molecular epidemiology
Molecular basis of virulence and pathogenicity
Pathogenesis of infection and development of mathematical models of the infection process
Sequencing of the variola virus genome
The following viruses are being studied:
Eastern equine encephalitis
Venezuelan equine encephalomyelitis
Tick-borne encephalitis
Hepatitis A, B, C, E
HIV-1, HIV-2, vaccinia
Cytomegalovirus, measles, rubella, Marburg, Ebola, Machupo, Lassa and many others
Biologically active preparations
Compilation and development of data bases and software for designing and optimizing their application
Using computer simulation and gene- and cell-engineering methods to develop a methodological base for obtaining these substances
Human genome
Sequencing the human genome nucleotides

The Experimental Agricultural Production Enterprise provides NPO Vector employees with foodstuffs (meat, milk, butter, vegetables). It also grows medicinal herbs and breeds reindeer for antler production for medicinal use.

IV. Challenges and opportunities

Until mid-1990 publications by NPO Vector were severely restricted because of so-called 'state interests'; even the list of pathogens being studied was classified (a similar situation existed in the field of nuclear physics research). Of course, some research results would be classified in any country because of defence requirements or commercial interest, but there was no real need to restrict most of this work. The situation began to change in 1989. For a long period the former state structures were antagonistic, but in 1989 the first group of scientists to be officially introduced as employees of NPO Vector participated in the International Arbovirus Symposium in Moscow. After that the author and two colleagues attended the 8th International Congress of Virology in West Berlin in 1990, and since then there has been routine participation in international scientific conferences, including the 9th International Conference of Virology in Glasgow, Scotland in 1993, where 11 employees of NPO Vector participated by invitation and on scholarships from the Organizing Committee.

In 1990 NPO Vector received its first Western visitors, from Oxford Virology PLC and the Institute of Virology and Experimental Biology, both of Oxford, England. Since then NPO Vector has been visited by many Western scientists and businessmen, among them representatives from Merck, Sharpe and Dohme and Ortho Diagnostic Systems (USA), Mérieux (France) and Pharmacia LKB Pribori (Finland). Most of them were invited with the object of discussing the organization of joint ventures and contract research. However,

Table 12.3. Applied research at the Institute of Molecular Biology

Diagnostics

Immunoenzyme assays or nucleic acid hybridization techniques (including a gene amplification method) for the following viruses:

- Hepatitis A, B, C, E and delta
- Tick-borne encephalitis
- Cytomegalovirus
- Herpesvirus
- Measles
- Mumps
- HIV-1, HIV-2, HIV-1+2, HIV-1+HBs
- Marburg
- Ebola

Vaccines

Live, killed and gene-engineered vaccines against the following viruses:

- Measles
- Mumps
- Hepatitis A, B, C
- Tick-borne encephalitis
- Marburg
- Ebola
- Lassa
- Crimean-Congo haemorrhagic fever
- Haemorrhagic fever with renal syndrome
- Eastern equine encephalitis
- Venezuelan equine encephalomyelitis
- Japanese encephalitis
- Machupo

Veterinary vaccines against the following viruses:

- Infectious enteritis of mink
- Canine distemper
- Infectious rhinotracheitis (bovine)
- Parainfluenza type 3 (bovine)

Gamma-globulins

Pilot production for treatment and emergency prophylaxis against:

- Hepatitis B
- Tick-borne encephalitis
- Marburg
- Ebola
- Crimean-Congo haemorrhagic fever and others

Drugs and biologically active substances

Peptide drugs, using classical peptide chemistry methods, including:

- Desmopressin
- Lutamin
- Somatostatin
- Carcinil and others

Cytokines using gene- and cell-engineering methods:

- Recombinant human erythropoietin
- Plasminogen tissue activator and others

Drugs derived from plant and animal raw materials

Purification using home-made sorbents

Expert analytical methods to test and correct immune status

Schemes for prophylaxis and treatment of viral infections and different pathologies

Tailor-made synthesis of oligonucleotides up to 80 nucleotides in length

Table 12.4. The Institute of Biologically Active Substances

Enzymes and reagents
Restriction endonucleases (more than 60)
Nucleotide exchange enzymes
Nucleic acids and their components
Biotin-streptavidin system
DNA amplification, sequencing, labelling and cDNA cloning kits
Non-radioactive hybridization diagnostic kits
Medicinal preparations
Cytokines (TNF-alpha, interleukin-2 and others)
Cytokine analogues (alpha-2 interferon, gamma-interferon)[a]
Recombinant alpha-2 human antitrypsin
Profesim (cellulose-immoblized proteolytic enzyme prosubtilin from *B. subtilis*)—for treatment of purulent necrosis of varying aetiology
Polyribonate (natural immunostimulant from *Saccharomyces cerevisiae* yeast)
Ridostine (interferon inducer based on double-stranded RNA from killer strain of *Saccharomyces cerevisiae* yeast)

[a] more stable than the natural product

Table 12.5. The Experimental Production Plant

Medicinal preparations
Recombinant alpha-2 human interferon
Surfagon (for veterinary use)
Immunoenzyme diagnostic systems
HBs antigen (hepatitis B)
Hepatitis A IgM
HIV-1 antibodies (to individual proteins)
Syphilis and many others
Laboratory products
Nutrient media for cell and virus cultivation (more than 60 items)
Sera (bovine foetal, cattle, swine, sheep, pregnant sheep)

international business is not developing as fast as could be wished and as yet no joint venture agreement has been signed, in spite of the interest shown by Western companies in NPO Vector's facilities and especially in its scientists.

The financial situation in the research departments of NPO Vector is lamentable in the extreme. Currently, conditions are such that the well-qualified scientific staff cannot conduct productive research work because of the lack of funds to buy chemicals; the experimental facilities, which are unique in Russia, are in only partial use. In 1992 and 1993 no foreign scientific literature could be bought; no hard currency was available for the purchase of reagents and materials that are not produced in Russia or the CIS. Minimal financial support (the average salary for scientists does not exceed $60 per month and is often paid out after a substantial delay in time) is now available for only one-third of the scientific personnel, even after significant staff reduction and the implementation of other administrative measures directed at reducing expenditure. By 1993 more than 20 talented scientists had left for Western institutions. This is not all bad, as they are becoming well-known in those places. However, recently at least two groups of NPO Vector scientists have received invitations from certain countries for contract work with dangerous pathogens. In the current situation of financing science in Russia they cannot be prevented from going abroad, but it must be obvious that this situation is not in the interest of the civilized world.

The Vaccines for Peace initiative is very topical and urgent. Most of the staff of NPO Vector are ready to support VFP, and to participate in the development of the programme. Every effort will be made to arrange a broad exchange of specialists with special competence in the field of dangerous viral infections, and to put the NPO Vector laboratories to work on the programme.

NPO Vector is prepared to collaborate with any foreign institution or company in basic research, R&D and production in the prophylaxis and treatment of human and veterinary virus diseases. NPO Vector is fully open for collaboration in both the scientific and production fields, and invites all interested parties to make contact.

13. Vaccines against dual-threat agents: regulation and quality, issues and constraints

JACK MELLING

I. Introduction

In considering the feasibility and utility of establishing a facility for the development and production of vaccines against dual-threat agents, many factors must obviously be taken into account. Among such will be the selection of appropriate vaccines in relation to the magnitude of the disease problem and the state of scientific knowledge about the particular vaccines. This chapter attempts to set out issues and constraints to be considered with respect to the regulatory, quality and ethical aspects pertaining to such vaccine production.

Vaccines belong to the class of medicinal products called biologics (or biologicals). The common feature of this class of products, which includes hormones and therapeutic proteins, is that, unlike other pharmaceutical products, biological products cannot be adequately tested for quality, safety and efficacy by chemical tests alone. Indeed, UK medicines legislation[1] defines biological products as such in that:

1. They may either have no clearly chemically defined composition or because of their tertiary or quaternary structure, simple chemical analysis is insufficient for effective characterization.
2. The only way of qualitatively or quantitatively evaluating them usually is by measuring their effect *in vivo.*
3. Quality cannot be guaranteed from a final test on random samples, but only from a combination of in-process and end-product tests that monitor the entire manufacturing process.

One consequence of this characteristic is that *in vivo* assays are required. Another and more far reaching one is that because of the interrelationship between the method of production and the characteristics of the final product, stringent control on all aspects of the production process is required in order to ensure reproducibility of the end-product. This contrasts with many chemical drugs where methods of manufacture can vary to a fairly wide degree so long as the end-product meets certain specifications. For biological products on the other hand, the same degree of certainty of quality can only be achieved by a much stricter control of the production process. For biologicals the product is indeed defined by the production process.

Most countries control the quality of medicines, and this is achieved by two mechanisms. First, for the licensing of products which are permitted to be supplied, licences are granted, usually by some government body, for those products which the licensee can demonstrate meet certain standards of quality, safety and efficacy (see below). Second, for a product that has been so licensed, it is

[1] *UK Medicines Act 1968* (Her Majesty's Stationery Office: London, 1968).

essential that all subsequent batches of the product meet the standards required. Hence, and especially for biologicals, there is a need to control the manufacturing process, which usually involves licensing the site of manufacture and inspection thereof, again by government agencies.

Vaccines which have been developed and/or licensed for one target population (e.g., adults) would require further evaluation if they were to be used in a different target population (e.g., children). It is just such a variation which would typify the change from defence to civil use. Furthermore, if changes are needed to manufacturing processes to accommodate increased scale of production, particularly if associated with changes in technology, additional determinants of quality, safety and efficacy will be required.

This chapter outlines some of the current regulatory requirements which apply to product licensing and manufacture in order to assess the issues which will need to be considered in establishing a vaccine programme. Although most comments are drawn from experience of the British and US requirements, these are similar to those of most developed countries and are used by many more. Clearly there can be no suggestion that lower standards should be applied to vaccines for developing countries.

There is a clear need for effective controls on the quality of medicines, including vaccines, and their manufacture. This need is exemplified *inter alia* by the toxicological effects shown by thalidomide, by the increased neurovirulance of vaccine strains of poliomyelitis virus on subculture and the need to establish limits on this[2] and by the incident when BCG vaccine (Bacille dilié de Calmette-Guérin, tuberculosis vaccine) contaminated with *Mycobacterium tuberculosis* caused the deaths of 73 children.[3]

To administer a vaccine which is either unsafe or lacking in efficacy is worse than giving none at all. In the first case it may cause more harm than it purports to prevent and, in the second, money spent on a useless product could be better used elsewhere. Third, a dangerous false sense of security could be engendered. It will therefore be an essential criterion of any vaccine programme that it be based on proper standards of quality, safety and efficacy.

II. Product licensing issues

Few vaccines developed or manufactured with a view to BW defence use have been subjected to the full rigour of the product licensing system. Where this has been done it was usually because a civil use for the product had already been identified (e.g., anthrax vaccine). Those products which are not currently licensed will have to be treated as would any new product. The most important criteria which such products must meet involve: (*a*) safety tests, including toxicological assessment, initially in animals, but then in man; (*b*) determination of efficacy, again initially using animal models, followed by human studies; and (*c*) assessment of product quality, involving data on all aspects of production designed to ensure not only that the product is acceptable according to current scientific standards, but also that the standard of quality can be maintained and reproduced from batch to batch during the life of the product.

[2] Minor, P., 'Comparative biochemical studies of type 3 poliovirus', *Journal of Virology*, vol. 34 (1980), pp. 73–84.

[3] Ryan, F., *Tuberculosis: The Greatest Story Never Told* (Swift: Bromsgrove, UK, 1992) p. 379.

Safety

A number of elements are involved in ensuring the safety of vaccines. Seed lots of the particular organism must be established and subjected to careful scrutiny as to the identity and provenance of the organism. This is not only important for live attenuated vaccines, but also for killed or subunit vaccines to ensure the presence of appropriate antigens.

The various ingredients used in growth media and materials with which the product comes into contact during processing must be selected with a view to their potential toxicity. This is especially so where carry-over of minute and undetectable amounts into the final product could have adverse consequences. For example, since the recognition of bovine spongiform encephalopathy (BSE), materials of bovine origin, particularly from BSE endemic areas, are excluded unless treated to inactivate the BSE agent. This has required re-formulation of many culture media for both bacteria and viruses, as well as re-appraisal of seed stocks which may have been produced using bovine products. A further example is the need to eliminate the use of toxic chemicals at the processing stage and to set limits for carry-over of other materials and determine that such limits are well below any toxic levels. Materials originating from living organisms which may be used in the production or purification processes (e.g., animal sera and monoclonal antibodies) must either be demonstrably free from adventitious micro-organisms or it must be shown that the procedures used would eliminate the risk of such organisms being carried through into the final product.

Depending upon the type of vaccine—killed, subunit or live, attenuated—appropriate tests including animal studies are required to validate the inactivation process or ensure effective attenuation. In the case of inactivation of organisms or toxoiding of toxins, the kinetics of inactivation must be determined to ensure a sufficient margin of safety is built into the process. Because any change in formulation or conditions (e.g., pH, temperature, ionic strength) of inactivation can radically alter the kinetics, great care is needed to ensure reproducibility.

Once a production process has been established and animal safety data established, tests in man would be the next stage.

Phase I studies in healthy adult volunteers would be required to show absence of unacceptable side-effects before proceeding to Phase II studies, again with informed consent, in larger numbers of people in the target population for the vaccine. Normally only after acceptable Phase II studies for safety would larger Phase III trials for efficacy be undertaken; these studies would also contribute to the data on adverse reactions.

A vaccine developed for BW defence is likely to have been tested only in healthy adults and if the target population for civil use is different, further studies would be essential. Before carrying out such further studies, it would be essential to review existing data and ensure their relevance to the current product and to the production process. If such data are not available, or if process changes have occurred, then a complete repeat of animal and human safety tests could be required.

Efficacy

Once the necessary safety criteria have been established, efficacy of vaccines has to be established usually in Phase III clinical trials. The number of people to be included and their age, sex and geographical distribution depend on the disease involved and its prevalence in particular populations. Such trials may take a number of years effectively to determine the value of a vaccine.

In the case of some potential BW agents, the natural (low) prevalence of the disease is such that no conclusive field trial of efficacy could be carried out.

Where any human experimentation is involved, voluntary, competent, informed and understanding consent is absolutely essential. This was one of the principles set out in the Nuremberg Code by the US judges in 1947.[4] A further requirement is that no experiment should be conducted where there is an a priori reason to believe that death or disabling injury will occur as a result.

Thus the efficacy of some vaccines cannot be determined in man because, even if consent could be obtained, it would be unethical and unacceptable to perform challenge tests, and in the case of some diseases field studies could not yield the necessary data on protection. Should any country have such data, they are unlikely to be made available since that would involve admitting the violation of human rights.

Human efficacy data are normally required for licensure. In the absence of this, for the reasons described above, a number of vaccines may not be licensable according to the usual criteria. This presents problems for production for civil use of defence vaccines. It would also be a major impediment to any international supply of vaccines for defence; although countries may have special procedures to license such vaccines, these would be harder to apply to non-indigenous products. It is worth noting that a number of such vaccines developed in the USA remain subject to restrictions as Investigational New Drugs and require the completion of detailed consent forms by recipients.

Where the precise mode of action of an agent is known and data are available on immunological protection (e.g., botulinum toxin) which allows effective prediction of the level of protection by determining amounts of antibody (IgG), there is a strong case to support licensing on the basis that no human *in vivo* challenge is needed to confirm the efficacy. In contrast, where more complex immune mechanisms are involved, such as pertain to other bacterial, viral or rickettsial infections, simple prediction without Phase III trials is not likely to be acceptable in the present state of our knowledge of immunity.

Quality

As mentioned above, the detail of the production process is a vital aspect in specifying a product. Thus in determining if a product should be licensed all aspects of the manufacturing process need to be considered to assess their impact on product quality and reproducibility.

[4] *Trials of War Criminals before the Nuremberg Military Tribunals, Tribunal 1, Case 1, The Military Case: United States of America v Karl Brandt et al.*, vol. 2 (US Government Printing Office: Washington, DC, 1950); Annas, G. J. and Grodin, M. A. (eds), *The Nazi Doctors and the Nuremberg Code: Human Rights in Human Experimentation* (Oxford University Press: Oxford, 1992), pp. 61–129, 188–208.

If vaccines are to be produced using recombinant DNA techniques and other new biotechnological methods, additional requirements may apply.

Biotechnology is not a new phenomenon; people have been making beer and wine for thousands of years and selective breeding of animals and plants is a form of genetic engineering that has also been going on for centuries. In recent years, particularly in the areas of recombinant DNA technology, fermentation and down-stream processing, biotechnology has become very much more sophisticated and has had an enormous impact on the development of antibiotics, hormones, vitamins and, to date at least, two human vaccines. Without biotechnological methods many therapeutic and prophylactic materials could not have been supplied in the quantities required, or could not have been produced economically (e.g., human insulin, human factor VIII, human growth hormone, human interferons, hepatitis A vaccine, hepatitis B vaccine and erythropoietin).

The rapid development of biotechnological processes, in particular those involving recombinant DNA, hybridomas and mammalian cell line technologies, has served to heighten some concerns in that: (*a*) products from genes expressed in foreign hosts may differ structurally, biologically or immunologically from their natural counterparts; (*b*) foreign genetic material might find its way into the end-product, thus adversely affecting man, animals or the environment; and (*c*) scale-up and unintended variation in culture during production may cause changes that favour expression of other host/vector genes, alter the product significantly, decrease yields of product or increase yields of impurities.

It has to be said that so far no such products made by any of these technologies have proved to be any more hazardous than those produced by more 'conventional' means. Nevertheless, the concerns are valid and to this end a number of additional analytical methodologies have been, or may be, brought into play as in-process and end-product tests to address: (*a*) identity, purity, specificity, stability and efficacy of the product; (*b*) characterization of source (seed) materials; and (*c*) validation of process procedures.

These procedures complement the more 'traditional' in-process and end-product safety and quality control tests, most of which remain as valid for the new methodologies as for the old. It is also apposite to qualify the word 'new' relating to these analytical methodologies—many are techniques that have been used for decades in specialized research applications, but have now been translated to production-associated activities consequent upon: (*a*) the advent and/or development of analytical equipment to perform the tests economically, and (*b*) the greatly increased purity of many of the products of modern biotechnological processes.

Seed source

Depending on the nature of the organism, bacterial, viral, eukaryotic or recombinant, a number of tests need to be applied to confirm the origin, purity or genotype. For eukaryotic cells used to grow viruses characterization would involve isoenzyme analysis, DNA fingerprinting and cytogenetics. In the case of recombinant organisms full details of the construct need to be confirmed involving preparation of the DNA segments, genes involved, origin of replication, fusion product (if present), characterization of the flanking regions, characterization of the promoter, enhancer and terminator regions and presence of antibiotic-resistance genes.

The DNA must be analysed by sequence analysis and restriction endonuclease digestion mapping and compared with the original gene sequence.

Master and submaster host/vector cell seed stocks will also require a similar range of tests to be applied, but in addition it is essential to monitor: (*a*) the physical state of the vector in the cell; (*b*) plasmid stability during storage, recovery and use; and (*c*) fidelity of the nucleotide sequence encoding the expression product, the copy number and effect of passage on that copy number.

Fermentation

The culture or fermentation process must also be specified in terms of medium composition, physical parameters, final yield and limits on contaminating organisms. Equine proteins and human blood components cannot be used in culture media and the Code of Federal Regulations (CFR) requires disclosure of sources of animal-derived products used in preparing products to be administered to humans.[5] Plasmid stability may be affected by a number of factors and is a potential problem in large-scale fermentations. It can be monitored by simple screening for antibiotic resistance markers, but this does not give any indication of copy number loss.

Purification or processing

Precise details are required of the further processing after the culture stage. These will include the identity and specifications of any added reagents and any materials with which the vaccine comes in contact, including, for example, chromatographic column matrices. Assays will be required and limits established in respect of potential carry-over of materials into the final product. Details of elution profiles from chromatographic columns, gel electrophoresis or other tests to determine purity of product are required. Other tests for potency and sterility may need to be specified at particular stages in the production process.

Various methods may need to be used to assess the identity and purity of the product, be it of 'natural' or 'recombinant' origin. In the latter instance there are very specific problems that can occur, viz—proteolytic clipping of N- or C-terminus sites, incorrect glycosylation, incorrect disulphide bond formation, amino acid substitution, oxidation, deamidation, incorrect folding after solubilization and aggregation.

The analytical methods employed to detect such deviations include: electrophoretic techniques, amino acid composition, sequence analysis, peptide mapping, nuclear magnetic resonance, circular dichroism and mass spectrometry.

Product finishing

A licensed product would have specified the nature of the finished product (e.g., lyophilized or liquid fill) which would include details of the formulation, the container, storage conditions and shelf life. Tests on the final product would

[5] Cox, C. B. and Hardegree, M. C., 'Diptheria and tetanus toxoids: results of assays for the presence of bovine antigens', *Journal of Biological Standardization*, vol. 4 (1976), pp. 81–89.

cover potency, identity, sterility (or freedom from adventitious agents), innocuity and limits on, for example, aluminium and formaldehyde.

III. Manufacture

The product licence, as has been described above, sets out in great detail the characteristics of the vaccine, the method of manufacture, the in-process controls and tests on the final product to ensure that the required standards can be met. Once a product licence has been granted, it is then necessary to ensure that during the months and years when the product may be made, the quality will be maintained.

The system by which this is achieved involves the application of good manufacturing practice (GMP) by the manufacturer.[6] The maintenance of GMP is reinforced by inspection and licensing of manufacturing plants by regulatory authorities.

GMP is based on the principle that quality cannot be 'tested in' at the end of a process and thus total quality assurance is an integral part of each stage of the manufacturing procedure. To achieve and maintain GMP involves every aspect of a production facility including buildings, equipment, personnel, raw materials and process documentation.

GMP is expensive to establish, costly to maintain and requires a discipline and rigorous adherence to written protocols which is anathema to most research scientists. Accordingly, to convert an R&D organization to a manufacturing site involves major expenditure, as well as retraining and replacement of staff. There is no place for the unbounded creativity of research workers in operating to GMP standards. A few examples will serve to emphasize the nature of GMP requirements.

Buildings

Buildings are usually purpose-built to ensure that clean air of specific quality in relation to particle counts can be supplied to the various manufacturing areas. The building layout should be such as to ensure a progression from raw materials to finished product without backtracking or cross-over. The aim is to avoid contamination of the final product with lower quality starting materials.

In many cases buildings are dedicated to production of a single product. Although production on a campaign basis is feasible, there are strict requirements for clean-up and decontamination between operations.

In the case of spore-bearing organisms the US Food and Drug Administration (FDA) operates to the CFR which specifically prohibits the use of facilities (buildings and equipment) with a non-spore-bearer if these have previously been used with spore-bearers.[7]

[6] *Guide to Good Pharmaceutical Manufacturing Practice* (Her Majesty's Stationery Office: London, 1983); *The Rules Governing Medicinal Products in the European Community*, vol. 4, *Guide to Good Manufacturing Practice for Medicinal Products* (Office for Official Publications of the European Communities: Luxembourg, 1992).

[7] United States of America Code of Federal Regulations, 21 CFR, 600.11(e) (3). 4.1.85 edn (Office of the Federal Register National Archives and Records Administration: Washington, DC, 1985).

Equipment

The key element concerning equipment is validation. This means that on a regular basis all equipment must be checked to ensure that it operates according to specification. This is especially so for autoclaves, incubators, hot air ovens and freeze-dryers, but extends to many other items. The checking is often at two levels, for example, daily checks on refrigerator temperatures and more thorough, but less frequent, checks to ensure that temperature distribution throughout the apparatus with a designated set of contents is within specified limits.

Personnel

Selection and training of personnel is a key element in GMP. Training is especially important and staff are involved in regular training in all aspects of GMP operations. Each person has to take responsibility for product quality to achieve total quality assurance and must not rely solely on others to ensure this.

Documentation

Every aspect of the production process is the subject of a standard operating procedure (SOP) which covers activities such as operating a piece of equipment (even a magnetic stirrer), weighing out ingredients, putting on protective clothing and carrying out validation checks. In many cases (e.g., making up culture media or buffer solutions), the SOP will be accompanied by a check sheet on which the operator (or sometimes two—one to check the other) will confirm that a particular activity has been carried out correctly according to the SOP.

From the examples given, it can be seen that establishing and maintaining GMP is a costly and time-consuming process. It requires a working culture involving attention to detail and self-criticism and which is reinforced by statutory controls and penalties for transgression.

IV. Conclusions

It is clear that much, if not all, of the published data on the safety and efficacy of vaccines developed against potential BW agents and which do not already have a civil use are restricted to healthy adult volunteers.

The creation of an effective R&D and production programme covering a number of agents would be a major task. It would have to comply with the high standards imposed on vaccine manufacturers generally and would require significant facilities for field testing in view of the agents involved and their geographical distribution. The vaccines would not be cheap to produce and in view of the target populations, continued financial support of a high order would be needed to procure the vaccines and to mount effective immunization campaigns.

Among the dual-threat agents which have been listed by various authors, a number of vaccines already exist that are in general civil use (including yellow fever, hepatitis A, Japanese encephalitis, tick-borne encephalitis). These are subject to the normal patent cover and/or commercial proprietary information.

It is questionable whether it would be justified to attempt, at not inconsiderable expense, to re-create these in a Vaccines for Peace programme when they are already available.

Where vaccines are already manufactured for civil use it is difficult to support any proposal that public funding, even on an international basis, should be used to duplicate such products. Vaccines derived from defence programmes and which have a potential civil use could be developed and produced providing a market existed and the operation could be commercially viable. In contrast, those vaccines which are essentially militarily oriented would, especially on an international basis, have to overcome the difficulties in meeting current regulatory requirements described above. Furthermore, to establish such an international programme would require the co-operation of many countries in technology transfer as well as financial support to a degree that is unlikely to be forthcoming. Any one vaccine is likely to cost many millions of dollars to reach the point of regulatory approval.

Part IV. Public health and biological defence

14. Vaccines for biological defence: defence considerations*

GRAHAM S. PEARSON

I. Introduction

The Persian Gulf conflict of 1990–91 has emphasized the importance of providing effective protective measures including the use of vaccines against the threat that chemical or biological weapons may be used against the armed forces of the United Kingdom. As the three key elements of such protective measures are detection, protection and medical countermeasures, it is timely to consider the role of vaccines in protecting the lives of those who may be exposed to an attack in which biological warfare agents are used so that they can maintain their operational effectiveness.

Consideration is given in this chapter to why biological defence is important, the types of protective measures are considered and then the requirements for medical countermeasures are explored. Criteria for effective vaccines are elaborated together with an appreciation of the objectives of such vaccination. Finally, the pros and cons of internationally available vaccines are considered. It is concluded that vaccines are an essential part of the range of protective measures needed to protect troops from biological weapon (BW) attack and that care needs to be taken that such vaccines are not available to potential aggressors. A defence that is freely available to a potential aggressor to examine and evaluate is no defence.

Finally, the ways in which the 1972 Biological and Toxin Weapons Convention (the BWC) can be strengthened are considered and, in particular, how the developing countries can benefit from exchange of information for peaceful purposes. The International Biological Monitoring Agency (IBMA) proposed by Marcovich in 1990[1] has the laudable aim of hastening and increasing the contribution of biology to peace, health and prosperity in the world. The contribution of Vaccines for Peace (VFP) proposed by Geissler[2] could be considered in the context of the Marcovich IBMA if VFP concentrated on countering endemic disease while leaving the IBMA to focus on preventing biological products being used for prohibited military purposes.

In this chapter, biological warfare agents are regarded as being pathogenic micro-organisms such as bacteria, rickettsia, viruses and fungi. Toxins, which are frequently regarded as a subset of biological warfare agents because they are naturally produced by bacteria and plants and are therefore included in the BWC, are non-living chemicals and now that the Chemical Weapons Conven-

[1] Marcovich, H., 'Proposal for an international biological monitoring agency', ed. E. Geissler, *Strengthening the Biological Weapons Convention by Confidence-Building Measures*, SIPRI Chemical & Biological Warfare Studies, no. 10 (Oxford University Press: Oxford, 1990), pp. 198–201.

[2] Geissler, E., 'Vaccines for Peace: an international program of development and use of vaccines against dual-threat agents', *Politics and the Life Sciences*, vol. 11, no. 2 (Aug. 1992), pp. 231–43.

tion (CWC) has been agreed ought to be regarded as also falling under the CWC. In this chapter, where the situation for toxins is different from that of the living micro-organisms, this will be indicated.

II. Why is biological defence important?

Biological weapons have been the subject of discussion and limited use through the ages. There is little evidence that biological weapons have been utilized in conflicts during the 20th century, particularly for the living biological agents, although it is more ambiguous when the toxins are taken into account as there have been allegations that tricothecene mycotoxins were used in South-East Asia.

It is important to remember that during this century many countries have considered the acquisition of BW capabilities. These countries included the United Kingdom in the 1940s and early 1950s, Canada, France, the former Soviet Union and the United States. The US programme which ended in 1969 resulted in the weaponization and type classification of a number of biological warfare agents and delivery systems. Although not used in war, there appears to be little doubt that such weapons systems have been demonstrated by all means short of actual use in modern conflict, and indeed, they have been demonstrated to a greater extent than nuclear weapons were before their first use at Hiroshima or Nagasaki.

The signing in 1972 of the BWC prohibited the development, production and possession of biological weapons. That Convention was hailed as the elimination of biological weapons. However, it has become clear that interests in biological weapons have continued. A particular example is the anthrax outbreak at Sverdlovsk (Ekaterinburg) on which additional information is increasingly becoming available as Russia becomes more open in its publication of what happened.[3] Finally, the Persian Gulf conflict of 1990–91 when Iraq was assessed to have a BW capability and the subsequent United Nations Special Commission inspections led to Iraq disclosing that it was indeed working on anthrax, botulinum toxin and perfringens toxins. The British Defence White Papers of 1991 and 1992[4] stated that some 10 states either have or are seeking a BW capability.

It is therefore clear that there is a potential threat from biological weapons. As authors such as Steve Fetter in *International Security* of summer 1991[5] have pointed out, the agreement by the Conference on Disarmament in Geneva in summer 1992 of the CWC, may result in biological weapons becoming the

[3] See, for example, Gumbell, P., 'The anthrax mystery', *Wall Street Journal*, 21 Oct. 1991. See also Zilinskas, R. A., 'Anthrax in Sverdlovsk: epidemic or BW?', *Bulletin of the Atomic Scientists*, vol. 39, no. 6 (1983), pp. 24–27; Meselson, M., 'The Biological Weapons Convention and the Sverdlovsk anthrax outbreak of 1979', *F.A.S. Public Interest Report*, vol. 41, no. 7 (Sep. 1988), pp. 1–6; see also Abramova, F. A., Grinberg, L. M., Yampolskaya, O. V. and Walker, D. H., 'Pathology of inhalational anthrax in 42 cases from the Sverdlovsk outbreak of 1979', *Proceedings of the National Academy of Sciences*, USA, vol. 90 (Mar. 1993), pp. 2291–94; Meselson, M., 'New evidence on the 1979 Soviet anthrax epidemic', *ASA Newsletter*, 93-2, no. 35 (8 Apr. 1993), pp. 1, 5.

[4] British Ministry of Defence, *Statement on the Defence Estimates 1991*, Cm 1559 (Her Majesty's Stationery Office: London, July 1991); *Statement on the Defence Estimates 1992*, Cm 1981 (Her Majesty's Stationery Office: London, July 1992).

[5] Fetter, S., 'Ballistic missiles and weapons of mass destruction: what is the threat? What should be done?', *International Security*, vol. 16, no. 1 (1991), p. 5.

Table 14.1. Comparison of conventional, chemical, biological and nuclear warheads[a]

Type of warhead	Number of dead	Number of injured
Conventional (1 tonne of HE)	5	13
Chemical (300 kg of GB)	200–3000	200–3000
Biological (30 kg of anthrax)	20 000–80 000	. .
Nuclear (20 kiloton yield)	40 000	40 000

. . = Data not available or not applicable

[a] Missile with 1 tonne warhead against large city with average population density of 30 unprotected civilians per hectare

Source: Fetter, S., 'Ballistic missiles and weapons of mass destruction: what is the threat? What should be done?', *International Security*, vol. 16, no. 1 (1991), p. 5.

agents of choice. He has also pointed out, as indeed did the UN Secretary-General in his publication of 1969,[6] biological weapons are strategic in nature and small quantities can attack large areas (see table 14.1) and because of their nature, they are easier to hide than nuclear or chemical weapon (CW) capabilities. Coupled with this, is the appreciation that delivery systems need not necessarily be complex or sophisticated.

Biological defence is therefore required to ensure that members of the armed forces can survive BW attacks and maintain their operational effectiveness. In addition, the maintenance of effective biological defence reduces the utility of biological warfare to a potential aggressor as it both reduces the range of materials that he may use and increases the uncertainties as to whether his use of biological weapons will be effective.

However, that is not to say that biological defence programmes should stand apart from the BWC. Everything possible must be done to strengthen the BWC by encouraging all States Parties to respond to the politically binding confidence-building measures (CBMs) agreed at the Third Review Conference in September 1991[7] to declare their programmes as required by those measures and to support the ongoing discussions about verification measures.[8] The future compliance monitoring regime[9] for Iraq is one designed to prevent and to deter Iraq from seeking to maintain or develop in the future a capability for biological warfare. There is a window of opportunity that should be used to do as much as possible to encourage states that have biological weapons or are

[6] United Nations, *Chemical and Bacteriological (Biological) Weapons and the Effects of their Possible Use*, Report of the Secretary-General, A/7575/Rev.1, S/9292/Rev.1 (United Nations: New York, 1969).

[7] United Nations, *Final Document of the Third Review Conference of the Parties to the Convention on the Prohibition of the Development, Production and Stockpiling of Bacteriological (Biological) and Toxin Weapons and on their Destruction*, BWC/CONF.III/22/Add.1, 27 Sep. 1991 (United Nations: Geneva, 1992).

[8] United Nations, 'Summary of the work of the *Ad Hoc* Group for the period 30 March to 10 April 1992', BWC/CONF.III/VEREX/2, 13 Apr. 1992. See also Tóth, Geissler and Stock, chapter 7, in this volume.

[9] United Nations, *Plan for Future Ongoing Monitoring and Verification of Iraq's Compliance with Relevant Parts of Section C of Security Council Resolution 687 (1991)*, Report of the Secretary-General, Security Council S/22871/Rev.1, 20 Oct. 1991 (United Nations: New York, 1991).

considering acquisition of biological weapons to judge that such acquisitions would be detected and would be politically unacceptable.[10]

III. Elements of biological defence

While the current situation continues, and into the foreseeable future, it is vitally important that States Parties maintain effective protective measures for their armed forces against the potential threat that biological weapons may be used against them. Indeed, provision of effective protective measures contributes to the web of deterrence made up of: (*a*) effective protective measures, (*b*) intrusive CW and BW arms control, (*c*) broad CW and BW export monitoring and control, and (*d*) a political commitment to react vigorously with a range of national and international response measures to violations of the BWC. The web should convince a potential aggressor that acquisition of a biological warfare capability is more of a liability than an asset. There are several key elements of an effective biological defence capability; they are discussed below.

An ability to evaluate the potential hazard

It is vital to be able to assess what challenge levels are likely to result in the event of a BW attack so that sensitivity criteria can be determined for detectors and protection factors for protective equipment and for medical countermeasures. In general, challenge levels in biological warfare attacks will be considerably greater than those that occur in natural outbreaks of disease. In addition, the main route of attack is through the respiratory system. Although biological warfare agents can be used to contaminate food and water supplies, or through infected fleas and other insects, such delivery systems are less suitable for military use. Such hazard evaluation capabilities are also necessary to assess the areas likely to be at risk in the event of any attack. Such a hazard evaluation capability is the essential forerunner to the provision of an effective portfolio of protective measures.

Detection and identification

The primary requirement of detection and identification is to detect a hazardous concentration of biological agent before a harmful concentration is inhaled by the target personnel so that warning can be given. Identification is of secondary importance but is required both for the prediction of downwind hazard areas and for the identification and deployment of the appropriate medical countermeasures. Identification may form an adjunct to a detection scheme as there is a valid argument for a detection scheme consisting of multiple technologies each with its own sensitivity and specificity.

Physical protection

Once a hazardous cloud has been detected, it is necessary to don appropriate physical protection consisting of a respirator and, depending on the information

[10] Pearson, G. S., 'Preventing biological warfare', *New Scientist*, 21 Mar. 1992, p. 8.

available, a protective suit or to enter collective protection facilities supplied with filtered air. The main route of BW attack of the human body by biological agents is through the respiratory system; respiratory protection is therefore the prime and essential requirement. Most biological agents have no effect against the intact skin and consequently full body protection may not be necessary especially if there is assessed to be no threat from chemical warfare agents such as mustard gas or the nerve agents which are effective through the skin as well as through inhalation. Once an alarm has been received of a biological attack, it will be necessary to wear respiratory protection until the hazard has decreased to a safe level.

Decontamination

Biological agents in general terms do not present a contamination problem. The most likely way in which such agents will be disseminated is through a line source which will be carried downwind. In broad terms, only about 1 per cent of the cloud will fall out onto the surface over which it is passing and the efficiency with which those particles which fall out on the surface may be reaerosolized is a further 1 per cent. Consequently, for there to be a reaerosolization hazard, the challenge level needs to be in excess of about 10 000 infective doses and this is unlikely to be the case except in the close proximity of the line source. There may, however, well be a problem in respect of public perception of residual contamination after a biological warfare attack. Since biological warfare agents are living micro-organisms, they are fragile in the environment and most will be killed through exposure to ultraviolet irradiation by sunlight and by ambient temperatures which promote biodegradation of the agents. Nevertheless, some would survive and there would be a few micro-organisms on the surface over which the attack cloud has passed even though these present no subsequent hazard to unprotected personnel. It would be important to mount a public information campaign to show that any residual living agent did not present a hazard. Such a campaign will need to emphasize that there are micro-organisms that occur in nature and are widely spread. For example, some micro-organisms pathogenic to man survive well in a natural environment (e.g., *Legionella* and *Listeria)*. These are opportunistic pathogens which frequent a man-made environmental niche such as cooling towers or silage and rarely cause disease although when such incidents occur there is considerable public reaction.

Medical countermeasures

Medical countermeasures fall into two broad areas, prophylactic and pre-treatment measures taken before exposure and therapeutic measures taken after exposure or after the development of signs and symptoms. Prophylactic pre-treatment measures generally require some advance knowledge of which agents are likely to be used, while therapy after exposure, and after symptoms develop, can be either generic or specific. These are considered in greater detail in the next section.

IV. Medical countermeasures

In contrast to chemical warfare agents, biological agents take time to infect the body and this enables additional approaches to be taken. These can be conveniently divided into three categories: (*a*) before exposure to the biological warfare agent, (*b*) after exposure and before development of symptoms, and (*c*) after development of symptoms.

Treatment before exposure

Vaccination can be used specifically to raise the level of antibodies in individuals within the target population prior to exposure to a biological warfare attack, and the immunity so generated can, depending on the challenge level, be effective in providing full or partial protection. Conventional vaccination requires weeks to months to develop full immunity. An alternative strategy is to administer passive antibody therapy which negates infection/intoxication prophylactically; these can be used immediately prior to or after an attack. In addition, antibiotics may be taken prophylactically against bacteriological warfare agents. Prolonged courses of antibiotics are not however advocated since they can result in antibiotic resistant strains of micro-organisms and may also produce adverse side effects. Vaccination is the preferred option.

Treatment after exposure and before development of symptoms

Antibiotic treatment may be the only option prior to the development of symptoms. In the case of toxins and viruses, the use of specific antisera is more appropriate. The effectiveness of a course of antibiotic treatments against a microbial disease may be augmented through a simultaneous course of immunizations so as to provide protection when the course of antibiotics ceases. It will be evident that identification of the biological warfare agent is essential to ensure optimum treatment prior to development of symptoms.

Treatment after development of symptoms

Treatment after development of symptoms is largely concerned with supportive therapy utilizing antibiotics, antivirals if appropriate, and specific antisera to toxins and viruses. The longer the interval between the attack and the start of treatment, the less successful treatment is likely to be.

V. The aim of biological defence

The aim of biological defence is to ensure that the armed forces can maintain their operational effectiveness despite being attacked by biological weapons. In other words, military personnel need to survive and to be able to use their weapon systems and platforms. Effective biological defence contributes to the web of deterrence which reduces the utility of biological warfare to a potential aggressor. However, as in all defence, a defence that is freely available to the potential aggressor to examine and evaluate is no defence as he will seek to and be able to circumvent that defence. The objective of an effective defence is to increase the uncertainty of the aggressor as to whether his biological warfare capability will be effective in achieving his military objective as well as to what response the use of BW will provoke. The goal is for the potential violator to judge that his acquisition of biological weapons would be militarily ineffective because of BW defence capabilities, prohibitively expensive because of export controls and arms control measures and liable to detection through verification or monitoring arrangements, and that the consequences would be politically unacceptable.

VI. The BWC

The States Parties to the BWC have undertaken never in any circumstances to develop, produce, stockpile or otherwise acquire or retain:

1. Microbial or other biological agents, or toxins whatever their origin or method of production, of types and in quantities that have no justification for prophylactic, protective or other peaceful purposes; [and]

2. Weapons, equipment or means of delivery designed to use such agents or toxins for hostile purposes or in armed conflict.[11]

These provisions have been incorporated into national legislation such as the Biological Weapons Act (1974) of the United Kingdom which makes it a criminal offence for any person within the UK to carry out work on offensive biological weapons.

Although the 1972 BWC had no requirements for declarations or provisions for verification, the Second Review Conference in 1986 saw the agreement of four politically binding CBMs which were subsequently strengthened in the 1991 Third Review Conference.[12] In addition, this conference mandated an *Ad Hoc* Group of Governmental Experts to consider possible verification measures from a scientific and technical viewpoint. The first meeting of this group took place in Geneva from 30 March to 10 April 1992 when a range of verification measures both off-site and on-site were identified,[13] and a second meeting took place on 23 November to 4 December 1992[14] to examine each measure to form the basis for evaluation at the next meeting held on 24 May to 4 June 1993.

Participation in the CBMs even though politically binding has been disappointing and much attention was given in the 1991 Third Review Conference to ways in which the developing countries could be encouraged to submit CBM returns and to participate. The response in 1992 was encouraging with 35 returns by September 1992 which compares well with responses from only 41 states over the four years since the Second Review Conference CBMs were agreed in 1987. Preparations for the 1991 Third Review Conference were assisted by the activities of non-governmental organizations (NGOs) such as the Federation of American Scientists (FAS) and the Stockholm International

[11] See the text of the BWC, annexe A, in this volume.
[12] United Nations (note 7).
[13] United Nations (note 8); see also Tóth, Geissler and Stock, chapter 7, in this volume.
[14] United Nations, 'Draft summary of the work of the *Ad Hoc* Group for the period 23 November to 4 December 1992', BWC/CONF.III/VEREX/CRP.25/Rev.2, 4 Dec. 1992.

Peace Research Institute (SIPRI) which produced useful papers and publications to stimulate national and international discussion.

One proposal put forward by Herbert Marcovich[15] was for the creation of an International Biological Monitoring Agency which would have the objective of striving to hasten and to increase the contribution of biology to peace, health and prosperity in the world. It would also ascertain that biological products were not utilized for prohibited military purposes and would consider the International Atomic Energy Agency as a model. This proposal would be costly but would facilitate the exchange of information for peaceful purposes. More recently, Erhard Geissler has developed the idea of Vaccines for Peace[16] as a further additional incentive for expanding participation in the BWC especially for developing countries. The proposed VFP programme would undertake research on and production of vaccines against pathogens that pose natural health threats and that also are putative biological weapons. VFP is intended to contribute to health care in developing countries, enhance international co-operation in biotechnology and reduce the danger of weapon proliferation. The programme would be administered by the World Health Organization. There would appear to be much benefit in considering Vaccines for Peace in the context of the proposed IBMA. Indeed, the work on verification measures for the BWC may lead to a requirement for an agency to implement whatever verification regime is agreed. The idea of an IBMA is thus timely and merits further consideration.

There is a range of potential benefits from some international monitoring regime ranging from standards for containment of pathogens, health and safety regulations, pollution standards, biosafety and genetic manipulation standards through to good laboratory and good manufacturing practice (GLP and GMP). These would be valuable for developing countries and would provide increased confidence that microbiological facilities were not being misused for prohibited purposes. This package of potential benefits could encourage developing countries to become States Parties of the BWC and implement the requirements of the CBM regime.

When considering how best the goal of increased international co-operation, collaboration and stability can be furthered it is important to consider whether the narrow focus on dual-threat agents is the most appropriate. This requires further consideration of the requirement of vaccines for biological defence and of to what extent the requirements for such vaccines are different from those required for protection against endemic diseases.

VII. Vaccines for biological defence

The objectives of vaccination in biological defence are to enhance the ability of the armed forces to survive and operate effectively should they be subject to a biological warfare attack and not have donned their respirators before inhaling a hazardous dosage. Vaccination of the armed forces will also be effective against contaminated food and water and other means of disseminating biological agents. In addition, the vaccination of the armed forces against the biological warfare agents that an aggressor is assessed to have will have the effect

[15] Marcovich (note 1).
[16] Geissler (note 2).

of reducing the utility of biological warfare to the aggressor. However, this reduced utility is dependent upon the aggressor being uncertain as to which agents the armed forces have been vaccinated against and just how effective that vaccine is against the challenge levels arising from his biological warfare attack. In addition, the vaccine used should not be freely available to the aggressor to examine and evaluate as this would facilitate the ability of the aggressor to defeat or circumvent the vaccine.

Evaluation of potential vaccines for use in biological defence requires consideration of a number of factors which are discussed below.

Effectiveness in providing protection against the likely challenge

In particular, the effectiveness of a vaccine against an aerosol challenge of the biological agent must be taken into account. Most public health vaccines are developed to provide protection against pathogenic organisms encountered through contact with body fluids or through ingestion rather than against pathogenic organisms in the respiratory system. There is a specific requirement that defence vaccines protect against aerosol challenge with agents at dose levels which are likely to be higher than those encountered naturally. In addition, defence vaccines should ideally provide effective long-term protection rapidly after a single immunization, and be compatible with other vaccines should there be a requirement to protect against a range of biological warfare agents. The development of recombinant vaccines based upon attenuated pathogens such as vaccinia and *Salmonella* mutants to produce simultaneous immunity against a range of biological warfare agents is a particularly exciting prospect for vaccines for biological defence.

Absence of side effects

The armed forces need to be able to maintain their operational effectiveness without this being impaired as a result of side effects associated with their being vaccinated or any undesirable interaction between vaccines simultaneously administered.

Degree of protection

The vaccine needs to be shown to provide an adequate degree of protection against the likely challenge levels to make vaccination worthwhile. The effectiveness of the vaccine will impact on the necessity of military personnel downwind from the attack having to don respiratory protection. The vaccination regime and the level of protection conferred need to be known so that the effectiveness of the vaccine can be judged and decisions taken as to whether to vaccinate the armed forces concerned.

Production, storage and issue

Vaccines require to be readily produced, stored and issued for immunization. Consideration of the advantages and disadvantages of attenuated live, killed or subunit vaccines and recombinant derivatives thereof need to be addressed to identify the most efficient way of ensuring that the armed forces are effectively protected.

Vaccines can either be licensed products or, in special circumstances, have an interim status such as the US IND (investigational new drug) status which can be given to personnel in an otherwise life-threatening situation. A licensed product is much the preferred option as it is a proven and approved product. However, for military vaccines it is frequently difficult to obtain a full licence as there is no target population suffering from the disease caused by the biological warfare agent. For products to be licensed in the UK, they must comply with certain standards including the requirement for a specific facility making a particular product which is bottled and dispensed in a specific way. Any deviation from the specified process will result in the product not being licensed. Consequently, there can be difficulties in an operational emergency when additional quantities of vaccines may be required at short notice.

VIII. Vaccines for civil use

Although many of the features of defence vaccines would be very beneficial for civil vaccines there are several significant differences between vaccines for civil use against endemic diseases and those for defence use. These range from the different route of challenge to the body, the different level of challenge, the different pathogens, the different licence status, the different scale of use, and the different storage requirements and the different time-scales under which protection is required. These difference are compared in table 14.2.

It is clear that while advances made for defence vaccines have application for civil vaccines and such defence spin-off should be encouraged, those advances need to be transferred to civil vaccines against endemic diseases. The proposals for an international programme of development and use of vaccines can now be considered to see how best such a programme can be devised to further international collaboration and security.

IX. International development and use of vaccines

The goal of vaccines against pathogens that pose natural health threats is a laudable one and is fully supported. The secondary objective of vaccines against putative biological weapons is doubtful on a number of counts. As already discussed, the characteristics of vaccines required for public health use are significantly different from those for biological defence not least because of the different pathogens and the different licence status.

The proposal to base VFP on so-called dual-threat agents is flawed on several counts. First, the diseases of prime concern to developing countries are those that threaten public health in those countries and are generally not the main putative biological warfare agents such as anthrax or tularaemia. Second, the emphasis on dual-threat agents will justifiably raise proliferation concerns as it would suggest that VFP would actually aid developing countries in acquiring the technology to produce such agents and to evaluate the effectiveness of the

Table 14.2. Vaccines for public health and defence

Vaccines for public health	Vaccines for defence
Endemic diseases	BW agents
Various routes of infection	Primarily aerosol
One or more ID_{50}	Multiple ID_{50}
	Rapid protection
Licensed product	Interim status
Produce and use	Long storage life
Large-scale use	Armed forces use
Freely available	Limited availability

vaccine against them. The increasing attention being given world-wide to improving export controls on biological agents and dual-use equipment would necessitate the imposition of tight controls on the VFP programme and might well defeat its aims.

Finally, the concept of internationally available vaccines for biological defence is also flawed. Effective biological defence is needed to maintain a web of deterrence so that potential aggressors judge that biological weapons are not worth acquiring; for this to be effective a defence vaccine must not be freely available to a potential aggressor to examine, evaluate and devise means of circumventing that defence.

The basic concept of VFP of converting past offensive biological warfare facilities into producing vaccines against public health threat is sound. The risk must be avoided that by seeking to also focus on putative biological weapons, VFP could actually promote proliferation. This must be a risk as it would bring biological weapons to the attention of developing countries through the international organization having to consider the nature of biological weapons in order to develop vaccines that were demonstrated to be effective against biological weapons. In addition, the conversion of past offensive biological warfare facilities into ones producing dual-threat agent vaccines could raise concern that such converted facilities might be changed back in a short space of time to offensive biological warfare facilities. This concern would be much reduced if the offensive biological warfare facility was converted to a facility producing public health vaccines which had no links to biological warfare or dual-threat agents.

There are other arguments for VFP concentrating on vaccines to counter public health threats; the quantities of vaccine required are much larger to protect populations against endemic diseases and the logistics of production, distribution and use are greatly eased for public health purposes. Both of these factors improve the practicality of the VFP proposals for countering public health threats.

X. Conclusions

Vaccines for biological defence are an essential component of the web of deterrence[17] aimed at leading a potential aggressor to judge that biological weapons

[17] Pearson, G. S., 'Prospects for chemical and biological arms control: the web of deterrence', *Washington Quarterly*, vol. 16, no. 2 (spring 1993), p. 145.

are not worth acquiring. To be an effective defence, these vaccines just as any other form of defence must not be available for a potential aggressor to examine, evaluate and defeat.

Defence vaccines will need to be produced by national facilities; such vaccines need to be shown to be effective against an aerosol challenge involving as wide a range of strains of the biological warfare agent as possible. There will be increased security in some duplication between such national facilities as it will increase the uncertainty for the aggressor state as to whether resorting to biological warfare will be militarily beneficial. The spin-off from defence vaccine technology to civil vaccine applications should be encouraged.

The BWC should be strengthened and States Parties encouraged to provide responses to the agreed politically binding CBMs and to participate in devising an appropriate verification regime to deter states from considering acquisition of biological weapons. An incentive for such increased participation by states in the BWC should stem from the benefits in improved standards for microbiological containment, health and safety, pollution, biosafety, genetic manipulation and good laboratory and good manufacturing practice which will provide increased confidence that a facility in a developing country is not being misused for a prohibited purpose.

The Vaccines for Peace proposal should as part of this concentrate on providing vaccines against public health threats and should be considered in the context of the International Biological Monitoring Agency with its aim of promoting the contribution of biology to peace, health and prosperity in the world.

15. Molecular aspects of the activity and design of antiviral agents

PETER LANGEN

I. Introduction

Measures to defend against diseases caused by bacteria, fungi, parasites and viruses include the development, production and use of drugs which are essentially designed to interfere with the pathogens, whether or not they are dual-threat agents (DTAs). One of the goals of military biological defence programmes is therefore the development of effective treatment capabilities.[1] The most important problem as regards DTAs is the development and production of antiviral substances, both for military and civilian purposes. These substances should act as selectively as possible with virus-specific targets (see table 15.1) in order to avoid damaging normal cellular structures and functions.

II. The current situation

The current situation for antiviral agents can be characterized in brief: poor but with bright prospects for future developments, although not necessarily with respect to DTAs. 'Poor' means that there are only very few selective agents in clinical use against some viruses[2] which are not DTAs. Two of these substances are antiherpetics—acyclovir and 5-(2-bromovinyl)-2'-deoxyuridine (BVDU)—both with almost unmatched selectivity. In addition, there are such agents as 3'-azido-3'-deoxythymidine, 2',3'-dideoxycytidine and 2',3'-dideoxyinosine for the treatment of AIDS with far less selectivity, owing in part to the fact that they have to be used for a longer period of time (i.e., for the entire life of a patient). However, the future appears bright because there are many molecular targets for which selective antivirals can be designed.

In molecular terms, there are two problems related to the design of chemotherapeutics: (*a*) the choice of molecular targets that are likely to exhibit selectivity when attacked, and (*b*) the design of compounds that are 'magic bullets' (a phrase coined by Paul Ehrlich, often considered the 'father of chemotherapy') which only hit their target and nothing else. Table 15.2 summarizes the current status of anticancer, antibacterial and antiviral agents.

Current anticancer agents are neither sufficiently selective to prevent severe side-effects nor are there any prospects of the future development of drugs which will have fewer side-effects. The reason is the great similarity between cancer cells and normal cells—the differences between both being in cellular regulation, which is only partially understood and not yet exploitable for cancer therapy.

[1] Huxsoll, D., testimony on 'Germ wars: biological weapons proliferation and the new genetics', 17 May 1989, in *Global Spread of Chemical and Biological Weapons*, Hearings before the Committee on Governmental Affairs and its Permanent Subcommittee on Investigations, US Senate (US Government Printing Office: Washington, DC, 1990), pp. 464–73, see especially p. 466.

[2] Bean, B., 'Antiviral therapy: current concepts and practices', *Clinical Microbiology Review*, vol. 5 (1992), pp. 146–82.

Table 15.1. Proteins encoded by virus genomes as targets for antiviral compounds

Type of protein
Without cellular counterparts
RNA-dependent RNA polymerase
RNA-dependent DNA polymerase (i.e., reverse transcription)
Envelope proteins
With cellular counterparts
DNA-dependent DNA polymerase
DNA-dependent RNA polymerase
Thymidine kinase
Proteases

The situation is better for antibacterial agents where safe compounds have existed since the middle of this century. Antibacterial agents are safer for two reasons. First, bacteria have a unique type of cell wall, which is completely different from that of animal cells. It is either itself a target (for antibiotics such as penicillin) or allows various compounds (e.g., sulfonamides) to be absorbed differently. Second, bacteria contain proteins coded by the bacterial genome which are either different from functionally identical proteins coded by the cellular genome, or are not present in animal cells. Of particular importance is the fact that at least some of the bacteria-coded proteins are more sensitive to certain compounds (e.g., antimetabolites) than their cellular counterparts.

For antiviral agents, virus-coded proteins have also been discovered which are different from functionally identical proteins coded by the cellular genome, or which are not present in animal cells. Again, at least some of these proteins are far more sensitive to certain drugs such as antimetabolites. However, for antiviral agents it is not possible to rely on a special cell wall. This creates a major obstacle to the design and detection of antivirals, a problem which does not occur with antibacterial compounds.

III. Antiviral agents

The development of specific antiviral agents has long been considered difficult because many processes of the life cycles of viruses depend on cellular biochemistry. Interference with these processes would destroy both viruses and cells, including uninfected cells. However, in recent decades advances in molecular virology have revealed many suitable targets, as discussed above. These are the virus-coded proteins.

Table 15.1 lists virus-coded proteins in two categories: (*a*) those which are present only in virus-infected cells, and (*b*) enzymes which occur with similar catalytic functions in normal cells.

If there are no cellular counterparts to the viral target proteins, compounds can be designed which react only with these targets, and which therefore do not harm cells. It will be more difficult to design compounds which differentiate between proteins coded by the virus genome and functionally identical proteins coded by the cellular genome. This is, however, feasible because of the greater

Table 15.2. Current status of chemotherapy against cancer cells, bacteria and viruses

Object of chemotherapy	Evaluation of response to chemotherapy
Cancer	Poor response owing to severe side-effects, lack of proper targets, great similarity between cancer cells and normal cells, future improvements uncertain
Bacteria	Very good response, selectivity of bacterial cell wall, greater sensitivity of bacterial proteins to drugs, main problem relates to the 'race' with development of resistance
Viruses	Poor response—only antiherpetics but with unmatched selectivity, greater sensitivity of virus-coded proteins to drugs, bright prospects

sensitivity of the virus-coded proteins (compared to that of the cellular proteins) and is best demonstrated with virus-coded enzymes and antimetabolite compounds. Antimetabolites are traditionally used in cancer chemotherapy and against bacteria; furthermore, all of the antivirals which are currently in clinical use are antimetabolites. Antimetabolites mimic the substrate structures of particular enzymes. The enzymes and substrates fit together like a lock and key (a comparison proposed by Emil Fischer[3]). Antimetabolites whose substrate structure has only slightly been modified also fit in this way to the enzyme. They mimic the substrate but block the enzyme reaction (owing to their structural alterations), or later spoil it (e.g., by incorporation of the altered compound into biopolymers such as DNA). If the structure of a substrate is chemically modified to a greater extent, it will no longer fit enzymes which have strict structural requirements for substrates, but it will still fit others with more relaxed requirements. These latter types of enzymes will be blocked, and fortunately these are the viral- or bacterial-coded enzymes. This occurs because the genome of 'lower' forms of life is often unable to code for highly sophisticated enzyme structures, unlike that of higher organisms.

Fischer's lock–key analogy can be taken a step further. Human and animal enzymes are similar to complex locks that can only be opened with a special key, while bacterial and viral enzymes are like very simple locks that can be opened with many things, even a bit of bent wire. The philosophy for an approach to selectivity by such antimetabolities (so-called 'non-classical antimetabolites') has been elaborated and described by B. R. Baker.[4] The feasibility of this approach is demonstrated by some antibacterials such as the antifolics, and by antiherpetic agents. An antimetabolite such as methotrexate—a drug that has been used in clinical cancer chemotherapy for approximately 40 years, and which differs in structure only slightly from folic acid (the substrate mimicked)—cannot be used selectively for bacteria such as *Staphylococcus aureus*. However, trimethoprin, a component of remedies against various

[3] Fischer, E., *Berichte der Deutschen Chemischen Gesellschaft*, vol. 27 (1894), p. 2985.

[4] Baker, B. R., *Designs of Active Site Directed Irreversible Enzyme Inhibitors* (J. Wiley and Sons: New York, 1967).

infections and an antimetabolite which bears little similarity in structure to folic acid, is highly selective against bacterial enzymes.[5]

In the case of the highly selective antiherpetic agent BVDU, it can easily be shown that as the size of the substituent in C-5 of 2'-deoxyuridine increases, so does selectivity—although activity diminishes if the substituent becomes too large.[6] However, the selective compound BVDU retains some similarity to the original substrate thymidine and the enzyme to which it fits: thymidine kinase. In contrast, it would not be expected that the guanine derivative acyclovir would fit the same enzyme, but this is in fact the case. This also demonstrates the limits of this approach. Serious consideration would never be given to designing compounds like acyclovir as substrates of viral thymidine kinase. Such compounds can be detected only if there is broad screening. Therefore, automated computerized evaluation and data collection continue to be necessary supplements to the rational, as opposed to empirical, approach. Naturally, the success of such screening will ultimately depend on the same differences in viral and cellular proteins which are exploited in the rational approach. It is necessary to screen for precisely the virus to be attacked, not just for a model virus because the selectivity of the agents can be striking. For example, BVDU only inhibits herpes simplex type 1 and varicella zoster virus, but not herpes simplex type 2, and neither BVDU nor acyclovir inhibit other herpes viruses such as, for example, cytomegalovirus.

IV. Antiviral agents and the Vaccines for Peace programme

A question of special importance for this volume is the development of antiviral agents on the basis of the above considerations as a useful supplement to the establishment of the Vaccines for Peace (VFP) programme. There are some factors which favour antiviral agents. Antiviral agents could take the form of stable compounds used in small quantities (e.g., as pills, taken orally). Antiviral agents can be developed in small chemical laboratories that do not have high safety levels, and their synthesis in kilogram amounts does not require special facilities. They can be tested in small laboratories using virus-infected cell cultures and only for pre-selected compounds. For a few compounds, animal experiments will be required.

Antiviral agents need not be prepared as solutions, which can be contaminated by pathogens or contain residual infectious viruses; this might, however, be the case with vaccines. Antiviral agents are also unaffected by antigen changes, and resistant strains are unlikely to develop within the short time they would be used after a biological warfare attack.

On the other hand, the development of such 'magic bullets' might be very time-consuming and possibly unsuccessful. This is best exemplified by the attempts to develop drugs against AIDS. In the case of AIDS, the selective targets are known (e.g., reverse transcriptases and proteases). There has also been political and financial support of AIDS drug research, as well as a great amount

[5] Burchall, J. J. and Hitchings, G. H., 'Inhibitor binding analysis of dihydrofolate reductases from various species', *Molecular Pharmacology*, vol. 1 (1965), pp. 126–36; Hitchings, G. H. and Burchall, J. J., 'Species differences among dihydrofolate reductases', *Federal Proceedings*, no. 25 (1966), pp. 881–83.

[6] Reefschläger, J., Bärwolff, D., Engelmann, P., Langen, P. and Rosenthal, H. A., 'Efficiency and selectivity of 5-(bromovinyl)-2'-deoxyuridine and some other 5-substituted 2'-deoxypyrimidine nucleosides as antiherpes agents', *Antiviral Research*, vol. 2 (1982), pp. 41–52.

of publicity. None the less, no drug has been found which cures AIDS, and there is also no vaccine just around the corner. However, HIV is a retrovirus which integrates into the cellular genome and is highly variable with regard to its antigens; it may be too formidable a virus to tackle first. In addition, HIV is not regarded as a DTA.

Nevertheless, there is no reason to assume that different demands or strategies are needed for the design, development, production and use of antiviral agents and other chemotherapeutic agents for civilian and military purposes with respect to vaccines as some suggest.[7] Accordingly, it is not necessary to conduct special military antiviral programmes. There is, however, a clear need to assist global activities in this area, not least as regards the treatment of diseases caused by DTAs. In any event, it would certainly be beneficial to develop not only vaccines but also antivirals for peaceful uses.

[7] See Pearson, chapter 14, in this volume.

16. Vaccines for public health: can Vaccines for Peace help in the war against disease?

STEPHEN S. MORSE*

I. Introduction

The disease agents suggested by Erhard Geissler[1] as targets for the Vaccines for Peace (VFP) programme include some of the most lethal agents known. This chapter assesses the value of a programme intended to make vaccines against geographically limited threats, including some that have been considered to be of interest as possible biological weapon (BW) agents.

II. Comparison of emerging diseases and BW agents

Given their high lethality and their relative obscurity (so that others are less likely to have *matériel* or experience to treat or prevent the infection), it is understandable that the agents involved have often been named as candidate BW agents. 'Exotic' agents indigenous to a particular region can also pose a threat to foreign troops sent there, a traditional justification for military research on these agents even if no offensive use is intended. However, their potential interest as BW agents should not obscure the fact that these agents were first identified when they caused naturally occurring outbreaks of disease. Natural disease outbreaks by such agents account for significant numbers of cases annually.

Many of these are also 'emerging viruses'. In recent years there has been a great deal of concern about emerging viruses, which can be defined as viruses that have recently increased in incidence and appear likely to continue increasing.[2] Included are viruses that have newly appeared in the human population, such as HIV (human immunodeficiency virus, the AIDS virus), or diseases that are rapidly expanding their range, with a corresponding increase in cases of disease. Table 16.1 shows several examples of emerging viruses. Besides being potential dangers to public health, the dramatic, seemingly random nature of their appearance makes emerging viruses psychologically devastating as well.

[1] Geissler, E., 'Vaccines for Peace: an international program of development and use of vaccines against dual-threat agents', *Politics and the Life Sciences*, vol. 11, no. 2 (Aug. 1992), pp. 231–43; see also Geissler (chapter 3) in this volume.

[2] Morse, S. S. and Schluederberg, A., 'Emerging viruses: the evolution of viruses and viral diseases', *Journal of Infectious Diseases*, vol. 162, no. 1 (July 1990), pp. 1–7.

* I thank the other participants in the Vaccines for Peace symposium for helpful comments and discussions. Special thanks for additional discussions to Erhard Geissler, Jack Woodall, Mark Wheelis and Barbara Hatch Rosenberg. I am supported by National Institutes of Health (NIH) grant RR 03121, US Department of Health and Human Services. Work on emerging viruses was supported by the NIH. I thank John La Montagne, Director of the Division of Microbiology & Infectious Diseases, National Institute of Allergy and Infectious Diseases, NIH for support in initiating work on emerging viruses and for valued discussions.

Table 16.1. Some examples of 'emerging' viruses[a]

Virus	Sign/symptoms	Distribution	Natural host
Orthomyxoviridae (RNA, 8 segments)			
Influenza[b]	Respiratory	World-wide (? from China)	Fowl, pigs
Bunyaviridae (RNA, 3 segments)			
Hantaviruses[b] (Hantaan, Seoul, others)	Haemorrhagic fever, renal syndrome, pulmonary syndrome	Asia, Europe, USA	Rodents (e.g., *Apodemus* for Hantaan)
Rift Valley fever[c]	Fever, ± haemorrhage	Africa	Mosquito, ungulates
Flaviviridae (RNA)			
Yellow fever[c]	Fever, jaundice	Africa, South America	Mosquito, monkey
Dengue virus[d]	Fever, ± haemorrhage	Asia, Africa Caribbean	Mosquito, human, monkey
Arenaviridae (RNA, 2 segments)			
Junin (Argentinian haemorrhagic fever) virus	Fever, haemorrhage	South America	Rodent (*Calomys musculinus*)
Machupo (Bolivian haemorrhagic fever) virus	Fever, haemorrhage	South America	Rodent (*Calomys callosus*)
Lassa fever	Fever, haemorrhage	West Africa	Rodent (*Mastomys natalensis*)
Filoviridae (RNA)			
Marburg, Ebola viruses	Fever, haemorrhage	Africa	Unknown, ? primate
Retroviridae (RNA and reverse transcriptase)			
HIV[b]	AIDS, etc.	World-wide	? Primate, human

[a] This list is offered as a set of examples only and is not meant to be exhaustive, or necessarily to predict causes of future disease outbreaks
[b] Virus of special concern for the near future
[c] Transmitted by arthropod vector
[d] Virus of special concern for the near future, transmitted by arthropod vector

Source: Adapted from Morse, S. S. and Schluederberg, A., 'Emerging viruses: the evolution of viruses and viral diseases', *Journal of Infectious Diseases*, vol. 162, no. 1 (July 1990), pp. 1–7, © 1990 by The University of Chicago, all rights reserved.

Emerging viruses and putative BW agents share many of the same characteristics, and many were first recognized when they caused sudden occurrences of severe disease. It is therefore hardly surprising that comparisons of various lists tabulating a number of putative BW or 'dual-threat' agents (DTAs) as suggested by various expert sources,[3] and lists of emerging viruses (such as table 16.1) reveal considerable overlap. Almost every agent on the list of emerging viruses, with the exception of the human retroviruses and some of the hepatitis viruses, has also been named at one time or another as a possible BW agent. These are the suggested targets of the Vaccines for Peace programme.

[3] Geissler, 'Vaccines for Peace: an international program of development and use of vaccines against dual-threat agents' (note 1); see especially the list in appendix 1, table A1, p. 239.

Therefore, one evaluation of the VFP programme could be based on its value as a public health programme to improve readiness against emerging infections. This consideration raises the following questions that are addressed in this chapter: Is it possible to be prepared for emerging infections, and is it important? What is the value of immunization in this regard? Finally, if immunization is of value, does the Vaccines for Peace approach help to fulfil this objective?

III. Is it possible to be prepared for emerging diseases?

In order to answer the above question, it is necessary to consider whether emerging diseases can be predicted. While this question appears impossible, in fact it can be answered. The present author has elsewhere analysed this question in more detail, and the results are only summarized here.[4] It is possible to be prepared for emerging diseases. However dramatic their first appearance, emerging diseases do not generally arise at random, but have identifiable causes. Most emerging pathogens probably already exist in nature and simply gain access to new host populations. This usually happens as a result of environmental changes that promote the transfer and dissemination of existing agents to new host populations (a process which may be called 'viral traffic' or, more broadly for both viral and non-viral diseases, 'microbial traffic'). In some cases there may be some evolutionary changes before emergence, but this is not usually a prerequisite. Some of the most lethal emerging viruses are zoonotic, naturally occurring infections of other species that are introduced into humans (see table 16.1). Other emerging viruses may exist in geographically restricted human populations for some time before they get the opportunity to spread to larger populations.

As table 16.2 shows, many of the factors that cause new diseases to emerge are social and environmental, such as agricultural development or movement from rural areas to cities. Thus, these emerging diseases often exist in nature, hidden in the environment, until appropriate factors allow them to be introduced into the human population and thence spread. Historically, emerging diseases are usually geographically isolated when they first emerge. Similarly, the causative agents (the viruses or organisms responsible for the disease) have often belonged to previously unknown or poorly studied families of microbes. HIV, for example, was the first lentivirus to be identified in any primate species (HIV is a member of the retroviral subfamily known as the lentiviruses). Before HIV was discovered in humans, only a handful of lentiviruses were known, and none of them was known to cause an AIDS-like immunodeficiency disease. Since then, the list of known lentiviruses has more than doubled and a number of other primate lentiviruses have been identified,[5] all the result of searching for additional lentiviruses in nature. As another example, the outbreaks of Marburg virus disease in 1967 and of Ebola virus in Africa in 1976 were the first recognition of a new family of viruses (still poorly understood), even though

[4] Morse, S. S., 'Emerging viruses: defining the rules for viral traffic', *Perspectives in Biology and Medicine*, vol. 34, no. 3 (spring 1991), pp. 387–409; Morse, S. S., 'Examining the origins of emerging viruses', ed. S. S. Morse, *Emerging Viruses* (Oxford University Press: Oxford, 1993), pp. 10–28.

[5] Myers, G., MacInnes, K. and Korber, B., 'The emergence of simian/human immunodeficiency viruses', *AIDS Research and Human Retroviruses*, vol. 8, no. 3 (Mar. 1992), pp. 373–85.

Table 16.2. Some emerging viruses and probable factors in their emergence

Virus family, virus	Probable factors in emergence
Arenaviridae	
Junin (Argentinian haemorrhagic fever) virus	Changes in agriculture (maize, changed conditions favouring *Calomys musculinus*, rodent host for virus)
Machupo (Bolivian haemorrhagic fever) virus	Changes in agriculture (changed conditions favouring *Calomys callosus*, rodent host for virus)
Bunyaviridae	
Hantaan virus	Agriculture (contact with mouse *Apodemus agrarius* during rice harvest)
Seoul virus	? Increasing population density of urban rats in contact with humans
Rift Valley fever	Dams, irrigation
Oropouche	Agriculture (cacao hulls encourage breeding of *Culicoides* vector)
Filoviridae	
Marburg, Ebola viruses	Unknown; in Europe and USA, importation of monkeys
Flaviviridae	
Dengue virus	Increasing population density in cities and other factors (e.g., open water storage) favouring increased population of mosquito vectors
Orthomyxoviridae	
Influenza	? Integrated pig–duck agriculture
Retroviridae	
HIV	Medical technology (transfusion), sexual transmission, other social factors (e.g., intravenous drug use)
Human T cell leukaemia virus (HTLV)	Medical technology (transfusion), sexual transmission, other social factors (virus is already naturally widespread in some populations)

Source: Morse, S. S., 'Examining the origins of emerging viruses', ed. S. S. Morse, *Emerging Viruses* (Oxford University Press: Oxford, 1993), pp. 10–28.

these viruses had undoubtedly existed in nature for quite some time. Because these pathogens have frequently escaped scientific notice before they emerged, medical science has often been poorly prepared to deal with them.

IV. The need for preparedness

Is it important to be prepared for emerging infections? This is a question of judgement, of course, but there are compelling reasons to be prepared, AIDS being only one. There is overwhelming evidence to indicate that emerging infections will continue and possibly even increase. Numerous recent episodes of emerging and re-emerging infections, including AIDS, Rift Valley fever in Africa, the continuing spread of dengue viruses, multidrug resistant tuberculosis and other antibiotic resistant bacteria, cholera in Africa and South America, and the resurgence of measles in cities in the United States, attest to mankind's continuing vulnerability to infectious diseases. A number of experts have warned that no part of the world is insulated from the possible introduction of 'new' diseases,[6] and many examples attest to this. A recent report from a committee of the Institute of Medicine (IOM) of the US National Academy of Sciences declared: 'Disease-causing microbes have threatened human health for centuries. . . . [The Committee] believes that this threat will continue and may even intensify in coming years. . . . Infectious diseases remain the major cause of death worldwide . . . and will not be conquered during our lifetimes.'[7]

However, it is now also possible to better anticipate disease emergence. Many of the factors responsible for disease emergence are now understood, and this information can be used to anticipate 'new' diseases. Awareness of 'microbial traffic' factors should make it easier to focus efforts more effectively. Especially in tropical areas, ecological or demographic changes including deforestation, dam building, changes in agricultural product or land use, and major demographic changes such as population migrations, often precipitate disease emergence. These are 'traffic signals' for microbial traffic: they should be seen as warning signals.[8]

Although emerging infections may often begin in geographic isolation, they increase their range as they emerge. Such is the history of most diseases that became global, such as smallpox, cholera, pandemic influenza and many others including (probably) HIV. As the types of environmental changes that cause disease emergence are still continuing, the incidence of emerging infections can be expected to increase. It would therefore seem wise to be prepared in the event new diseases emerge.

V. Possible defences against emerging diseases

At a practical level, there must be mechanisms in place for recognizing disease emergence and for initiating appropriate action.[9] Global infectious disease (epidemiologic) surveillance is one most urgently needed first step.[10] Mark Wheelis has noted that such public health programmes would also strengthen BW verification by increasing transparency, detecting unusual outbreaks of disease and facilitating investigations of alleged BW use.[11] In the United States, the IOM committee of the National Academy of Sciences, quoted above, has also endorsed recommendations to establish a global infectious disease surveillance system for early warning against emerging infections.[12]

Immunization will have to play a key role in efforts at control and prevention. This conclusion is based on the following considerations. Once an emerging

[6] Lederberg, J., Shope, R. E. and Oaks, Jr, S. C. (eds), *Emerging Infections: Microbial Threats to Health in the United States* (National Academy Press: Washington, DC, 1992); and Lederberg, J., 'Medical science, infectious disease, and the unity of humankind', *Journal of the American Medical Association*, vol. 260, no. 5 (5 Aug. 1988), pp. 684–85.

[7] Lederberg, Shope and Oaks (note 6), p. 1ff.

[8] Morse, S. S., 'Regulating viral traffic', *Issues in Science and Technology*, vol. 7, no. 1 (fall 1990), pp. 81–84; Morse, S. S., 'Global microbial traffic and the interchange of disease', *American Journal of Public Health*, vol. 82, no. 10 (Oct. 1992), pp. 1326–27.

[9] See note 8.

[10] Henderson, D. A., 'Surveillance systems and intergovernmental cooperation', ed. S. S. Morse, *Emerging Viruses* (note 4), pp. 283–89; Wheelis, M. L., 'Strengthening biological weapons control through global epidemiological surveillance', *Politics and the Life Sciences*, vol. 11, no. 2 (Aug. 1992), pp. 179–89; Morse, S. S., 'Regulating viral traffic' (note 8); and Morse, S. S., 'Epidemiologic surveillance for investigating chemical or biological warfare and for improving human health', *Politics and the Life Sciences*, vol. 11, no. 1 (Feb. 1992), pp. 28–29.

[11] See Wheelis, chapter 17, in this volume, and Wheelis (note 10).

[12] Lederberg, Shope and Oaks (note 6), p. 137.

infection is identified, what is the armamentarium for dealing with it? As with any infectious disease, there are a few feasible areas of attack. Infected individuals can be treated with antimicrobials, such as antibiotics, if appropriate. Otherwise, medical intervention is limited to supportive therapy, treating the symptoms and damage caused by the infection in order to help the patient recover. For protecting the uninfected, public health measures include prophylactic antimicrobials in some cases, epidemiologic investigation and control of transmission (often involving environmental measures), and immunization. Each has its place and its characteristic limitations. Prophylactic antibiotics are possible in principle, but are often not practicable and are not always efficacious. The effectiveness of measures to control transmission will vary with the local situation and the specific means of transmission. For the majority of infections that cannot be controlled solely by hygienic measures, immunization traditionally has been at the fore, both the most effective and the most economical public health measure. This is particularly true of viruses, where there often is no antimicrobial therapy available, as there are few antiviral agents comparable in usefulness to the antibiotics used to treat bacterial infections, and the drugs are generally more toxic. Environmental measures alone in many cases may be insufficient or difficult to apply. Therefore, they will often need to be coupled with other measures, such as immunization. The effectiveness of immunization as a strategy is well documented, and it has long been a mainstay of disease control programmes. The eradication of smallpox was achieved through strategies largely based on immunization, together with surveillance of cases,[13] and the present programme to eradicate polio relies on a similar approach with immunization as the centrepiece.[14] The conclusion to be drawn is that immunization has long been a leading weapon (in some cases, the only one) in controlling infectious diseases. There is nothing on the horizon to suggest that the essential role of immunization will change in the foreseeable future.

VI. Constraints on developing vaccines for emerging diseases indicate a role for new programmes

For many infections, immunization is therefore a most important defence, and in some cases the only feasible measure. Unfortunately, many factors militate against the ready availability of vaccines for emerging diseases. Some of these are economic. Although these diseases already cause illness and death in significant numbers, many of them are too restricted geographically or currently affect too few people to be attractive for commercial vaccine efforts. In general, commercial vaccine development is expensive, and the relatively few companies that produce most of the world's vaccines are reluctant to produce new vaccines without assurances of a sufficient market to balance the costs and per-

[13] See Fenner, Wittek, F. R. and Dumbell, K. R., *The Orthopoxviruses* (Academic Press: New York, 1989), chapter 5, which refers to the vaccine as 'the tool for smallpox eradication'. Chapter 11 ('The global spread, control, and eradication of smallpox', pp. 317–52) in the same volume discusses how this was accomplished. For the latter, see also Fenner, F. *et al.*, *Smallpox and Its Eradication* (World Health Organization: Geneva, 1988).

[14] de Quadros, C. A. *et al.*, 'Polio eradication from the western hemisphere', *Annual Review of Public Health*, vol. 13 (1992), pp. 239–52; Wright, P. F. *et al.*, 'Strategies for the global eradication of poliomyelitis by the year 2000', *New England Journal of Medicine*, vol. 325, no. 25 (19 Dec. 1991), pp. 1774–79.

ceived risks. A number of experts have noted that few companies would consider developing a vaccine unless the market exceeded 40 million potential vaccinees able to pay full market price.[15] Furthermore, many of these diseases are perceived as 'exotic' and therefore of little concern to the industrialized countries that would necessarily have to provide most of the money for developing and purchasing the vaccines. As a result, it is difficult to develop new vaccines that might be desirable now, let alone to consider vaccines against currently restricted but potentially emerging threats. In the event of an emergency, it is almost impossible to develop new vaccines rapidly, and there is very limited capacity to increase production should the need suddenly arise.[16] Thus, the armamentarium against emerging infections is very limited, a potentially dangerous situation should any of these diseases emerge rapidly.

This is true generally of all infections that are geographically restricted. In addition to the potential of some as emerging diseases, many of these exotic, or geographically restricted, infections cause considerable illness and death. Japanese encephalitis is estimated to affect over 30 000 people annually, and Korean haemorrhagic fever over 100 000 in China alone. In 1977–78 Rift Valley fever caused an epidemic in Egypt with an estimated 200 000 cases and at least 598 known deaths.[17] Dengue virus, which already affects millions annually, is becoming more frequent. On the other hand, vaccine economics make it difficult to develop new vaccines or to generate capacity for stockpiling vaccines against currently limited diseases. By using existing facilities and expertise, available in several places, and aiding transfer of low-cost vaccine production capability, as the VFP programme proposes, the cost of developing and producing these vaccines could be greatly reduced, making it possible to develop vaccines that are otherwise not economically feasible. In the immediate future, at least, a programme like VFP would therefore appear to be the most practical possibility for building up vaccine stocks and capacity against emerging diseases. This would provide at least a little margin of safety in preparing for emerging infections and simultaneously contribute to improving regional public health.

Given the fact that commercial vaccine economics are rather forbidding, most of the target vaccines for the VFP programme, with smaller markets, are also not likely to compete with industry. Less industrialized countries could receive public health benefits from the vaccines and could also benefit economically from the development of an indigenous biotechnology industry making vaccines. In addition, there are a number of facilities in the former Soviet Union that have long worked to produce various vaccines, most using strains they have themselves developed.[18] Some are directed to emerging agents for which other vaccines are currently not readily available. These facilities could be well employed in a programme like VFP, and would benefit economically from it. It would also prevent the diversion of trained personnel to countries that might consider developing a BW programme.

There are of course fundamental issues involving public health programmes generally, and vaccines specifically; and in the longer run, there might be hope

[15] See Woodall, chapter 20, in this volume.

[16] Lederberg, Shope and Oaks (note 6), pp. 150–59.

[17] Meegan, J. M, and Shope, R. E., 'Emerging concepts on Rift Valley fever', ed. M. Pollard, *Perspectives in Virology*, vol. 11 (Alan R. Liss: New York, 1981), pp. 267–87.

[18] See Drozdov, chapter 11, in this volume.

for additional improvements. It has been noted that such major diseases as malaria, tuberculosis, schistosomiasis and even measles, are desperately in need of control.[19] Despite the future promise of advanced biotechnology, most vaccines are still developed and made by traditional methodologies,[20] and this is likely to continue. Even once the promise of biotechnology is fulfilled, an event perhaps in the foreseeable future but not imminent, there are still likely to be serious limitations imposed by safety, regulatory and legal requirements and by market considerations that would continue to inhibit the optimal availability and use of vaccines. Delivery also remains a weak link. It is to be hoped that these problems will be resolved soon, but past experience suggests that it will take some time. Until then, any capability to respond to new infectious disease threats is far better than no capability at all. Since the costs are likely to be relatively low, it represents cheap insurance. It should also be noted that the ready availability of effective vaccines on a world-wide basis can remove some of the incentive for having a BW programme, as potential adversaries could be assured of protecting themselves even against obscure agents.

In the ideal world, there would never have been any interest in devising biological weapons, and all potentially life-saving measures such as immunization would be universally available. The realities of life make it possible only to work gradually towards these goals. Any plan that could turn past interest in biological weapons towards inexpensively producing vaccines—vaccines that could be important but the production of which is not economically compelling—could help make a real step towards that goal.

[19] See Fenner, chapter 18, and Thränert, chapter 5, in this volume.

[20] See Ajjan, Saliou and Valette, chapter 10; Horaud, chapter 9; Melling, chapter 13; and Drozdov, chapter 11, in this volume.

17. The Global Epidemiological Surveillance System and Vaccines for Peace: complementary initiatives in public health and weapon control

MARK L. WHEELIS*

I. Global epidemiological surveillance

The present author has recently proposed[1] that a Global Epidemiological Surveillance System (GESS) of human, veterinary and crop diseases be developed and implemented under multinational supervision. The impetus of this suggestion was the conviction that clandestine use of biological agents is a possible, and arguably the most likely, form of biological warfare.[2] Since clandestine use requires that the resulting disease outbreak be misunderstood as a natural occurrence, this kind of biological warfare can only be seriously contemplated if such misunderstanding is probable. The comprehensive understanding of disease ecology that would be the result of the GESS, including the ability to recognize the geographical and temporal origin of aetiological agents, would make this kind of misunderstanding very much less likely, and would consequently act as a powerful deterrent to the hostile use of biological agents. In this way it would act to bolster the international treaty regimes that control biological weapons (BW): the 1972 Biological Weapons Convention (BWC)[3] and the 1925 Geneva Protocol;[4] the GESS is essential to verify the latter, and would be an important confidence-building measure for the former.

Although the proposal for the GESS grew out of weapon control considerations, it is clear that the principal benefits of such a system would be in the arena of public health more generally. Implementation of the GESS would catalyse a dramatic improvement in global public health (if for no other reason than the expanded clinical facilities that would be necessary for diagnostic purposes), and, if it were also implemented for both veterinary and crop organisms, would lead to a similar increase in veterinary health and agricultural productivity, with consequent human health benefits. It would also offer much

[1] Wheelis, M. L., 'Strengthening biological weapons control through global epidemiological surveillance', *Politics and the Life Sciences*, vol. 11, no. 2 (Aug. 1992), pp. 179–89.

[2] The term biological warfare is here used quite loosely to include all forms of hostile use of biological agents by one group of people against another, be these groups subnational, national, supranational, ethnic, political or geographic, and independently of whether the attack is direct (using human pathogens) or indirect (using plant or animal pathogens to cause economic or other harm).

[3] Convention on the Prohibition of the Development, Production and Stockpiling of Bacteriological (Biological) and Toxin Weapons and on their Destruction, signed at Washington, London and Moscow, 10 Apr. 1972, entered into force 26 Mar. 1975 (see annexe A in this volume).

[4] Protocol for the Prohibition of the Use in War of Asphyxiating, Poisonous or Other Gases, and of Bacteriological Methods of Warfare, signed at Geneva, 17 June 1925, entered into force 8 Feb. 1928; see Geissler, E. (ed.), SIPRI, *Biological and Toxin Weapons Today* (Oxford University Press: Oxford, 1986), appendix 1.

* Supported by grant 049-3 from the US Institute of Peace (USIP). The opinions, conclusions and recommendations expressed here are those of the author and do not necessarily reflect those of the USIP.

greater assurance than now exists that emerging diseases would be detected early enough to contain their spread;[5] in the light of the human immunodeficiency virus (HIV) epidemic, such an early-warning capability might in itself be sufficient to justify even a very expensive version of the GESS.

The synergy between BW control and public health is not coincidental. Both biological warfare and public health programmes aim to manipulate microbial populations to increase or decrease, respectively, the extent to which humans (or their domestic animals and crop plants) are burdened by microbial parasitism. Both are hence aspects of applied microbial ecology, differing largely in their reciprocal intents. This close relationship has long been recognized; indeed, biological warfare has been termed '[public health] upside down'.[6]

The ecological nature of infectious disease can be considered at two levels. Each infected host organism can be considered the habitat for the population of microbes that parasitizes it, the symptoms of disease representing alterations of the habitat that may be either beneficial or harmful to the microbial populations. In the extreme, death of the host represents the ultimate degradation of the habitat, and leads to extinction of the parasitizing microbial populations unless they were able to first colonize another host. Mechanisms of microbial pathogenesis and of host defences are thus aspects of microbial ecology.

At the level of populations of host organisms, disease patterns are the result of the interaction of populations of two or more organisms—host and parasite plus, if relevant, vectors and alternate hosts. Epidemiology is the study of these patterns of interaction. It is important to note that such interactions are always dynamic, and the patterns constantly change; however, the rate of change can be quite variable. At one extreme, some patterns can be very stable, as in some instances of endemic disease, in which the levels of parasitism and the geographical ranges of the interacting populations remain stable for decades, even centuries. Such stable interactions may be disturbed principally by ecological disruption from without, as by climatic shifts that affect the ecology of the host, or the invasion of a competing species of host or parasite. At the other extreme, epidemic diseases can represent instances of extreme changes in the level of parasitism, and the size and geographic range of parasite populations as in global pandemics.

It is the ability of some infectious diseases to undergo such dramatic shifts in their frequency (i.e., for the population of their aetiologic agents to multiply explosively and colonize many new hosts/habitats) that makes infectious disease so often unpredictable, and that makes microbial agents attractive as weapons. It also explains the attraction of clandestine biological warfare, since a very small, easily concealed and transported, initial population can under the right conditions cause widespread harm. It is a principal goal of public health programmes to contain as much as possible the increase and spread of populations of aetiologic agents. It is a principal goal of biological warfare to facilitate that increase and spread, hence the close and antagonistic relationship between

[5] See, for example, Morse, S. S., 'Emerging viruses: defining the rules for viral traffic', *Perspectives in Biology and Medicine*, no. 34 (1991), pp. 387–409; Institute of Medicine, *Emerging Infections: Microbial Threats to Health in the United States* (National Academy Press: Washington, DC, 1992); and Morse, chapter 16, in this volume.

[6] Rosebury, T., *Peace or Pestilence: Biological Warfare and How to Avoid It* (Whittlesey House: New York, 1949). Rosebury use the term 'bacteriology' instead of 'public health', but it is clear that in this context the terms are used as synonyms.

the two. Consequently, the conclusion can be drawn that the best defence against biological warfare is an effective public health programme.

Epidemiological surveillance is an essential component of any comprehensive public health programme. An effective surveillance system would also, even by itself, be sufficient to deter most attempts at clandestine BW, and should give some assurance that new diseases will be detected fairly early in their emergence. It is thus reasonable to contemplate implementing the GESS as an early step towards these three goals. Jack Woodall of the World Health Organization (WHO) has observed[7] that significant progress could be made towards the goals of the GESS by simply linking existing epidemiological centres together with an effective telecommunication and data base system. Since such a linkage is a critical component of the GESS, it would be reasonable to make it the first step.

Organization of the GESS needs to be multilateral for a variety of reasons. Since the distributions of pathogens, vectors and alternate hosts often overlap national boundaries, infectious diseases are almost always at least a regional problem. Also, modern air travel and commerce make virtually every spot on the globe accessible to every other within the incubation period of most diseases; novel pathogens (or for that matter long-standing ones) can thus cause sudden and unexpected outbreaks far from their point of origin.[8] All nations of the world thus have a stake in an effective system of global epidemiological surveillance, and in ensuring multinational co-operation in its implementation. Furthermore, the resources necessary to implement the GESS are not evenly distributed, and its implementation will therefore require that the wealthier countries, with the greatest concentration of medical and scientific expertise, provide the bulk of the resources. Their great stake in early detection of emerging diseases should constitute sufficient incentive to do so.

From the perspective of arms control, a multilateral perspective for the GESS is essential to inspire confidence in the results of epidemiological investigations.[9] Clearly, when biological warfare is suspected, neither the victim nor the suspected aggressor should have control of the investigation; otherwise, its results will have little credibility. However, the multilateral political structures that must be in place to guarantee the integrity and credibility of an epidemiological investigation carried out in the highly charged atmosphere of an accusation of biological attack may be too cumbersome for routine surveillance in the absence of such adversarial context. Probably the GESS should be implemented in a more casual fashion, with the understanding that accusation or suspicion of biological warfare (or of other activities prohibited under the BWC) will trigger a more rigorous and systematic process of international oversight.

[7] Woodall, J. P., Personal communication, Dec. 1990.

[8] For instance, the first known manifestation of the lethal African filoviruses (Marburg and Ebola viruses) was an outbreak in Germany in which 31 people became mysteriously ill, with 7 dying. The source of the outbreak was traced to infected monkeys imported for use in vaccine production (all monkeys died of the disease). Similarly, HIV (probably also of African origin) was first recognized in the USA, where epidemiological surveillance detected a cluster of unusual cases of *Pneumocystis* pneumonia and Kaposi's sarcoma.

[9] Wheelis, M. L., 'The role of epidemiology in strengthening the Biological Weapons Convention', eds E. Geissler and R. H. Haynes, *Prevention of a Biological and Toxin Arms Race and the Responsibility of Scientists* (Akademie Verlag: Berlin, 1991), pp. 277–83.

II. Relationship to the Vaccines for Peace programme

The Vaccines for Peace (VFP) programme is an initiative proposed by Erhard Geissler[10] simultaneously with the proposal for the GESS made by the present author. It proposes that vaccine development and production be placed under the supervision of the WHO and sited in the developing world or in the states of the former Soviet Union, when the vaccines are directed against 'dual-threat' organisms: organisms that are both public health problems and potential biological warfare agents. The benefits of such a system are potentially numerous: elimination of the suspicion that necessarily attends military development of vaccines, and hence more secure and stable biological arms control; peaceful technology transfer to the developing world; public health benefits from wider availability of vaccines and productive employment of scientists and technicians from former Soviet BW laboratories (giving them an alternative to continued employment as weapon developers in other states).

The VFP programme and the GESS are both multilateral public health initiatives that would make a significant contribution to arms control; they are thus largely compatible, indeed complementary initiatives. There is, of course, a possibility that they will compete for the same resources (personnel or money), and some care will have to be taken to ensure that neither is pressed forward in an overly ambitious manner, to the detriment of the other. However, with care and co-ordination it should be possible to implement both initiatives in an effective manner.

In the arena of arms control, both initiatives seek to reduce the uncertainty surrounding biological arms development and use. The VFP programme would remove vaccine development from military control, and thus reduce the suspicion that such development might have an offensive function. The GESS would make the natural origin of most disease outbreaks clear, and thereby reduce the suspicion that some epidemics might be deliberate, or the accidental result of prohibited weapons development. Both would contribute to the stability of the BWC, whose lack of verification provisions makes it quite vulnerable to the corrosive effects of suspicion.

There is another way in which these initiatives bolster the BWC. As with a number of multilateral arms control treaties in which a major objective is to reduce arms proliferation, the BWC offers the promise of international co-operation and technology transfer as an inducement to forgo the development and possession of biological weapons. Article X states in part:

> The States Parties to this Convention undertake to facilitate, and have the right to participate in, the fullest possible exchange of equipment, materials and scientific and technological information for the use of bacteriological (biological) agents and toxins for peaceful purposes. Parties to the Convention in a position to do so shall also cooperate in contributing individually or together with other States or international organizations to the further development and application of scientific discoveries in the field of bacteriology (biology) for prevention of disease, or for other peaceful purposes.

[10] Geissler, E., 'Vaccines for Peace: an international program of development and use of vaccines against dual-threat agents', *Politics and the Life Sciences*, vol. 11, no. 2 (Aug. 1992), pp. 231–43.

As with similar commitments in other treaties, there has been little progress in implementing Article X of the BWC, with the predictable result that many developing nations have not become parties to it, and many of those that are States Parties have not participated in the periodic Review Conferences or the information exchanges designed to increase confidence in the level of treaty compliance.[11] Among those that have participated in the Review Conferences, the notable lack of implementation of Article X has been an issue of great importance.[12] There are probably additional, less obvious consequences; the cavalier attitude of the developed countries towards their obligation under the BWC to co-operate in the peaceful applications of microbiology invites a similar attitude from the developing nations towards their non-proliferation commitment. Substantial efforts to implement Article X might therefore be quite important. Both the GESS and the VFP programme do this in a dramatic and highly visible way.

The GESS and the VFP programme address complementary areas: disease detection and disease prevention. Accurate, world-wide epidemiological information is essential to a rational vaccine development strategy: to help decide which organisms pose the most significant public health and military threats; their range of antigenic variation; the frequency and locations of emergence of new strains; whether humans or reservoir populations should be immunized and so on. For instance, influenza vaccines change yearly, based on epidemiological information on the strains that appear to present the most serious immediate hazard. Similarly, epidemiological surveillance is being used to monitor the efficacy of the European attempt to control rabies by vaccination of wild populations of host animals. It is worth remembering that the vaccination strategies used so successfully in the campaign to eradicate smallpox were predicated on the known epidemiology of the disease, and required an effective (albeit primitive) mechanism of global epidemiological surveillance for smallpox cases.[13]

[11] Geissler, E., 'The first three rounds of information exchanges', ed. E. Geissler, *Strengthening the Biological Weapons Convention by Confidence-Building Measures,* SIPRI Chemical & Biological Warfare Studies, no. 10 (Oxford University Press: Oxford, 1990), pp. 71–79.

[12] For instance, the final documents of all three BWC Review Conferences (1980, 1986 and 1991) contain nearly identical wording in the section discussing Article X that says in part 'The Conference emphasizes the increasing importance of the provisions of Article X, especially in the light of recent scientific and technological developments . . . which have vastly increased the potential for cooperation between States to help promote economic and social development, and scientific and technological progress, particularly in the developing countries, in conformity with their interests, needs and priorities. The Conference, while acknowledging what has already been done towards this end, notes with concern the increasing gap between the developed and the developing countries in the field of biotechnology, genetic engineering, microbiology and other related areas. The Conference urges all States Parties actively to promote international cooperation and exchange with States Parties in the peaceful uses of biotechnology, and urges the developed countries possessing advanced biotechnology to adopt positive measures to promote technological transfer and international cooperation on an equal and non-discriminatory basis . . .' (Third Review Conference of the Parties to the Convention on the Prohibition of the Development, Production and Stockpiling of Bacteriological (Biological) and Toxin Weapons, and on their Destruction, *Final Document*, part II, *Final Declaration*, BWC/CONF.III/23, 27 Sep. 1991, p. 21. That the States Parties could leave this wording largely unchanged over the course of three successive reviews of performance is an indication of the lack of effective implementation of the provisions of this article.

[13] See Fenner, chapter 18, in this volume; Fenner, F., Henderson, D. A., Arita, I., Jezek, Z. and Ladnyi, I. D., *Smallpox and Its Eradication* (World Health Organization: Geneva, 1988).

III. Conclusion and recommendations

The VFP programme and the GESS are complementary initiatives in global public health and weapons control. They are closely related in their broad goals and in their implementation strategies. Both should be implemented by the international community, under the aegis of the United Nations, in a co-ordinated fashion. Both should be implemented in such a way as to maximize their contribution to global public health, national development and weapons control.

In implementing the VFP programme, the list of dual-threat agents should not be restricted to the agents that have traditionally been identified as potential military biological warfare agents. The recognition of the threat posed by clandestine use for destabilization or harassment of a non-belligerent state, or among subnational groups involved in civil wars or ethnic separatist movements, implies that the list of potential biological warfare agents is much broader than traditionally defined. In addition to including non-lethal human pathogens, it would include plant and animal agents as well.[14]

[14] Meryl Nass has made a plausible case for the use of anthrax by the Rhodesian forces of Ian Smith against cattle (with attendant human cases as well) in guerrilla-controlled territory. See Nass, M., 'Anthrax epizootic in Zimbabwe, 1978–80: due to deliberate spread?', *Physicians for Social Responsibility Quarterly*, vol. 2, no. 6 (Dec. 1992), pp. 198–209, a possible example of both the use of an animal pathogen and of use in a civil conflict. Another example of the possible use of an animal agent is the swine fever epidemic among Cuban pigs in 1971, an epidemic attributed by the Cuban Government, with some corroboration by the US investigative press, to hostile action by the USA, see Fetherston, D. and Cummings, J., 'Cuban outbreak of swine fever linked to CIA', *Newsday*, 9 Jan. 1977, p. 5.

Part V. International programmes for prevention of disease

18. The WHO global smallpox eradication programme: vaccine supply and variola virus stocks

FRANK FENNER

I. Introduction

There is sometimes confusion between the virus that caused smallpox and the virus used to control it. This chapter is therefore prefaced with a few explanatory comments. Smallpox was a disease caused by a virus referred to by virologists as variola virus (incidentally, the past tense is used because the disease is extinct). The terms smallpox virus and variola virus are synonyms. The other virus to be discussed here is vaccinia virus, which is a different virus but one which is related to variola virus. It is essentially a brother virus, another species in the same genus. In this respect, the original vaccine, developed by Edward Jenner in 1796, is different from all the other viral vaccines—poliovaccine, measles vaccine, yellow fever vaccine, and so on. These vaccines are attenuated variants of the virulent disease-causing viruses. Vaccinia, on the other hand, is a different virus from variola virus, and was first derived from lesions on cows (which cannot be infected with variola virus). Jenner's great discovery was to show that inoculation in the skin with material from the skin lesion of a person infected with this cow virus gave protection against smallpox.

Variola virus as a dual-threat and single-threat agent

Until the eradication of smallpox, variola virus was a dual-threat agent. A group of WHO consultants to the United Nations report on chemical and bacteriological weapons[1] commented as follows:

> Because of the effectiveness of the vaccine and the relative ease with which it can be produced and administered, it is unlikely that smallpox virus would be used as an agent for a large-scale biological attack against countries systematically practising periodic vaccination.
>
> The variola virus, however, can easily be employed for acts of sabotage. Such acts, at selected points within a country, could have serious socio-economic effects unless efficiently dealt with by the public service.[2]

Variola virus is now a unique 'single-threat agent', because since 1978 it has never caused a case of smallpox, but since no country is now 'systematically practising periodic vaccination' [against smallpox], it could be used quite effectively as an orthodox biological weapon agent. More likely, however, would be its clandestine use, for terrorism. The kind of impact that it might have, if so used, can be gauged from some experiments carried out in the United States in

[1] United Nations, *Chemical and Bacteriological (Biological) Weapons and the Effects of their Possible Use*, UN Report S/9292/Rev.1 (United Nations: New York, 1969).

[2] World Health Organization, *Health Aspects of Chemical and Biological Weapons: Report of a WHO Group of Consultants* (World Health Organization: Geneva, 1970), pp. 69–70.

1964 and 1965 and made public in 1984.[3] Tests were made with aerosols containing *Bacillus subtilis* as a marker, secretly disseminated in a crowded airport in Washington, DC. The idea was to test the possibility that variola virus might be released in this way and thus cause 'inexplicable' cases or outbreaks of smallpox a few weeks later in the diverse local and overseas places to which the infected passengers travelled, a result that would cause much public alarm.

The persistence of the idea that variola virus might be used for biological warfare between armies is reflected in the long period during which military personnel of several nations continued to be vaccinated against smallpox after civilian vaccination had ceased in most countries in 1981, and in all countries by 1985. At least until the end of 1991 smallpox vaccination was still the policy of the US armed forces and, according to a leading expert in that field, presumably also of the Soviet armed forces.[4] The possibility of the clandestine use of variola virus emphasizes the need for 'military' as well as microbiological security in laboratories holding variola virus stocks, as is discussed below.

II. The early history of vaccination

Immunization against smallpox has a long history. It began with variolation (i.e., inoculation with smallpox virus itself), used in China and India since about the 11th century and spreading to Europe early in the 18th century. In 1796 Edward Jenner, who had himself been variolated as a child and as a physician practised variolation, carried out his classic experiments with cowpox virus.[5] This new method of immunization—called vaccination to denote its association with the cow (*vacca*)—spread around the world with remarkable speed, a fact that attests to the widespread and justified fear of smallpox and the severe nature of the skin lesions produced by variolation, to say nothing of the cases of smallpox that it sometimes caused in contacts and the occasional death it caused in those inoculated (1–2 per cent of inoculations). Within three years of its publication in 1798, Jenner's pamphlet had been translated into five languages; by 1802 vaccination had been adopted throughout the Western world of the time. Vaccine had also been successfully sent to Bombay, and by 1805 it had been introduced into the Spanish and Portuguese colonies in China, the Philippines and South America.

Until the second half of the 19th century smallpox vaccine was maintained by human-to-human passage, usually in children. This practice had not infrequently transmitted syphilis as well,[6] and at least one well-reported outbreak of what is now recognized as hepatitis B.[7] It was therefore a great advance when first

[3] Young, S. and Lenarcic, A., 'Army conducted germ warfare tests in Washington's National Airport', *Freedom*, Dec. 1984, pp. 1–3; Cole, L. A., *Clouds of Secrecy: The Army's Germ Warfare Tests over Populated Areas* (Rowman & Littlefield: Totowa, N.J., 1988).

[4] Dalrymple, J. M., 'DoD-sponsored virus vaccine development: an investigator's perspective', ed. R. A. Zilinskas, *The Microbiologist and Biological Defense Research: Ethics, Politics and International Security*, Annals of the New York Academy of Sciences, vol. 666 (1992), pp. 202–17, see particularly p. 212.

[5] Jenner, E., *An Inquiry into the Causes and Effects of the Variolae Vaccinae, a Disease Discovered in Some of the Western Counties of England, Particularly Gloucestershire, and Known by the Name of the Cow Pox* (London, 1798), reprinted in Camac, C. N. B. (ed.), *Classics of Medicine and Surgery* (Dover: New York, 1959), pp. 213–40.

[6] Grön, K., 'Syphilis-Endemien', ed. J. Jadassohn, *Handbuch der Haut- und Geschlechtskrankheiten*, vol. 17/3 (Springer: Berlin, 1928), pp. 283–350.

[7] Lürman, (–), 'Eine Icterusepidemie', *Berliner klinische Wochenschrift*, vol. 22 (1885), pp. 20–23.

the Italians, then the French and finally the health services of all other countries successfully produced smallpox vaccine by passage on the skin of cows.[8]

By 1950 endemic smallpox had been eliminated from most countries in Europe and North America by the systematic use of liquid vaccine produced by scarification of the skin of cows. However, in tropical countries liquid vaccine was not sufficiently heat stable under the conditions then obtaining. Tests with liquid vaccine revealed a take rate of only 27 per cent in India and 7–20 per cent in central Africa. The next major advance came in the early 1950s, when a commercially practicable method of freeze-drying was introduced.[9]

The WHO standards for smallpox vaccine

In 1958 WHO standards were developed for vaccine potency, heat stability and bacterial content (bacterial contamination was inevitable because most vaccine was produced in animal skin). These standards were revised and strengthened in 1965 and remained in force throughout the Intensified Smallpox Eradication Programme (see below). In the 1965 revision, the initial potency was set at 10^8 pock-forming units per ml (since pock counting on the chorioallantoic membrane of the developing chicken egg was and remained the usual method of assay of vaccinia virus), maintenance of minimal acceptable potency (10^8 pock-forming units per ml of the reconstituted vaccine) after heating for 4 weeks at 37°C, and a bacterial count of <500 per ml, with no pathogenic bacteria.

III. The WHO Smallpox Eradication Programme, 1959–66

After an unsuccessful attempt in 1953 by the first Director-General of the WHO, Dr Brock Chisholm, to persuade the World Health Assembly to accept a proposal for the global eradication of smallpox, a proposal made by the Soviet Union in 1958 was accepted.[10] As outlined in the planning document submitted by the Soviet scientists, the proposed strategy relied entirely on vaccination, using freeze-dried vaccine in such a way as to vaccinate or revaccinate 80 per cent of the population within a period of four to five years. It was thought that such a programme would so enhance herd immunity to smallpox that all chains of transmission would be interrupted.

With acceptance of the Soviet proposal by the World Health Assembly in 1959, freeze-dried vaccine was supplied to many developing countries, through bilateral programmes (mostly with the Soviet Union) or through the WHO, and many of the larger endemic countries produced freeze-dried vaccine themselves. This programme was successful in eliminating smallpox from several countries in Asia and South America and north Africa (see table 18.1). A largely unheralded success, since it was then outside the UN system, was the eradication of smallpox from the People's Republic of China during the period 1950–65.[11] However by 1966 it was clear that the '80 per cent vaccination'

[8] Fenner, F. *et al.*, *Smallpox and its Eradication* (World Health Organization: Geneva, 1988), pp. 265–67.

[9] See Fenner *et al.* (note 8), pp. 286–89.

[10] See Fenner *et al.* (note 8), pp. 366–71.

[11] See Fenner *et al.* (note 8), pp. 339–43.

Table 18.1. Countries believed to have endemic smallpox in 1959 and 1967: summary by continent

	Countries with endemic smallpox in 1959[a]		Countries with endemic smallpox in 1967[b]	
Continent	Number	Population (thousands)	Number	Population (thousands)
Africa	34	198 490	23	215 914
Americas	6	115 198	1	88 737
Asia	19	1 421 233	7	774 124
Total endemic	**59**	**1 734 921**	**31**	**1 078 775**
World population		2 958 143		3 463 145

[a] 59% of world population living in endemic areas
[b] 31% of world population living in endemic areas

Source: Fenner, F. *et al.*, *Smallpox and its Eradication* (World Health Organization: Geneva, 1988), p. 395, courtesy of the World Health Organization.

strategy would never succeed in eliminating smallpox from the densely populated countries of the Indian subcontinent, for reasons first clearly enunciated by Arita *et al.*[12] Attainment of even an 80 per cent vaccination rate was very difficult in such countries and in many countries of sub-Saharan Africa, and attainment of higher rates was impractical—some other strategy was needed if global eradication was to be achieved.

IV. The WHO Intensified Smallpox Eradication Programme, 1967–80

During 1966 a new strategic plan was developed by Donald A. Henderson and Dr Isao Arita, working in the WHO Headquarters in Geneva, with two principal operational components: (*a*) mass vaccination with freeze-dried vaccine of assured quality, followed up by assessment of the success of vaccination by special teams; and (*b*) the development of a surveillance system for the detection and investigation of cases and the containment of outbreaks. In contrast to the 1959 programme, a commitment for continuing research was built into the Intensified Programme, which was supervised and co-ordinated by a small Smallpox Eradication Unit located at the WHO Headquarters in Geneva and with direct access to the Director-General.

V. Assuring the quality of vaccine

In any immunization programme it is clearly of the utmost importance to use potent vaccine; it is worse than useless (because it gives a false sense of security) to use vaccine with too low a content of viable virus to immunize. One of the first initiatives of the Smallpox Eradication Unit was therefore to devise ways of assuring that enough vaccine was available in every country requiring

[12] Arita, I., Wickett, J. and Fenner, F., 'Impact of population density on immunization programmes', *Journal of Hygiene* (Cambridge), vol. 96 (1986), pp. 459–66.

it, and that all vaccine used in the programme came up to WHO standards of quality.

Financing the programme

The budget of the Intensified Programme was set by the World Health Assembly at $2.4 million a year for 10 years. Before the programme began, it was estimated that about 300 million persons would need to be vaccinated annually in the endemic countries and countries adjacent to them. Thus even at the low cost of 1–2 US cents per dose and assuming no wastage, the vaccine alone would cost US $3-6 million, significantly exceeding the budget if the WHO provided all the vaccine required. Fortunately three other sources of vaccine were available: (*a*) production in endemic countries; (*b*) donations to the WHO by producer countries; and (*c*) vaccine supplied to developing countries through bilateral aid programmes. It was therefore decided to expand these sources so that no vaccine needed to be purchased out of the regular budget, which was used for maintaining the small central Smallpox Eradication Unit and for technical assistance, consultants, training and research and equipment, including transport.

Shortfalls in vaccine quality and quantity

When the actual situation was assessed it turned out that the WHO was faced, not with the relatively small problem of closing what was thought to be a small gap between the total requirement and supplies obtained from existing vaccine donors and existing local production in endemic countries, but with the much larger task of developing a production–donation system to serve most of the endemic countries and their neighbours. Further, the only vaccine subjected to quality-control testing by an authority independent of the producer was the small amount of vaccine supplied through the WHO, which was at that time seven million doses per year. The problems of quantity and quality control were compounded by the complicated and slow methods then used for testing vaccine and for shipping it from producer to recipient countries, since the WHO had no supplies of vaccine for immediate shipment in an emergency. The administrative problems were overcome when distribution was centralized through the Smallpox Eradication Unit in Geneva, but there remained problems of unknown dimensions in relation to both the quantity and quality of vaccine.

The WHO survey of vaccine producers

To provide a factual basis for introducing the changes needed to ensure that sufficient quantities of vaccine of suitable quality were available for the global eradication programme, a questionnaire was sent world-wide to all current or planned production facilities for freeze-dried vaccine. This requested information on the method of freeze-drying, the strain of vaccinia virus used, the number of doses in each vial or ampoule and the results of recent quality-control tests for potency, heat stability and bacterial content. Of 77 production laboratories contacted in 52 countries, 59 laboratories in 44 countries replied. The results of this initial survey were as set out below.

Methods of vaccine production

It was found that vaccinia virus was harvested from the skin of calves in 39 laboratories, from sheep in 12, and from water buffaloes in 6. In 3 laboratories smallpox vaccine was produced on the chorioallantoic membrane of developing eggs and 3 laboratories used tissue culture; some laboratories used more than one method. The survey showed that animal skin was by far the most extensively used method throughout the world, including both developing countries and countries such as the former Soviet Union, the United Kingdom and the United States. In 1967 tissue-culture methods had long been in use for poliovaccine production and inoculation of chick embryos for the production of yellow fever vaccine, both methods of preparing vaccines free of bacterial contamination. However, the Smallpox Eradication Unit took the pragmatic view that because of the urgency of the programme and the difficulty of quickly introducing a new method, especially in developing countries, it would encourage all producers to use the method of smallpox vaccine production that they were used to (in most cases scarification of calves or sheep), if necessary improving its performance.

Strains of vaccinia virus

By 1967 smallpox vaccine had been in use all over the world for over 150 years, so it was inevitable that many different strains of vaccinia virus were being used, although several strains with different names might have had a common origin and several with the same name had different passage histories and different biological properties. In 1968 a survey showed that 19 differently designated strains, plus 9 strains of unknown origin, were being used in 71 production laboratories. If there were questions from producers, the WHO recommended the use of either the Lister strain or the New York City Board of Health strain; by 1971 40 laboratories were using the Lister strain, seed virus being supplied by the International Reference Centre in the Netherlands, and 4 laboratories (all in the Americas) were using the New York City Board of Health strain.

Number of doses per container

Since it was much less expensive to freeze-dry vaccine in large containers, it was found that most producers used vials containing about 100, or even 500 doses. Such containers posed major logistic problems for field staff since reconstituted vaccine in large ampoules was either kept for a prolonged period, with consequent deterioration in quality, or in sparsely populated rural areas, discarded after use of only a few doses, thus wasting large quantities of a scarce resource.

Vaccine quality

Information was also sought on the initial potency, heat stability and bacterial contamination of the last three batches of vaccine. Many producers did not supply data on one or more of these tests. The results obtained from producers who did reply are shown in tables 18.2, 18.3 and 18.4; they represent the results of assays by the producers themselves, not by an independent testing authority.

In all categories, the results were not encouraging. Only 31 of 59 reporting laboratories reported that the initial potency met WHO standards in all three batches, and only 16 of 59 laboratories recorded satisfactory results for heat stability on all three batches (see tables 18.2 and 18.3).

Of the 50 lots for which a bacterial count of zero (per ml) was recorded, 10 were produced on the chorioallantoic membrane or in tissue culture, in three countries. All the other batches were produced in animal skin; 12 were unsatisfactory by WHO standards (see table 18.4).

VI. The WHO Reference Centres for Smallpox Vaccine

From these results it was clear that the WHO needed a mechanism for the periodic testing of vaccine supplied to the eradication programme, whether by donation to the WHO, through bilateral assistance agreements or by local production in endemic countries. Since the WHO does not operate laboratories, contractual arrangements were made with the Connaught Laboratories in Toronto, Canada, for the Americas, and with the National Institute of Public Health at Bilthoven, the Netherlands, for the rest of the world.

The two International Reference Centres undertook to provide the following services: (*a*) to test smallpox vaccines submitted to the WHO from different production laboratories, (*b*) on the basis of the results of tests and special studies, to advise appropriately on the improvement of vaccine production methods, (*c*) to collect, maintain and study strains of vaccinia virus from different parts of the world, (*d*) to provide seed virus and national reference vaccine when required, (*e*) to conduct research which could contribute to the improvement of vaccine production and testing methodology, and (*f*) to train virologists in the production and testing of smallpox vaccine.

Shortly after the survey just described, 20 laboratories in 20 different countries submitted samples of their vaccine to the Bilthoven centre for testing. Six of these laboratories were producing vaccine intended for use in the programme, through donation to the WHO or as bilateral assistance; 14 laboratories supplied material manufactured in experimental production runs. The results were disturbing (see table 18.5).

Of the 35 batches actually proposed for use in the eradication programme, 22 failed the initial potency or heat-stability requirements, and some of these batches came from potential donors in industrialized countries. Of the 39 batches from producers intending to develop freeze-dried vaccine for use in their own (endemic) countries, 25 failed to meet WHO requirements.

Table 18.2. Initial potency of three production lots of vaccine, 1967

Continent	Number reporting	Three lots satisfactory	Some lots satisfactory	No lots satisfactory	Rabbit skin only (unsatisfactory assay)
Africa	8	4	2	1	1
Americas	12	6	4	1	1
Asia[a] and Oceania	13	9	2	1	1
Europe	20	12	6	–	2
Total	**53**	**31**	**14**	**3**	**5**

– = Nil
[a] Excluding the People's Republic of China

Source: Fenner, F. *et al.*, *Smallpox and its Eradication* (World Health Organization: Geneva, 1988), p. 546, courtesy of the World Health Organization.

Table 18.3. Heat stability (4 weeks at 37°C) of three production lots of vaccine, 1967

Continent	Number reporting	Three lots satisfactory	Some lots satisfactory	No lots satisfactory
Africa	7	2	1	3
Americas	7	2	2	3
Asia[a] and Oceania	9	5	3	1
Europe	17	7	5	5
Total	**40**	**16**	**11**	**12**

[a] Excluding the People's Republic of China

Source: Fenner, F. *et al.*, *Smallpox and its Eradication* (World Health Organization: Geneva, 1988), p. 546, courtesy of the World Health Organization.

Table 18.4. Bacterial counts of three production lots of vaccine, 1967

			Bacterial count per ml[a]				
Continent	Number reporting	Number of batches	0	1–9	10–99	100–499	>500[b]
Africa	8	19	2	–	2	12	3
Americas	12	31	22	2	2	2	3
Asia[c] and Oceania	13	33	7	3	10	10	3
Europe	20	55	19	5	14	14	3
Total	**53**	**138**	**50**	**10**	**28**	**38**	**12**

– = Nil
[a] Viable non-pathogenic bacteria
[b] Unacceptable by WHO standards
[c] Excluding the People's Republic of China

Source: Fenner, F. *et al.*, *Smallpox and its Eradication* (World Health Organization: Geneva, 1988), p. 547, courtesy of the World Health Organization.

Table 18.5. Testing of production batches by the International Reference Centres, 1967

	Proposed for donation			Experimental production batches		
Continent	Number of producers	Number of batches	Number of batches unsatisfactory	Number of producers	Number of batches	Number of batches unsatisfactory
Africa	1	1	0	5	21	19
Americas	1	1	1	0	0	0
Asia[a]	2	11	9	3	6	4
Europe	2	22	12	6	12	2
Total	**6**	**35**	**22**	**14**	**39**	**25**

[a] Excluding the People's Republic of China

Source: Fenner, F. *et al.*, *Smallpox and its Eradication* (World Health Organization: Geneva, 1988), p. 549, courtesy of the World Health Organization.

VII. Development of improved vaccines

The finding that so much of the smallpox vaccine then in use was unsatisfactory called for urgent measures. The Smallpox Eradication Unit made a number of arrangements to overcome these problems: (*a*) organization of a Travelling Seminar on Vaccine Production and production of a comprehensive manual, *Methodology of Freeze-dried Smallpox Vaccine Manufacture*, (*b*) visits to production laboratories by WHO staff and consultants, (*c*) establishment of a reference vaccine, (*d*) production of seed lots of Lister strain by the International Reference Centre for Smallpox Vaccine at Bilthoven, (*e*) development of a rapid heat-stability test, and (*f*) regular checking of vaccine potency and stability by the WHO Reference Centres for Smallpox Vaccine.

Most of these procedures are self-explanatory, but the supply of seed lots of vaccine and the rapid heat-stability test require some explanation. Because of the great number of different strains of vaccinia virus initially in use and the unacceptable number of complications following the use of some of them, the Bilthoven Reference Laboratory supplied seed lots of Lister strain vaccine, which had a good history as a satisfactory vaccine strain, from which not more than five production runs were made before going back to another seed lot. The standard heat-stability test required four weeks exposure at 37°C, then a few days for the assay, and greatly delayed the provision of the results of vaccine testing. A rapid test was developed which proved equally satisfactory; namely, maintenance of a titre of $>10^{7.5}$ pock-forming units per ml after heating a vial of freeze-dried vaccine at 100°C for one hour.

It may not be appreciated now how revolutionary some of these proposals were in the 1960s, especially the proposal to test vaccine other than that donated to the WHO, for at that time UN agencies regarded national sovereignty as inviolate. The Intensified Smallpox Eradication Programme marked the first time in history that an effective world-wide quality-control programme for biological products had been established that looked at *all* vaccine used in the programme, both that produced locally and donated via bilateral programmes, as well as donations made through the WHO. Its global reach is indicated in figure 18.1.

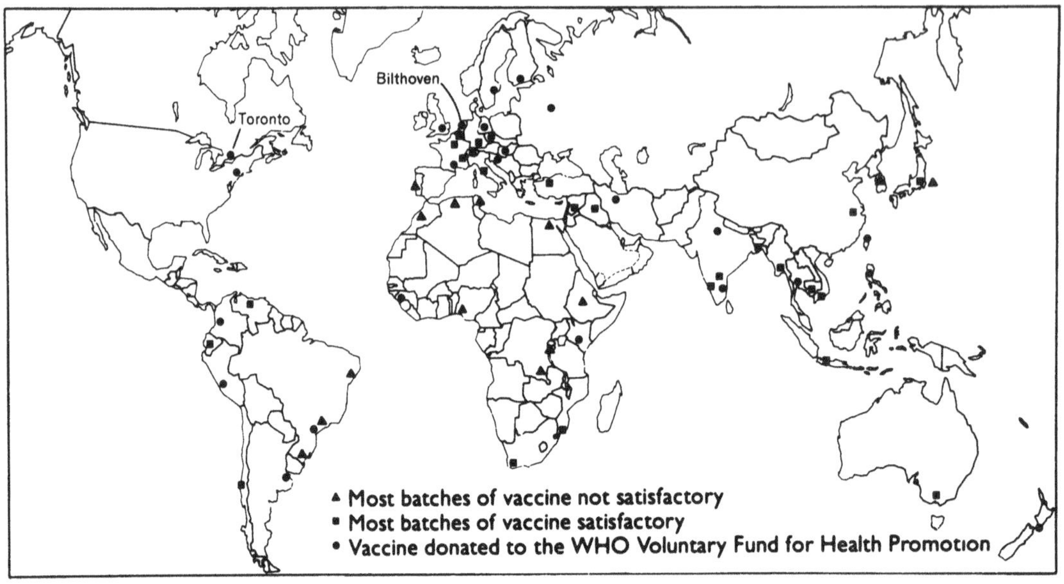

Figure 18.1. Locations of various categories of producers of freeze-dried smallpox vaccine, 1967–79; and of the WHO Reference Centre for Smallpox Vaccine for the Americas (Toronto, Canada) and the WHO International Reference Centre for Smallpox Vaccine (Bilthoven, the Netherlands).

Source: Fenner, F. *et al.*, *Smallpox and its Eradication* (World Health Organization: Geneva, 1988), p. 560, courtesy of the World Health Organization.

By 1969 these measures were in place, and there was a dramatic improvement in the quality of the vaccine, from 36 per cent satisfactory batches in 1967 to 78 per cent in 1969, and over 9 per cent from 1973 onwards (see table 18.6).

Vaccine production in endemic countries

Although in the interests of self-sufficiency many endemic countries wished to embark on the production of freeze-dried smallpox vaccine, the WHO could not afford the investment in manpower and training resources to offer assistance to all. Since vaccine production in a country with a population of less than 10 million would be uneconomic, it was rarely supported in small developing countries; Kenya, which became an exporter to its neighbours, was an exception. However, local production was essential in the large developing countries, and such countries produced very large amounts of vaccine (see table 18.7).

Donations of vaccine

Annually from 1967 to 1979 between 15 and 45 million doses of vaccine were dispatched by the WHO to endemic countries, in addition to the much larger quantities that were produced locally or donated through bilateral aid programmes. In all, 465 million doses of vaccine, worth US $8.5 million, were donated to the WHO for the Intensified Smallpox Eradication Programme, by 27 countries. The major donors were the former USSR (298 million doses),

Table 18.6. Results of quality-control testing by the International Reference Centres, 1967–80

Year	Number of producers	Number of batches	Number (%) of batches satisfactory	Number (%) of batches unsatisfactory	Unsatisfactory Initial potency	Unsatisfactory Heat stability	Unsatisfactory Bacterial count
1967	20	74	27 *(36)*	47 *(64)*	32	12	8
1968	23	136	74 *(54)*	62 *(46)*	26	36	5
1969	30	164	128 *(78)*	36 *(22)*	23	12	5
1970	27	380	312 *(82)*	68 *(18)*	27	35	13
1971	32	206	154 *(75)*	52 *(25)*	31	23	5
1972	27	311	241 *(77)*	70 *(23)*	32	39	1
1973	30	392	367 *(94)*	25 *(6)*	5	20	0
1974	28	231	199 *(86)*	32 *(14)*	11	20	1
1975	21	167	139 *(83)*	28 *(17)*	15	10	6
1976	16	213	203 *(95)*	10 *(5)*	2	7	3
1977	11	114	101 *(89)*	13 *(11)*	1	12	1
1978	9	59	57 *(97)*	2 *(3)*	0	2	0
1979	10	85	82 *(96)*	3 *(4)*	3	1	0
1980	5	46	46 *(100)*	0 *(–)*	0	0	0
Total		**2 578**	**2 130** ***(82.6)***	**448** ***(17.4)***	**208**	**229**	**48**

– = Nil

Source: Fenner, F. *et al.*, *Smallpox and its Eradication* (World Health Organization: Geneva, 1988), p. 560, courtesy of the World Health Organization.

Table 18.7. Smallpox vaccine production in densely populated endemic countries

Year	Production in thousands of doses: Bangladesh (70.4 million[a])	India (577.4 million[a])	Indonesia (126.2 million[a])
1966	..	21 223	..
1967	..	21 173	..
1968	..	34 675	7 506
1969	..	53 493	20 057
1970	..	42 398	22 149
1971	..	40 291	16 720
1972	8 585	52 853	7 377
1973	20 175	87 898	4 180
1974[b]	24 088	132 112	1 763
1975	18 254	141 364	..
1976	11 469	107 603	..
1977[c]	17 590	84 485	..

.. = Data not available or not applicable

[a] Population in 1972

[b] Indonesia certified smallpox-free

[c] Bangladesh and India certified smallpox-free

Source: Fenner, F. *et al.*, *Smallpox and its Eradication* (World Health Organization: Geneva, 1988), p. 563, courtesy of the World Health Organization.

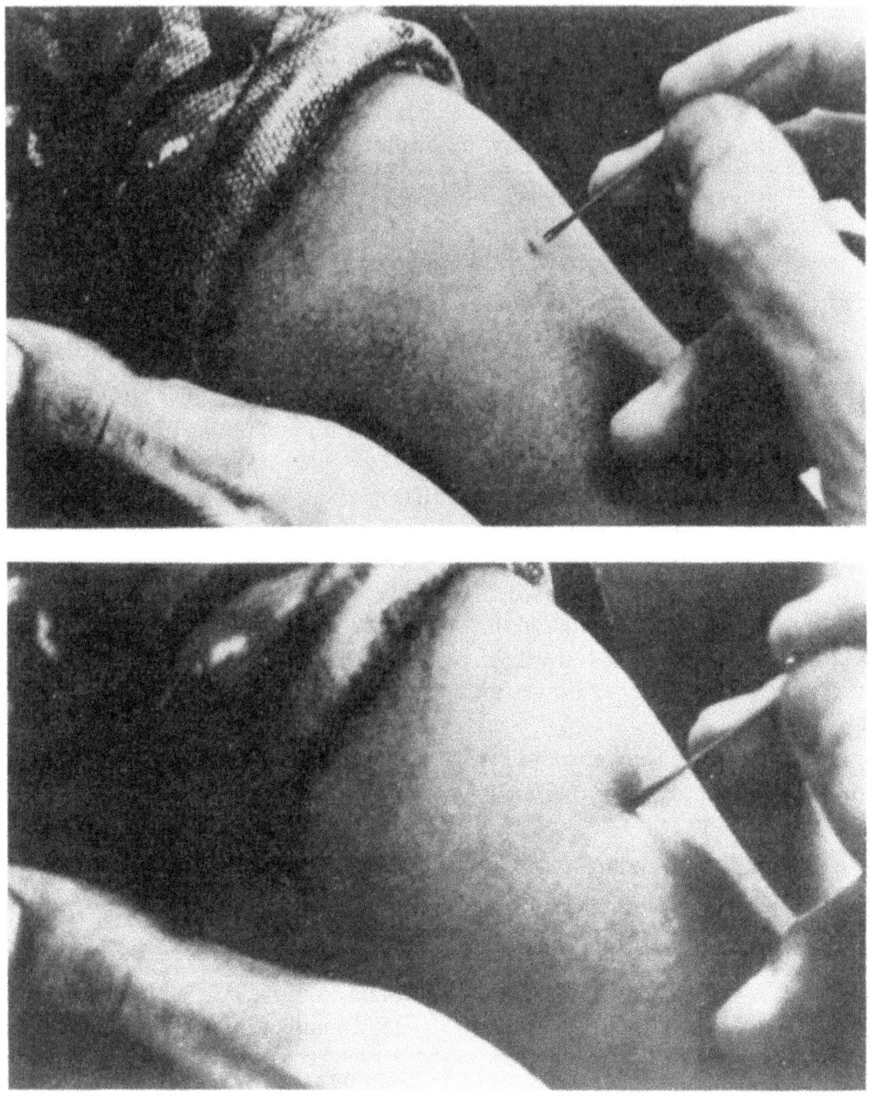

Figure 18.2. Vaccination with the bifurcated needle. The requisite amount of reconstituted vaccine (about one-quarter of the amount used in scratch or multiple-pressure vaccinations) is held between the prongs of the needle and vaccination done by multiple puncture. The procedure usually used consisted of 15 strokes, at right angles to the skin, over the deltoid muscle, in an area about 5 mm in diameter.

Source: Fenner, F. *et al.*, *Smallpox and its Eradication* (World Health Organization: Geneva, 1988), p. 570, courtesy of the World Health Organization.

Canada (41 million doses), Iran (26 million doses), Switzerland (18 million doses), India (15 million doses), Kenya (15 million doses), Belgium (13 million doses) and the Netherlands (11 million doses).

Although the bulk of the vaccine came through local production or bilateral aid programmes, the vaccine donated to the WHO was critical in ensuring that emergency requirements could be met. Between 1958 and 1966 there had been problems in effectively distributing the small amounts of vaccine that were donated to the WHO. These were resolved by centralizing distribution through the

Smallpox Eradication Unit, which rented cold-storage space in Geneva. Special arrangements were made over Christmas and Easter holidays to ensure that vaccine, if urgently required, could be sent on the earliest possible flight. Even so, there were difficulties when there were unexpected large demands, as occurred when smallpox spread across Iran, Iraq, Syria and into Yugoslavia in 1972. Although vaccine was usually sent from Geneva, donations to the WHO from Kenya were sent direct to other African countries, from Iran to Pakistan, and from India to Bangladesh, Nepal and Sri Lanka.

VIII. Methods of vaccination

Before 1967 vaccination was carried out either by a scratch method or by a multiple-pressure technique. During the Intensified Programme two new methods of vaccination were introduced: the jet injector and the bifurcated needle. The jet injector was used in early campaigns in Brazil and some countries in western and central Africa, but was inefficient unless large numbers of vaccinees were assembled in one place. Further, the machines were difficult to maintain, especially in rural areas of developing countries. They were little used after 1969, when the bifurcated needle (see figure 18.2) came into universal use. Besides its simplicity and efficiency, the bifurcated needle used only one-quarter as much vaccine as the traditional multiple-pressure method, and much vaccine was saved by using this method of vaccination and vials containing only a few doses when carrying out vaccinations in rural areas.

IX. Reasons for the success of the Intensified Smallpox Eradication Programme

A number of factors contributed to the success of the smallpox eradication campaign; those listed in table 18.8 were important. From the current point of view, the provision of adequate supplies of high-quality vaccine at the site of use was clearly of major importance. Smallpox vaccine was unique among vaccines in being unusually heat stable so that cold chain requirements were much less critical than for many other vaccines. Also, it could be administered very efficiently with a bifurcated needle, thus obviating the need for syringes and needles.

Application of these lessons to other immunization programmes

The WHO Expanded Programme on Immunization (EPI) is a direct outcome of the smallpox programme, and was conceived by Dr D. A. Henderson, then Chief of the Intensified Smallpox Eradication Programme, in 1974, when it seemed likely that smallpox eradication would be achieved, and there was the potential of using for other health programmes the many health workers, at all levels, who had served in the smallpox programme. It was approved by the World Health Assembly in 1977. As a result of an intensive effort by the WHO to set up vaccine delivery systems, supported by the contributions from the United Nations Children's Fund (UNICEF) to vaccine procurement, the vacci-

Table 18.8. Biological and socio-political features of smallpox that made its global eradication possible

Type of feature	Characteristics
Biological	It was a very serious disease, with high mortality and serious after-effects.
	Because of the characteristic rash, cases were easily recognized.
	There were very few subclinical cases.
	Cases did not become infectious until the onset of the rash, which was a day or so after the onset of fever, so that control by containment and ring vaccination was possible.
	Recurrent infectivity was unknown.
	There was only one serotype.
	An effective heat-stable vaccine was available.
	There was no animal reservoir of variola virus.
Socio-political	Earlier country-wide elimination demonstrated that global eradication was an attainable objective.
	There were few social or religious barriers to the recognition of cases (compare sexually transmitted diseases).
	The costs of quarantine arrangements and vaccination of travellers provided a strong incentive for wealthy, smallpox-free countries to assist financially.
	The WHO Smallpox Eradication Unit had inspired and inspiring leaders and enlisted devoted health workers.
	The Smallpox Eradication Unit ensured that adequate supplies of high-quality vaccine were always available.

nation coverage in most developing countries increased from less than 5 per cent in 1980 to about 80 per cent in 1992. In September 1990, at the Children's Summit, the United Nations launched the Children's Vaccine Initiative (CVI).

The person responsible for establishing the smallpox vaccine quality-control regime just described was Dr Isao Arita, who was a member of the Smallpox Eradication Unit from its inception and Chief from 1977 to 1985. After serving as Director of the National Hospital at Kumamoto for several years, he now devotes himself full time to a small Japanese non-governmental organization called the Agency for Cooperation in International Health (ACIH). Among its main projects is an effort to introduce into the EPI and the CVI the same standards of attention to all vaccine, not only that procured through UNICEF, so that sufficient quantities of certified high-quality vaccines can be provided on a global scale, as was achieved during the smallpox eradication campaign. The author of this chapter attended the two small meetings on this matter that the ACIH held in April 1991 and August 1992, and the value of this approach, supported by financial help from international and national donor agencies, seems apparent. It is essential that some such plan should be established for the EPI and similar global immunization programmes, and any contribution that the ideas developed at the Biesenthal meeting can make to ensuring the provision of adequate quantities of high-quality vaccines is of the utmost importance.

X. The use of variola virus as a biological warfare agent

The elimination of smallpox in countries and regions was followed up, after an interval of not less than two years after the last known case, by 'certification of eradication', a process carried out by visits to the countries or countries concerned by independent international teams of experts, called International Commissions for the Certification of Smallpox Eradication. In all there were 22 such Commissions and they operated between 1973 (South America) and 1979 (Somalia). All countries visited made intensive efforts during the two years that followed the 'last known case' to ensure that there were no hidden pockets of continuing transmission, and members of each Commission made extensive visits to critical areas. Eventually all the International Commission reports were examined by the Global Commission for the Certification of Smallpox Eradication, which after a preliminary meeting in 1977 met again in 1978, and in December 1979 issued its Final Report, with 19 recommendations for post-eradication strategies.[13] The report and all its recommendations were endorsed without change by the World Health Assembly in May 1980.

The International Commissions in various countries paid special attention to laboratories doing diagnostic or poxvirus research work, asking whether they held stocks of variola virus. In 1975, to supplement these enquiries, the Smallpox Eradication Unit distributed a questionnaire to laboratories around the world requesting information on holdings of variola virus stocks, with a request that unless there were special reasons, all such stocks should be destroyed. The response was both disturbing, in that in 1975 no fewer than 75 laboratories replied that they held such stocks, and encouraging, in that the number had dropped to 18 two years later (see table 18.9). However, it was difficult to feel that the situation was secure with variola virus stocks being held in 18 laboratories in as many different countries; much remained to be done.

After extensive correspondence and visits by the Smallpox Eradication Unit staff and consultants, by 1983 all laboratories had disposed of their virus stocks except the two major WHO Collaborating Centres, the Centers for Disease Control (CDC) in Atlanta, Georgia, USA and the Institute for Viral Preparations in Moscow, where they are stored in liquid nitrogen under conditions of microbiological and military security (see table 18.10). Some laboratories did not destroy their stocks but transferred them to the laboratory at the CDC. It was decided to retain stocks in the two WHO Collaborating Centres as an insurance policy; it was argued that if any disease resembling smallpox were ever to occur again, it would be useful to compare the virus isolated from such cases with a known strain of variola virus.

The destruction of the remaining stocks of variola virus

During the early 1980s scientists had cloned the DNA of several strains of variola virus in *Escherichia coli.* Because by this time comparison of restriction patterns had become the most reliable way of identifying orthopoxviruses, there

[13] World Health Organization, *The Global Eradication of Smallpox: Final Report of the Global Commission for the Certification of Smallpox Eradication,* History of International Public Health, no. 4 (World Health Organization: Geneva, 1980).

Table 18.9. Laboratories holding variola virus in 1975, and the reduction in numbers as of July 1977

	Number of countries		Number of laboratories		By July 1977	
WHO region	Information requested	Responded to WHO	Responded to WHO	Had variola virus in 1975	Disposed of virus	Retained virus
Africa	46	43	15	5	4	1
Americas	34	34	506	18	13	5
South-East Asia	11	11	57	13	13	0
Europe	36	36	185	29	19	10
Eastern Mediterranean	23	23	25	3	3	0
Western Pacific	31	29	35	6 (7)[a]	5	1 (2)[a]
Total	**181**	**176**	**823**	**74 (75)**	**57**	**17 (18)**

[a]Although China did not respond to the WHO letter of request, stocks of variola virus were then held at the Institute for the Control of Drugs and Biological Products, Beijing.

Source: Fenner, F. *et al.*, *Smallpox and its Eradication* (World Health Organization: Geneva, 1988), p. 1340, courtesy of the World Health Organization

Table 18.10. Laboratories holding variola virus stocks at the end of calendar years 1977–83

Continent	1977	1978	1979	1980	1981	1982	1983
Africa	1	1	1	1	1	1	0
America	5	3	2	1	1	1	1[a]
Asia	2	1	1	1	0	0	0
Europe	10	8	3	3	2	1	1[b]
Total	**18**	**13**	**7**	**6**	**4**	**3**	**2**

[a] WHO Collaborating Centre at the Centers for Disease Control, Atlanta, Georgia, USA
[b] WHO Collaborating Centre at the Moscow Research Institute for Viral Preparations

Source: Fenner, F. *et al.*, *Smallpox and its Eradication* (World Health Organization: Geneva, 1988), p. 1340, courtesy of the World Health Organization

was now no need to preserve strains of variola virus for comparison; the cloned variola virus DNA would serve this purpose just as well. In 1980 the WHO had set up a Committee on Orthopoxvirus Infections to oversee the implementation of the recommendations of the Global Commission on Smallpox Eradication. In 1986 this Committee recommended that all remaining stocks of variola virus (i.e., those at the CDC and at the Institute for Viral Preparations) should be destroyed, but that the international health community should be consulted before activating this recommendation.[14] Many responses were received, but no further action was taken by the WHO until December 1990, when another meeting of the same expert group, now with the status of an *Ad Hoc* Committee, was held.[15] By this time methods of rapid nucleotide sequencing were so advanced that this meeting recommended that all stocks of variola virus, and all clones of

[14] World Health Organization, 'Committee on Orthopoxvirus Infections: report of the fourth meeting', *Weekly Epidemiological Record*, vol. 61, no. 38 (Sep. 1986), pp. 289–93.
[15] World Health Organization, 'Post-smallpox eradication policies', *Weekly Epidemiological Record*, vol. 67, no. 1/2 (Jan. 1992), pp. 3–4.

variola virus DNA, should be destroyed, but that by the end of December 1993 four representative strains of variola virus should be sequenced. This operation, which is being carried out in the Collaborating Centres in Atlanta and Moscow, is proceeding well. However, another problem has now arisen. Some of the strains of variola virus in the repository at the CDC were deposited there in 1979 by the American Type Culture Collection (ATCC), on the understanding 'that the material would be preserved indefinitely, but would be returned [to ATCC] if CDC decided at some later date to abandon its programs on smallpox'. The ATCC is committed to the preservation of these (and all other) microbial cultures, and has twice brought its concerns about the possible destruction of its stock of variola virus to the attention of the CDC and the WHO. Resolution of this problem has been deferred until the final meeting of the *Ad Hoc* WHO Committee on Orthopoxvirus Infections, early in 1994.

Philosophical considerations regarding the 'eradication' of variola virus

During the meeting at Biesenthal the question was raised as to the morality of destroying any form of life, including variola virus. This was not a new question. The position of the present author is the same now as it was when the book *Smallpox and its Eradication* was written.

> From time to time commentators in scientific journals have questioned the moral rectitude of destroying all known stocks of variola virus, on the grounds that man should not knowingly cause the extinction of any living thing. With the cloning of variola virus DNA [or the sequencing of its DNA] this raises some interesting philosophical questions. Are variola virions, in an ampoule, 'living things'? In fact they are inert until their genetic potential can be expressed, and the only 'natural' form of living variola virus would be that found in an [infected] human being, since man was the only known host of the virus. Presumably, the periodic occurrence of cases of smallpox is not what conservationists have in mind when they argue that variola virus stocks should never be totally destroyed.
>
> . . .
>
> When viewed against the regrettable but wholesale extinction of species that results from human interventions in natural ecosystems, concern about the preservation of variola virus seems to us misplaced. The only criterion by which to judge the necessity for the preservation of the virus, we believe, is whether it is necessary for scientific work.[16]

Comments made during the Biesenthal meeting emphasized the real possibility that variola virus might be used for clandestine terrorism (state or 'private'). This adds another dimension to the request by the ATCC that its strains of variola virus should not be destroyed. If not destroyed, they will have to be maintained *forever*, and under conditions of microbiological *and military* security. By whom, and for how long? Logically, by the ATCC, alternatively, they could be kept at their current location at the CDC. In view of the fact that the virus stored in this way will remain forever in liquid nitrogen, could not the money required to preserve variola virus be better spent?

During 1993 there were further developments. In April 1993 the ATCC wrote to the CDC indicating that it would release the CDC from its obligation to

[16] See Fenner *et al.* (note 8), p. 1339.

maintain the variola virus strains deposited by the Collection, noting that 'the elimination of smallpox virus stocks should be considered a special case . . . and not a precedent for future decisions regarding retention or elimination of other organisms'. Following a round table discussion at the International Congress of Virology in Glasgow on 11 August 1993, in November the journal *Science* published a Policy Forum comprising two papers summarizing the views of prominent virologists supporting and opposing the destruction of the remaining variola virus stocks, and a few weeks later Nobel laureate David Baltimore published a letter supporting the case for destruction.[17]

At about the same time a short account was published outlining some of the significant findings emerging from the complete sequencing of the genome of an Asian variola virus strain;[18] the genome of another strain of variola major virus and that of one strain of variola minor virus have been almost completely sequenced. The proposed date of destruction, December 1993, was symbolic and designed to indicate the time available for the sequencing effort. The matter of whether and when destruction will be recommended by the WHO (rather than by one of its committees) is expected to be decided at the meeting of the World Health Assembly in May 1994.

XI. Summary

The Intensified Smallpox Eradication Programme is of particular relevance to the topics discussed in this volume. It provides an object lesson in the need, and the feasibility, of ensuring that all vaccine used in any immunization programme is potent. It also points up the difficulty of ensuring the provision of adequate amounts of high-quality vaccine for any global programme. Finally, it provides an example of the kind of problems to be faced if decisions are made to eliminate forever the risk of any particular microbe being available for use as an agent for biological warfare.

[17] Mahy, B. W. J. *et al.*, 'The remaining stocks of smallpox virus should be destroyed', *Science*, vol. 262 (1993), pp. 1223–24; Joklik, W. K. *et al.*, 'Why smallpox virus should not be destroyed', *Science*, vol. 262 (1993), pp. 1225–26; Baltimore, D., 'Smallpox virus stocks', *Science*, vol. 263 (1994), p. 13.

[18] Massung, R. F. *et al.*, 'Potential virulence determinants in terminal regions of variola smallpox virus genome', *Nature*, vol. 366 (1993), pp. 748–51.

19. Options for the development and transfer of vaccine technology

DEVAGUPTAPU SUBRAHMANYAM*

I. Introduction

This volume addresses the development of an international programme for the development and use of vaccines against dual-threat agents: agents that threaten the health of humankind during peace, and biological weapons (BW) that endanger populations during conflict. BW agents also include several pathogenic organisms that normally should be guarded against.[1] Some examples of these are dengue, influenza, Japanese encephalitis and yellow fever viruses, and bacteria such as *Salmonella typhi* and *Vibrio cholerae*. Furthermore, many of the antigens that are included as a 'core group' and as 'regional antigens' in children's vaccines could be used in biological warfare. This chapter is an overview of the current state of research and development (R&D) and production of vaccines against human pathogens and the need for a long-term strategy for making vaccines available to developing countries.

II. The role of the United Nations Industrial Development Organization

The pioneering efforts of United Nations agencies such as the World Health Organization and the United Nations Children's Fund (UNICEF) in this area are well known. The United Nations Industrial Development Organization (UNIDO) is involved in promoting these efforts owing to its mandate to assist the economic development of developing countries through industrialization. In this context, UNIDO pays special attention to industry's contribution to meeting the basic needs of the populations of the developing countries. One of the most basic needs is the improvement of health-care facilities. The Industrial Operations, Industrial Development and Promotion divisions of UNIDO, in particular, have actively promoted strengthening science and technology in developing countries, which UNIDO believes will have an impact on the improvement of health care. Accordingly, UNIDO established an Advisory Panel on Preventive Medicine in 1984 which periodically advises UNIDO on the technological and economic aspects of the establishment of a programme on industrial production of biologicals, including vaccines. UNIDO promoted the establishment of the International Centre for Genetic Engineering and Biotechnology (ICGEB) to strengthen the biotechnology capabilities of developing countries. This is vital for their involvement in producing new and improved vaccines. These initiatives are dealt with in greater detail below.

[1] Geissler, E., 'Vaccines for Peace: an international program of development and use of vaccines against dual-threat agents', *Politics and the Life Sciences*, vol. 11, no. 2 (Aug. 1992), pp. 231–43.

* The views expressed in this paper are those of the author and do not necessarily reflect the views of the Secretariat of the United Nations Industrial Development Organization.

III. Health-care problems in developing countries

Over 70 per cent of the world's population live in developing countries where more than 5 million children die each year, largely from measles, pertussis and neonatal tetanus. This figure increases to almost 14 million children if the other major causes of mortality are included such as diarrhoeas, lower respiratory infections, malaria, meningitis, tuberculosis and typhoid. In addition, these diseases cause disability to untold millions of children and prevent their normal development. Among the other infections that afflict the developing world are the parasitic diseases such as filariasis, leishmaniasis, schistosomiasis and trypanosomiasis. Most of these diseases also affect adults causing considerable morbidity and loss of man-hours. Many of these non-parasitic infections can be prevented by vaccines that are already available or at an advanced stage of development.[2] The development of vaccines for parasitic infections is still at the laboratory research level[3] or, in some cases, still at an early conceptual stage.

IV. International efforts for controlling infections through vaccination

Immunization is perhaps the most important, inexpensive, practical and cost-effective single tool to prevent the above infections. With the impetus gained from the eradication of smallpox,[4] the WHO, in collaboration with UNICEF and other international agencies, launched the Expanded Programme on Immunization (EPI) with the aim of immunizing 60 million children annually against six major causes of mortality: diphtheria, pertussis and tetanus (DPT), measles, polio and tuberculosis. According to the WHO, globally nearly 80 per cent of all children have been immunized against these diseases under the EPI. Estimates show that yearly the lives of two to three million children are saved by the EPI. This momentum should be maintained and improved upon. In addition, the WHO has pledged that polio will be eradicated by the year 2000. These objectives require a steady source of the relevant vaccines and the raising of adequate funds by UN agencies to meet the vaccine requirements of the next decade.

Currently, the vaccines needed to contain these infections are largely obtained from firms located in developed countries. Owing to low profitability, most vaccine-manufacturing firms in the developed countries have little interest in producing the vaccines needed for the EPI, let alone those needed by developing countries against regional-specific diseases. At present, the EPI obtains vaccines at reasonable prices by open bidding from the few manufacturers in Canada, Europe and Japan that still produce these vaccines. There is increasing concern that sooner or later, as profits dwindle, these few producers may review their policies and opt to produce more profitable vaccines. In addition, a few developing countries themselves manufacture vaccines against a limited range of infections in government-owned or supported companies and institutions.

[2] Warren, K., 'New scientific opportunities and old obstacles in vaccine development', *Proceedings of the National Academy of Sciences* (USA), vol. 83 (1986), pp. 9275–77.

[3] Playfair, J. W. L., Blackwell, J. M. and Miller, H. R. P., 'Modern vaccines: parasitic diseases', *The Lancet*, vol. 2 (1990), pp. 1263–66.

[4] See Fenner, chapter 18, in this volume.

V. The current vaccine-production scenario in the developing countries

Many countries in Asia[5] and Latin America[6] do manufacture vaccines, particularly some of those used in the EPI. In Asia, China and India have a long and good record of production of a few vaccines. India is currently involved in expanding production facilities for DPT, measles, polio and rabies vaccines with appropriate international collaborative agreements. Indonesia has also been successful to a limited extent; it produces DPT vaccine and plans to expand its output of this triple vaccine to meet increasing demand. Myanmar, Pakistan, the Philippines and Thailand make few of the EPI vaccines. Bangladesh, Malaysia, Singapore and Sri Lanka have practically no vaccine-manufacturing facilities.

In Latin America, 11 countries produce BCG (Bacille dilié de Calmette-Guérin, tuberculosis vaccine) and DPT vaccine, and three countries produce measles and polio vaccines. Brazil, Cuba, Mexico and Venezuela are among the major producers of a few of the EPI vaccines.

At their request, UNIDO has commissioned consultants to assist some countries in Asia and Latin America to review their vaccine requirements and production facilities. According to the consultants, none of the vaccine-producing countries is self-sufficient in the production of vaccines, even those used in the EPI. Over 50 developing countries receive the EPI vaccines from external sources. Facilities for regional vaccine production in these countries are inadequate; there is not a dependable supply of EPI vaccines which meet the WHO quality requirements and good manufacturing practice (GMP) standards. There is a need for trained personnel and for modernization of equipment and manufacturing processes in these countries.

With the possible exceptions of Egypt and Tunisia, there are practically no vaccine-manufacturing facilities in Africa.[7] The UNIDO Advisory Panel of Preventive Medicine studied the production of vaccines in Africa, taking into consideration the Lagos Plan,[8] and recommended that activities be initiated to promote the creation of vaccine-manufacturing facilities in the region. With the assistance of the National Institute of Public Health and Environmental Hygiene (RIVM) of the Netherlands, a technical paper was prepared which addressed problems related to the manufacture of seven vaccines—BCG, diphtheria, measles, pertussis, polio, rabies and tetanus—including vaccine-production technology, quality control, economic aspects, building layout and personnel training requirements.[9] UNIDO also established a demonstration and train-

[5] United Nations Industrial Development Organization (UNIDO), 'Supply of EPI vaccines in the Asian countries', UNIDO Technical Report no. UC/RAS/83/234, 19 Feb. 1987, pp. 1–158.

[6] UNIDO, 'Production of vaccines in Latin America including a survey of production facilities, ancillary services and manpower', UNIDO Technical Report no. UC/RLA/87/276, 19 Feb. 1990, pp. 1–196.

[7] UNIDO, *Proceedings of the Meeting of the Advisory Panel on Preventive Medicine, Garoua, Cameroon* (UNIDO: Vienna, 1991), pp. 1–97.

[8] The Lagos Plan of Action for the Economic Development of Africa, 1980–2000, was developed at the meeting of the Heads of State and Government of the Organization of African Unity (OAU) in Lagos, Nigeria, on 28–29 April 1980, at the second extraordinary session of the OAU Assembly. The meeting was devoted to African economic problems, and the participants adopted a Plan of Action aimed at rapidly achieving self-reliance, self-sustaining development and economic growth in Africa. Elements of the plan included the development of human resources and science and technology, self-sufficiency in food production and supply, protection of the environment and industrial development in Africa.

[9] UNIDO, 'Model programme for the production of vaccines in developing countries', UNIDO Technical Report no. UC/GLO/84/120, 4 Nov. 1986, pp. 1–178.

ing unit at the National Veterinary Laboratory at Garoua-Bokle, Cameroon, with facilities for the production of tetanus vaccine.[10]

VI. The need for a long-term strategy

Poor sanitary and hygiene conditions in many developing countries allow infectious diseases to continue to play havoc, and there is a constant and sustained need for quality vaccines to combat these infections. Long-term strategies are needed to ensure an uninterrupted supply of vaccines. Furthermore, some existing vaccines need improvement to eliminate occasional unwanted side-effects (pertussis and polio vaccines); to develop more effective vaccines (tuberculosis and cholera vaccines); and to achieve effective immunization with a single dose rather than multiple doses, as is currently the case with DPT and polio vaccines. There are also other diseases in developing countries that are not covered by the EPI for which vaccines have been developed or are under development. For reasons of poor financial return, these vaccines are unlikely to be manufactured by companies in industrialized countries. During the next decade many new vaccines may be developed including those against parasitic diseases—a major problem in the developing countries—and potential manufacturers have to be identified for these vaccines.

VII. New research developments

The phenomenal advances in biomedical sciences in general and in molecular biology and hybridoma technology, in particular, have opened new vistas for developing safe, heat-stable and more effective vaccines against infectious diseases. The WHO programmes such as the Children's Vaccine Initiative (CVI) and the Programme for Vaccine Development and Tropical Diseases Research have promoted application of these developments to the production of new and improved vaccines. The advent of recombinant DNA technology has facilitated the elimination of harmful genes and the cloning of protective genes into appropriate vectors. A few of these developments are discussed below.

The immunogenic components of several pathogens have been characterized. In many cases the genes coding for protective antigens and for toxins have been identified. The genes that encode A (toxin) subunit were deleted from *Vibrio cholerae* strain 569B to make it well-tolerated and more immunogenic.[11] Ty21a, an attenuated strain of *Salmonella typhi*, was found to be safe and protective as a live oral vaccine.[12] The capsular polysaccharide Vi antigen of *S. typhi* was shown to protect against typhoid,[13] with the added advantage of not requiring a cold chain.

[10] See note 7.

[11] Levine, M. M. *et al.*, 'Safety, immunogenicity and efficacy in man of recombinant live oral cholera vaccine CVD 103 and CVD 103-HgR', *The Lancet* vol. 2 (1988), pp. 467–70.

[12] Levine, M. M., Taylor, D. N. and Ferreccio, C., 'Typhoid vaccines come of age', *Paediatric Infectious Diseases Journal*, vol. 8 (1989), pp. 374–81.

[13] Acharya, I. L. *et al.*, 'Prevention of typhoid fever in Nepal with the Vi capsular polysaccharide of *S. typhi*: a preliminary report', *New England Journal of Medicine*, vol. 17 (1987), pp. 1101–4.

For malaria, several candidate antigens having B and T cell epitopes of sporozoites, merozoites and gametocytes have been identified by cloning techniques.[14] Similar advances have been made with schistosomiasis.[15]

Attempts are under way to engineer a novel, live attenuated polio virus by making a chimeric organism with epitopes of type 3 inserted into a receptive region of type 1 virus.[16] A recombinant yeast-cell-derived vaccine against hepatitis B virus (HBV) is already on the market. Significant progress is being made in developing third-generation synthetic peptide vaccines consisting of immunogenic components of S and preS2 of the virus.[17]

More recent developments aim at evolving multi-vaccine vehicles using bacterial or viral vectors to immunize simultaneously against multiple antigens. Attenuated *S. typhi* is being used as a live 'carrier' for other foreign antigens which facilitate oral delivery of vaccines. An example of this is the attempt to express by recombinant techniques the concerned antigens of *V. cholerae* in attenuated *S. typhi*.[18] BCG, which induces cell-mediated immunity and also acts as an effective adjuvant, is being examined as a vehicle for immunogens. A number of attenuated viruses such as polio, vaccinia and the yellow fever 17D strain are being studied for expression of foreign antigens.[19] Another concept which shows promise is the use of anti-idiotype vaccines. These types of vaccines dispense with the continuous need for antigens for immunization and may be particularly useful when dealing with antigens with carbohydrate epitopes.

Among the other advances that are taking place are novel methods of vaccine delivery with pulsed antigen-release systems using biodegradable microcapsules, new adjuvants and immune enhancers and vaccines that are effective when administered orally. Research in vaccine development is also directed at inducing heat stability, thus producing a longer shelf-life for the vaccines.[20]

VIII. Vaccine-production problems and possible solutions

It is evident that much effort will be required to evolve a long-term strategy for the development and transfer of the necessary technologies and the creation of facilities to meet the need for existing, improved and new vaccines in the developing countries. An undertaking of this magnitude requires a sound technological and industrial infrastructure, and adoption of GMP in the production of

[14] See Playfair *et al.* (note 3); Cox, F. E. G., 'Malaria vaccines: the shape of things to come', *Nature* vol. 333 (1988), p. 702.

[15] Balloul, J. M. *et al.*, 'Molecular cloning of a protein antigen of schistosomes', *Nature*, vol. 326 (1987), pp. 149–53; Goudot-Crozel, V. *et al.*, 'A major parasite surface antigen associated with human resistance to schistosomiasis is a 37 KD G-3-P dehydrogenase', *Journal of Experimental Medicine*, vol. 134 (1989), pp. 2065–80.

[16] Burke, K. L. *et al.*, 'Antigen chimeras of polio virus as potential new vaccines', *Nature*, vol. 332 (1988), pp. 81–82.

[17] Zuckerman, A. J., 'Bioengineering of hepatitis B vaccine', *Journal of Chemical Technology and Biotechnology*, vol. 43 (1988), pp. 57–67; Emini, E. A. *et al.*, 'Protective effect of a synthetic peptide comprising the complete preS2 region of hepatitis B virus surface protein', *Journal of Medical Virology*, vol. 28 (1989), pp. 7–12; Rao, K. V. S., Panda, S. K. and Manivel, V., 'Macromolecular self-association of a synthetic peptide derived from the hepatitis B surface antigen: construction of a quaternary epitope', *Vaccine*, vol. 10 (1992), pp. 204–8.

[18] Forrest, B. D. *et al.*, 'A candidate live oral typhoid/cholera hybrid vaccine is immunogenic in humans', *Journal of Infectious Diseases*, vol. 159 (1989), pp. 145–46.

[19] Brown, F., 'From Jenner to genes: the new vaccines', *The Lancet*, vol. 335 (1990), pp. 587–90.

[20] World Health Organization/United Nations Development Programme, *Programme for Vaccine Development*, report no. MIM.PVD/91.8 (WHO/UNDP: Geneva, 1991), pp. 1–34.

vaccines. The products should be subject to strict quality control in established centres. In addition, there should be efficient distribution systems to ensure the timely delivery of vaccines to the target population under optimal conditions of stability, such as maintenance of the required cold chain at all times. Furthermore, the production units should be at the forefront of developments in the application of new technologies to upgrade the potency and increase the shelf-life of existing vaccines. Facilities to manufacture new vaccines must be created which avail themselves of the state-of-the-art advances in the field. As summarized in the previous section, several new developments—primarily the result of the application of recombinant DNA technology—are on the horizon which will lead to the evolution of new and better vaccines against many infections, including those caused by parasites. Most of these advances are taking place in academic and other research institutions in the developed countries, and there is a need to devise mechanisms for technology transfer of these developments to production centres. New vaccines should also be cost-effective since they will be bought by developing countries.

Various options have been suggested to produce these vaccines and to ensure a guaranteed supply.[21] Among these are:

1. Sufficient funds might be raised by the United Nations to purchase vaccines at market price. Manufacturers in developed countries that are now hesitant to produce such vaccines might become interested to undertake this task owing to its profitability.
2. Sufficient funds might be raised by the United Nations, specifically to manufacture particular 'orphan vaccines'[22] deemed important for many developing countries and to induce public sector institutes and private companies to develop such vaccines and to supply them at or near the cost of production.
3. The United Nations might create international centre(s) for the development and manufacture of the vaccines.
4. Small and relatively specialized facilities for the production and quality control of vaccines that currently exist in developed countries might be entrusted to undertake this venture. This might involve expansion and scaling up of facilities.
5. Vaccine-development and production units might be established in developing countries that have sufficient scientific and industrial infrastructure.

Each of the above suggestions has its merits and drawbacks as regards implementation. The first and second suggestions entail continuous effort by the UN to raise funds for the purchase of vaccines, which experience shows is not easy. The third suggestion calls for the establishment of international centre(s) to ensure the supply of quality vaccines. However, this may be too expensive. The fourth suggestion aims at the expansion of existing specialized facilities in developed countries. It is uncertain whether these facilities are willing and able

[21] Robbins, A. and Freeman, P., 'Obstacles to developing vaccines for the Third World', *Scientific American*, vol. 258 (1988), pp. 90–95; Morehouse, W., 'Vaccine production in the Third World: the search for alternatives', Report to UNIDO under Special Service Agreement, report no. CLT 89/225, 12 Nov. 1989, pp. 1–52; Salk, J., as reported by W. Morehouse in 'Creating international facilities for technical development and production of orphan vaccines in developing countries', Report to UNIDO under Special Service Agreement, report no. CLT 89/550, 24 Jan. 1990, pp. 1–10.

[22] The term 'orphan vaccines' designates vaccines that have no significant market in the industrialized countries. See Morehouse (note 21), p. 15.

to manufacture the required quantities of the vaccines which are primarily needed by developing countries. The fifth suggestion envisages production of vaccines at several centres in the developing countries that have a scientific and industrial infrastructure of a high calibre.

It seems appropriate to encourage the developing countries (where the need is greatest) to strive to produce adequate quantities of vaccines to meet their own demands and those of other developing countries. It may be most feasible to produce vaccines at economical prices in the quantities desired by decentralized production in developing countries, and there are several developing countries which have the necessary scientific, technological and industrial infrastructure to do so. International agencies could assist by strengthening science and technology support to these countries so that they could continuously upgrade the coverage, potency and safety of these vaccines by using the latest advances in research for production of better vaccines. While this might be a suitable long-term strategy for ensuring an adequate supply of vaccines, a mechanism would also have to be devised to ensure high quality and GMP standards of production at the various centres.

IX. Technical support to vaccine-manufacturing centres

Significant technological support to raise standards should be provided to the vaccine-manufacturing centres if they are located in the developing countries. In this context, a consultancy entity (which could be a company, a foundation or an extension of a vaccine development institution) could be established which could facilitate technology transfer to the production centres. The following could be among its functions: (*a*) monitoring and technological intelligence (through multi-client studies and other means) of trends in technology development and transfer, and of facilities involved in vaccine manufacture; (*b*) preparation and feasibility studies for the production of new vaccines, upgrading of established technologies and establishment of new facilities; (*c*) advisory services and trouble shooting; (*d*) help in quality control and quality-control surveillance of vaccines; and (*e*) upgrading of the technology infrastructure, assistance in the transfer of new technologies and fostering of collaborative ventures.

The consultancy unit might require initial funding but should be designed to be self-financing eventually through payments by the manufacturing centres for the various services rendered.

X. Biotechnology development in developing countries

In order to take advantage of modern biotechnology R&D leading to new and improved vaccines and their production, developing countries must strengthen their capabilities in this respect.

Recognizing the vast potential of genetic engineering and biotechnology for industrial development, in 1981 UNIDO began to disseminate these frontier technologies to developing countries. This initiative resulted in the creation of the International Centre for Genetic Engineering and Biotechnology, as mentioned above.

On the initiative of UNIDO, representatives of more than 40 governments agreed in a December 1982 meeting at Belgrade, Yugoslavia, to establish the ICGEB. It is devoted to training and R&D in genetic engineering and biotechnology with a view to enhancing human health, food and nutritional levels and to promoting industries in developing countries. The Statutes of the ICGEB were agreed in September 1983 at Madrid, Spain. In April 1984 it was decided to establish the Centre at two locations—in Trieste, Italy, and in New Delhi, India.

In 1987 the ICGEB began its work; it has shown itself to be a unique intergovernmental centre engaged in research in biotechnology and genetic engineering that has reached a high level of scientific excellence within a short time. Research at New Delhi focuses on mammalian biology, plant biology and structural biology. At Trieste, studies are carried out on the molecular biology of the human papilloma virus, the microbial degradation of lignin and on protein structure and function, including molecular modelling, pathology and immunological aspects.

Currently 46 countries are members of the ICGEB; 29 of them have ratified its Statutes. The ICGEB is assisted by a panel of high-ranking scientists and also has affiliations with national institutions in 20 countries.

The ICGEB has reached an important stage in its development with the adoption of a rolling five-year programme which has enabled the recruitment of highly qualified scientists and imparted a sense of stability to the Centre's operations. The ICGEB has a budget of US $72 million for the period 1992–96, and it has a network of activities such as colloquia, seminars, workshops and funding of collaborative research projects and 'bioinformatics'. The magnitude of the training efforts of this nascent institution can be gauged by the fact that over 350 scientists from 25 developing countries have already been trained in approximately 40 short-term training activities. Since 1989 one million dollars have been disbursed yearly by the Centre on collaborative research projects to member country institutions. Owing to its multilateral character and its pursuit of excellence in biotechnology research, the ICGEB can play a key role in strengthening the biotechnology capabilities of developing countries as regards the safe handling of bacterial and biological toxins and their use for peaceful and beneficial purposes. In fact, Article 2 of the ICGEB Statutes states that one of the objectives of the Centre is to promote international co-operation in developing and applying peaceful uses of genetic engineering and biotechnology particularly for developing countries.

The Centre has published a number of good papers in reputable scientific journals.[23] Steps are being taken to patent the products of ICGEB research, and a number of industrial enterprises have approached the ICGEB for funding of collaborative ventures. The ICGEB is gaining increasing international attention and recognition. Reference was made to the ICGEB in relation to Article X of the BWC at the Third Review Conference of the BWC.[24] States Parties were urged to increase their technical co-operation and assistance to developing countries in the use of biosciences and genetic engineering for peaceful pur-

[23] UNIDO/International Centre for Genetic Engineering and Biotechnology (ICGEB), *Activity Report* (UNIDO: Vienna, 1991), pp. 1–113.

[24] United Nations, Final document of the Third Review Conference of the Parties to the Convention on the Prohibition and Stockpiling of Bacteriological (Biological) and Toxic Weapons and on their Destruction, part II, *Final Declaration*, BWC/CONF.III/23, 27 Sep. 1991.

poses through active association with UN organizations, including the ICGEB. Similar calls for support of the ICGEB were made at the Third Sessions of the Preparatory Committees of both the UN Conference for Environment and Development (UNCED)[25] and the Biodiversity Convention of the United Nations Environment Programme (UNEP),[26] respectively.

UNEP has entered into joint sponsorship with the ICGEB for training courses and meetings, and the WHO and the Rockefeller Foundation have awarded grants to the ICGEB for research in specified areas. The Centre is also becoming increasingly involved in harmonizing legislation and control of biotechnology safety, intellectual property rights and patenting policies in its member countries.

The ICGEB Statutes have been ratified by a greater number of member states than the minimum required, and the ICGEB will soon become autonomous. At that time, a Governing Body consisting of representatives of member countries will be constituted to administer the Centre. The ICGEB is keen to expand its membership, particularly as regards industrialized countries. Many developed countries are already considering joining the ICGEB. There is a great need to strengthen the ICGEB and its affiliated centres in order to provide the manpower needed to meet effectively the strategies proposed in the Vaccines for Peace programme.

UNIDO is also actively involved in the safe handling of genetically modified organisms (GMOs) which are used in a variety of areas such as vaccine production and which have also been released into the environment in connection with industrial development. In order to promote the safe use of GMOs, UNIDO—together with UNEP, the WHO and the Food and Agricultural Organization (FAO)—developed a Voluntary Code of Conduct for the release of GMOs into the environment.[27] Other activities include assisting developing countries, on request, in matters related to biosafety regulations via an International Network and Advisory Service and offering training courses on biosafety through the ICGEB. It is hoped that the Voluntary Code of Conduct will be the basis for countries to establish biosafety guidelines to meet their own requirements.

Another initiative being pursued by UNIDO is the creation of a Consultative Group on Biotechnology, patterned on the model of the Consultative Group on International Agricultural Research (CGIAR); this is being done as the result of a recommendation in a UNIDO-commissioned study[28] on the contribution of biotechnology to sustainable development within the framework of the UN system.

[25] United Nations Conference on Environment and Development, 'Report of the meeting of the Third Session of the Preparatory Committee', document no. A/CONF.151/PC/66, 9 July 1991, pp. 1–16.

[26] United Nations Environment Programme (UNEP), 'Biodiversity Convention: report of the meeting of the Third Session of the Preparatory Committee', document no. UNEP/Bio.Div/WG.2/3/5, 29 Apr. 1991, pp. 1–12.

[27] UNIDO/UNEP/WHO/FAO Working Group on Biosafety, *Voluntary Code of Conduct for the Release of Organisms into the Environment* (UNIDO: Vienna, 1992), pp. 1–22.

[28] UNIDO, Swaminathan, M. S., 'Contribution of biotechnology to sustainable development within the framework of the United Nations system', UNIDO, IPCT (Industrial Promotion, Consultations and Technology) document no. 148 (spec.), 4 Feb. 1992, pp. 1–88.

XI. Conclusions

The development and transfer of technology for vaccine manufacture to meet the long-term needs of developing countries is a complex, wide-ranging and challenging undertaking. It will need to be dealt with in a series of steps but with a concentrated effort. UN agencies such as the WHO and UNICEF are making commendable efforts in securing the resources to meet the needs of developing countries. Additional and complementary initiatives are essential to build on this foundation in order to ensure the availability of human resources and production facilities for a sustained, long-term supply of existing, improved and new vaccines. A plausible solution to this problem appears to be the creation or augmentation of the facilities of regional or national centres in the developing countries that currently possess the science and technology infrastructure to manufacture high-quality vaccines for all developing countries. However, as mentioned above, the GMP conditions and the current technology infrastructure of the few manufacturing centres in the developing countries which are engaged in vaccine production are such that there is a need for considerable strengthening of current efforts. It is therefore vital that international organizations such as the WHO, UNICEF and UNIDO join forces to promote the upgrading of technology and the transfer of knowledge, and that they support existing centres via a consultancy device that enables such centres to use and implement advances in the development of new and better vaccines in their production units. A feasibility study for this purpose is needed which extensively reviews the various available options to find workable solutions. The issues discussed in this chapter, together with others, could form the basis for an in-depth discussion by a few experts in the field, together with policy- and business-oriented development specialists, with the aim of arriving at a concrete strategy for addressing this important and vital public health need.

20. Funding and managing international programmes in biosciences and health care

JOHN P. WOODALL*

I. Funding

Biotechnology funding is in a critical phase. Although there was never a geographical 'DNA valley' in the same sense as 'silicon valley', the industry has been going through some of the same stages as the computer industry, although it did not start in a garage—the equipment required is too expensive for that. However, the hundreds of small genetic engineering companies that sprang up in the beginning, supported by large amounts of venture capital, are facing a shake-out, and industry analysts predict that only a handful will survive, in the same way that most small computer companies have gone out of business.

So in the private sector, venture capital is drying up and only the largest or most innovative companies will survive. In the public and non-profit sectors, the recession has forced cut-backs in spending, and for the time being grandiose development projects are on hold. Also the World Bank is currently less free with soft loans and grants to establish production facilities in developing countries where a good return on investment cannot be foreseen in the short term.

However, first, development has to be seen in the context of the recent revolution in the vaccine industry. Take-overs and mergers have left only seven European vaccine manufacturers in the market, all of them owned by multinational pharmaceutical companies. No longer will major vaccine R&D funds be available to them; the parent companies will be concentrating their R&D money on new drugs, and cutting back on the production of all but the most profitable vaccines. This may result in time-tested vaccines being removed from the market and replaced by much more expensive versions with marginally improved freedom from side-effects or other advantages.

Market size will determine everything. The rule of thumb in the industry is that a population base of 40 million is the minimum for commercial viability for a vaccine—and that is in the industrialized world where a relatively high price can be charged. The market for dengue vaccine, for example, in the Far East, Latin America and the Caribbean, is much larger than that, but most of those countries will not be able to afford a price that will give a rapid enough return on investment. Industry estimates that the average cost of bringing a new vaccine to market was $100 million to $160 million in 1992, and one can be sure that today the higher figure is the more likely. The research costs are, paradoxically, the smallest part of this; it is the development, namely the clinical

* The views expressed here are those of the author, and do not necessarily represent those of the World Health Organization.

trials for safety, efficacy and dosage limits, and the scaling up to mass production while maintaining quality control, that incurs the highest costs.[1]

The same problem will confront the eventual marketers of the newly developed malignant melanoma vaccine, which is a treatment rather than a preventive measure. Unless the ozone hole becomes much larger or more permanent, only an estimated 32 000 people in the USA will contract that virulent form of skin cancer each year, not enough to ensure a profitable market.

What does all this mean for the prospects of yet another vaccine initiative? There are at least four possible mechanisms for supporting this.[2] One is the traditional approach of bulk ordering by multinational aid agencies such as the WHO and UNICEF, through a revolving fund or similar mechanism. The problem is, manufacturers demand firm orders for quantities, preferably for more than one year ahead. While it is possible to calculate the number of children who will need immunization over the next five years, it is not possible to be sure of the income of UN agencies over that period. The charitable organization Rotary International was able to pledge for five years ahead to the poliomyelitis eradication programme, and other foundations may be able to do the same, although their income has also been affected by the recession.

A second approach is the development of a United Nations institute to develop and produce its own vaccines. Under current UN pay regimes it would be difficult to recruit and retain the best qualified staff for such a project, and although the institute might not be required to show a profit, at least for several years, it would take a long time to set up and get going, and would certainly be complicated by international politics. The UN Industrial Development Organization (UNIDO) has experienced such complications while setting up its twin biotechnology centres in Trieste, Italy, and New Delhi, India. In the first five years not one product was able to be put forward.

A third alternative is to establish vaccine production centres in developing countries with a large enough population base to provide an internal market, with the added prospect of increasing production further for export to smaller countries at affordable prices, possibly paid for in soft currencies. However, in spite of this incentive India, for example, has not been able to meet its own vaccine needs, let alone produce for export. Also some vaccine and serum institutes in the developing countries and the former USSR have experienced quality control problems, which complicate exportability. For a relatively small outlay, however, it might be possible to rehabilitate selected former Soviet institutes and retain experienced staff to restart production that meets international standards. The WHO's Regional Office for the Americas, the Pan American Health Organization (PAHO), has had some success with strengthening vaccine production facilities in Latin America, and has organized a vaccine surveillance system and network of quality control laboratories to assure the quality of vaccines used in that region.

[1] The WHO-initiated Programme for Vaccine Development (PVD) has estimated the costs of developing a combination vaccine for cholera/shigella/enterotoxigenic *E. coli*, and a tetravalent dengue vaccine as $20–30 million each, and for Japanese encephalitis as $10–15 million. These micro-organisms are of interest as DTAs; new or improved vaccines for them are in the process of development by the PVD, and are expected to become available by 1999. See 'Ten years of progress 1984–1993: the Programme for Vaccine Development, a WHO/UNDP partnership working for the world's children', WHO document WHO/MIM/93.1, 1993.

[2] Robbins, A. R. and Freeman, P., 'Obstacles to developing vaccines for the Third World', *Scientific American*, vol. 259, no. 5 (Nov. 1988), pp. 90–95.

A fourth approach would be to extend the existing system by which UN agencies such as the World Bank and the UNDP fund biotechnology research—including vaccine research—to vaccine development, giving money to commercial manufacturers to put to a designated use, such as developing a haemorrhagic fever vaccine. The manufacturers would apply for a development grant just as, at present, academic institutions compete for research grants. The companies would, of course, generally be in the industrialized countries, but they could be required to hire scientists from developing countries to join their teams and gain experience for a future when they could handle such a project in their home country. A step in this direction has been taken by the WHO/UNDP/ Rockefeller Foundation Programme for Vaccine Development (PVD).

Since infectious diseases have a tendency to spread world-wide, as shown most recently by the extension of the cholera pandemic to the Americas, it must be in the interest of donor nations to fund the development of vaccines against them, even if those diseases do not yet cause a problem within their own borders. The potential cost-benefits of such an investment are considerable.[3]

In the final analysis, however, a funding mechanism has to be foreseen whereby the largest developing countries can gradually take over responsibility for producing enough of the appropriate vaccines for their own needs and those of their smaller, regional neighbours, so that they do not remain locked into the problem of having to spend hard currency to import bulk or finished vaccines to protect their own population. Some innovative means such as a debt-for-health swap might help, as would also liberalization of trade laws.

II. Managing

The model for managing programmes in biotechnology, and especially vaccine development, is well seen in the PVD.[4] A Scientific Advisory Group of Experts (SAGE) decides on the general orientation of the programme and reviews its implementation. The members of the SAGE are scientists from all over the world, internationally recognized for their expertise in microbiology, molecular biology, immunology, epidemiology or vaccinology. For each vaccine or group of vaccines there is a Steering Committee consisting of two members of the SAGE plus relevant specialists from the WHO Secretariat and support staff. These decide on strategy, recommend projects and promote collaborative work. The relevant section of the WHO (in this case, the Microbiology and Immunology Support Services within the Division of Communicable Diseases at the WHO, Geneva) is responsible for the operational management and administration of the PVD.

There is close collaboration within the WHO Geneva with those other programmes directly related to the PVD, including the Expanded Programme on Immunization (EPI), the Diarrhoeal Disease Control Programme (CDD), Control of Acute Respiratory Infections (ARI), the Special Programme for Research and Training in Tropical Diseases (TDR), the Division of Control of

[3] See chapter 21, section XVI, in this volume.

[4] See note 1; see also WHO/UNDP, *Moving Towards New Vaccines*, brochure (WHO: Geneva, Dec. 1991); WHO/MIM/PVD, *WHO/UNDP Programme for Vaccine Development, 1991–1992: Progress Report* (WHO: Geneva, Dec. 1992).

Tropical Diseases (CTD), the Biologicals Unit (BLG) and the Global Programme on AIDS (GPA).

The cost of all necessary meetings of the SAGE and seven Steering Committees, including Task Force meetings, covering travel and per diem for the members, related administrative costs and temporary support staff, came to only $280 000 for the 12 months 1 July 1992–30 June 1993. For a total budget of $5.74 million, that represents only 4.8 per cent, but the WHO takes another 13 per cent for general administrative support, while contributing 5 per cent of the budget, for a net total management charge of about 13 per cent.

In summary, the WHO has the structure and system for managing another vaccine initiative, but it would have to be closely co-ordinated with the EPI and the PVD, both of which are currently administered through the WHO. If a sufficient number of countries demand that a new vaccine initiative be supported, and vote the necessary seed money, and a policy decision is taken by the WHO executive management to support it, the structure already exists in the WHO to administer it.

Part VI. Final discussion

21. From BVI to VFP: towards a system of global biological security

ERHARD GEISSLER, FÉLIX C. CALDERÓN and JOHN P. WOODALL

I. The Biesenthal Vaccine Initiative

Discussing the Vaccines for Peace (VFP) proposal at the Biesenthal workshop there was unanimous agreement that at least a *modified* VFP programme should be established. The modified programme was designated the Biesenthal Vaccine Initiative (BVI).

As stated in the Biesenthal Consensus,[1] the key objectives of the BVI should include:

* strengthening the BTWC through implementation of Article X and increased mutual transparency in activities related to the Convention,
* prevention of diseases, especially in developing countries,
* enhancement of peaceful international cooperation in molecular medicine and biotechnology and prevention of misuse,
* conversion, where appropriate, of biological warfare (BW) facilities to peaceful purposes under civilian control,
* increasing world capacity to produce vaccines, [and]
* expanding participation in the BTWC and its confidence-building measures.

Implementation of the BVI would contribute significantly to improving health care on a global scale, to strengthening the international norm against biological and toxin warfare, and to reducing the (bio)technology gap between North and South.

Discussing the Vaccines for Peace proposal at the Biesenthal workshop and in several articles[2] there was no consensus, however, regarding some other recommendations of the original VFP proposal. Some participants in the discussions expressed concern that: (*a*) the *title* of the programme should be changed; (*b*) the VFP programme might increase rather than decrease the risk of *proliferation*; (*c*) vaccines for public health are *different* from those for biological defence; and (*d*) *conversion* of former BW facilities to institutions developing vaccines against dual-threat agents (DTAs) might be dangerous; and it was proposed that (*e*) the VFP programme should not deal with or even concentrate on *DTAs*.

[1] See the Biesenthal Consensus, annexe C, in this volume.

[2] Leitenberg, M., 'A note on the proposal by Dr. Erhard Geissler: "Vaccines for Peace: an international program of development and use of vaccines against 'dual use' agents"', Paper distributed among the members of the Federation of American Scientists (FAS) Working Group on Biological and Toxin Weapons Verification, Aug. 1992; Pearson, G., 'Vaccines for Peace: an incentive for developing countries', *Politics and the Life Sciences*, vol. 12, no. 1 (Feb. 1993), pp. 87–89; Thränert, O., 'The "Vaccines for Peace" program: does it really help to strengthen the Biological Weapons Convention?', *Politics and the Life Sciences*, vol. 12, no. 1 (Feb. 1993), pp. 89–90; Woodall, J., 'An exceptional window of opportunity: comments on "Vaccines for Peace"', *Politics and the Life Sciences*, vol. 12, no. 1 (Feb. 1993), pp. 91–92.

After considering important publications issued after the Biesenthal workshop[3] and following the conclusion of the Chemical Weapons Convention (CWC), the authors of this chapter remain convinced that a comprehensive VFP programme would contribute much more to strengthening the BWC and to enhancing health care than the BVI alone, for the reasons discussed below.

II. VFP vs. Atoms for Peace

The title Vaccines for Peace was criticized by some participants of the Biesenthal workshop because the term *peace* was heavily misused by communist leaders, states and institutions during the past 75 years. This criticism is not valid because, of course, the word 'peace' describes one of the long-lasting supreme goals of humankind, and it has by no means lost its content despite misuse. The authors of this chapter refer to this goal in the title of the proposed programme because we are convinced that the VFP programme would contribute to peace, not only as a programme to facilitate disarmament but also via its contributions to reducing tension and to improving North–South relations.

Another criticism of the programme and its title was that 'the essential character of the proposal is analogous to the US Atoms for Peace programme of the late 1950s and 1960s (even in its name, "Vaccines for Peace"), and for precisely the same reasons it is misdirected and risks potentially disastrous consequences'.[4] Although the existence of the Atoms for Peace proposal launched by President Dwight D. Eisenhower in 1953[5] did not play a role in redesignating *our* proposal analogies can, of course, be drawn between VFP and Atoms for Peace. In fact, President Eisenhower's appeal to the international community, 'to help solve the fearful atomic dilemma—to devote its entire heart and mind to find the way by which the miraculous inventiveness of man shall not be dedicated to his death, but consecrated to his life',[6] could be an appeal made by the authors of this chapter, with the only change being the substitution of 'bioweapons' for 'atomic'.

Although Atoms for Peace and Vaccines for Peace are similar not only in name but in intention, there are at least four major differences between them:

1. Atoms for Peace was launched at the beginning of the cold war, during the Korean War. Vaccines for Peace would be established after the end of the cold

[3] Lederberg, J., Shope, R. E. and Oaks, Jr, S. C. (eds), *Emerging Infections: Microbial Threats to Health in the United States* (National Academy Press: Washington, DC, 1992); *Arms Control: US and International Efforts to Ban Biological Weapons*, Report to the Hon. Albert Gore, Jr, US Senate, GAO/NSIAD-93-113 (US General Accounting Office: Washington, DC, Dec. 1992); *Countering the Chemical and Biological Weapons Threat in the Post-Soviet World*, Report of the Special Inquiry into the Chemical and Biological Threat of the Committee on Armed Services, US House of Representatives, 102nd Congress, 2nd session, 23 Feb. 1993 (US Government Printing Office: Washington, DC, 1993); Roberts, B. (ed.), *Biological Weapons: Weapons of the Future?* (Center for Strategic and International Studies: Washington, DC, 1993); Zilinskas, R. A. (ed.), *The Microbiologist and Biological Defense Research: Ethics, Politics, and International Security*, Annals of the New York Academy of Sciences, vol. 666 (New York Academy of Sciences: New York, 1992).

[4] Leitenberg (note 2).

[5] Hewlett, R. G. and Hall, J. M., *Atoms for Peace and War, 1953–1961: Eisenhower and the Atomic Energy Commission* (University of California Press: Berkeley, Calif., 1989), pp. 209–37; Pilat, J. F., Pendley, R. E. and Ebinger, C. K. (eds), *Atoms for Peace: An Analysis After Thirty Years* (Westview Press: Boulder, Colo., 1985).

[6] Eisenhower, D. D., *Public Papers of the President of the United States, Dwight D. Eisenhower, 1953* (US Government Printing Office: Washington, DC, 1955), p. 332.

war and in a completely new geopolitical situation when confrontation must be replaced by co-operation.

2. The starting point for Atoms for Peace was the division of the world into a few nuclear 'haves' and a majority of nuclear 'have nots'. Its main intention was to interfere with further nuclear armament by the Soviet Union and to prevent an increase in the number of nuclear 'haves'. For a variety of reasons, neither of these goals was attained. The Soviet Union was interested in nuclear balance, if not in superiority. Some of the nuclear 'have nots' sought access to nuclear weapons, not least for reasons of prestige. Finally, Eisenhower's serious purpose was obstructed by senior members of his Administration who did not believe in the programme.[7]

3. Regarding the availability of biological weapon (BW) and toxin weapon (TW) agents, which are all DTAs,[8] a division of the world into 'biological haves' and 'biological have nots' is impossible. The world is full of DTAs—more or less equally distributed. All countries and, in fact, all people are 'biological haves', inhabited to varying extents by myriads of microbes including DTAs. The military consequences of this are that limited amounts of BW and TW agents, small but sufficient for sabotage and terrorist use, can be developed from agents which cause natural outbreaks of disease. As mentioned above,[9] it is more efficient for BW development purposes to isolate a virulent naturally occurring DTA from natural sources than to order it from, for example, the American Type Culture Collection (ATCC). In addition, it is the right of member states of the World Health Organization (WHO) to request pathogens—regardless of whether they are DTAs or not—from WHO Reference Centres without being obliged to explain the purpose for which the strain requested will be used. According to US estimates, 'perhaps as many as 100 countries have the means of making their own biological weapons without depending on exports from the advanced industrial countries'.[10]

The public health consequence of the fact that humans are all 'biological haves' is that people in all countries, whether civilians or military personnel, are threatened by 'dual-threat' biological and toxin agents. It is the legitimate right of people to defend themselves against these agents whether they occur naturally or after hostile dissemination. In addition, it is not only the legitimate right but the duty of all governments and health services to request that they be provided with the necessary means to fight diseases and with the know-how, technology and equipment to develop such means, if needs be from developed countries.

Of course, the world is divided with respect to the means and know-how necessary to handle DTAs and to provide protection against them. The world is also divided into 'biotechnology haves' and 'biotechnology have nots'. For reasons of humanity—or, more pragmatically, in order to implement the obligations of Article X of the BWC—the 'biotechnology have nots' must be sup-

[7] Bundy, M., *Danger and Survival: Choices About the Bomb in the First Fifty Years* (Random House: New York, 1988), p. 303.

[8] See Geissler, chapter 3, in this volume.

[9] See Thränert, chapter 5, in his volume.

[10] Roberts, B., 'New challenges and new policy priorities for the 1990s', in Roberts (note 3), pp. 68–101, p. 77. Roberts refers here to testimony by Thomas Welch, Deputy Assistant Secretary of Defense, as reported in *Defense Week*, 9 May 1988.

ported so that they have access to the means to protect their populations from infections and intoxinations caused by DTAs.

4. Independently of nuclear disarmament activities, the need for nuclear explosives for peaceful purposes and the need for nuclear energy are also under debate—not for security but for safety and environmental reasons. DTAs must be handled, however, if not for basic research purposes[11] then at least in order to provide health care. The possibility of military misuse of dual-use biotechnologies, of DTAs and of the vaccines against them notwithstanding, industrialized countries have no right to deny other countries access to them.

III. Conversion

One of the key objectives of Vaccines for Peace is the proposal to make use of an international programme for the development and use of vaccines to assist in the process of conversion of former BW facilities. The proposal was included in the BVI although some experts criticized the proposal to convert former BW institutions to civilian facilities involved in R&D and production of vaccines against *inter alia* DTAs. Their basic assumption was that 'if existing BW facilities are converted, it is clearly beneficial from the disarmament and arms-control standpoint the more "distance" there is in the projects chosen for the converted facility from those that might have BW relevance as well . . . simply [to] allay suspicion of intent'.[12] It was also argued that 'the conversion of past offensive biological warfare facilities into ones producing dual threat agent vaccines could raise concern that such converted facilities might be changed back in a short space of time to offensive biological warfare facilities'.[13]

These arguments cannot explain why vaccine R&D in a converted facility might raise more suspicion of intent than vaccine R&D in military institutions (permitted by the BWC), or comparable activities carried out in truly civilian institutions which have never been involved in either offensive or defensive BW activities. Both biological defence research programme (BDRP) facilities and facilities involved in the development and production of 'public health vaccines' can easily be 'reconverted' into offensive BW facilities. Although reconversion cannot be completely prevented, it would be much more difficult to do so if the facility were subject to the VFP programme's verification system (see section X below).

Critics of Vaccines for Peace seem to assume that it is a proposal to disable Western military BW defence capabilities, while in reality the ultimate goal of the proposal is to deal with *all* corresponding capabilities of at least (but not only) States Parties to the BWC.

In view of the current global economic situation, not least that in the former Soviet Union, it is not feasible to convert former BW facilities and their personnel to institutions which will carry out quite different activities while simultaneously establishing new facilities and training new staff for the development of vaccines, including those against DTAs. However, the VFP proposal would

[11] In basic research, at least, it is sometimes possible to substitute a non-DTA simulant for an extremely dangerous DTA.

[12] See Leitenberg, chapter 8, in this volume.

[13] See Pearson, chapter 14, in this volume.

permit former BW facilities to also develop vaccines against non-DTAs and to conduct other biomedical projects.

Facilities and personnel currently not engaged in defence activities should also be involved in the research and production of vaccines against DTAs. As a result, the net yield of products would be much greater than before. Since these vaccines would also be available for military purposes, the VFP programme would enhance biological defence capacities and would even allow establishment of a global defence system similar to other proposed global systems (see section VII below). For this reason, it is not possible to agree that 'the proposed conversion of biological defence activities to public health ones . . . would reduce national and international security'.[14]

Measures should be taken to ensure that vaccine R&D, production and use under the VFP and BVI programmes are carried out in complete openness and transparency. This would also hold true for facilities which are being converted and for their personnel (see section X on verification, below).

IV. Dual-threat agents

During discussion at the Biesenthal workshop and on other occasions it was suggested that the term 'dual-threat agent' might be ambiguous and subject to misinterpretation. Hence reference is not made to DTAs in the Biesenthal Consensus[15] or in the Mission Statement[16] adopted by the BVI Steering Committee. The original proposal was designated An International Program of Development and Use of Vaccines Against 'Dual-*Use*' Agents (emphasis added). During preparation of a manuscript to be published in *Politics and the Life Sciences* (PLS) the PLS editor correctly noted that dual-use agent is an incorrect description of agents that are both natural enemies of living organisms and putative warfare agents. Mother Nature does not 'use' endemic pathogens to infect people, animals or plants.[17] The term dual-threat agent thus seems more apt.

It was argued, for example, that 'the proposal to base VFP on so-called dual-threat agents is flawed on several counts',[18] especially because of their relatively minor public health importance and because of proliferation concerns. It would perhaps be advisable to make the VFP programme subject to export controls (see section XIII on proliferation, below). It was also stated that 'every precept of arms control would suggest that an emphasis on vaccine production for "dual use" agents in particular should be avoided at all costs'.[19] Instead, 'the disease agents selected against which vaccines should be prepared should follow the priority of diseases which most seriously affect developing nations'.[20]

It is correct that DTAs such as the causative agents of anthrax and tularaemia do not cause the most serious diseases in the South or elsewhere. However,

[14] See Pearson (note 2).

[15] See the Biesenthal Consensus, annexe C, in this volume.

[16] See the BVI Mission Statement, annexe D, in this volume.

[17] However, some putative TW agents are simultaneously DTAs and dual-use agents. They may threaten people by natural intoxinations. They have dual-use as research tools in neurobiology or drugs used in cancer therapy and ophthalmology on the one hand, and as TW agents on the other.

[18] See Pearson, chapter 14, in this volume.

[19] See Leitenberg, chapter 8, in this volume.

[20] See Leitenberg, chapter 8, in this volume.

Table 21.1. Diseases in developing countries ranked by total disease burden

Disease	Total disease burden value in infant mortality equivalence (IME) units
Streptococcus pneumoniae	6 612 261
Hepatitis B virus	2 394 256
Plasmodium spp.	2 111 795
Salmonella typhi	1 308 121
Escherichia coli	978 248
Rotavirus	925 042
Shigella spp	828 068
Streptococcus Group A	811 477
Mycobacterium leprae	657 349
(*Escherichia coli*)	(550 248)[a]
(Rotavirus)	(488 542)[a]
Haemophilus influenzae type b	471 336
Respiratory syncytial virus	183 326
Parainfluenza virus	145 954
Neisseria meningitidis	68 252
Rabies virus	67 821
Dual-threat agents	
Vibrio cholera	229 217
Dengue virus	34 365
Yellow fever virus	32 887
Hepatitis A virus	30 229
Japanese encephalitis virus	18 075

[a] The anticipated disease burden from certain diarrhoeal pathogens, if a plausible increase in oral rehydration therapy is assumed

Source: Institute of Medicine, *New Vaccine Development, Establishing Priorities: Diseases of Importance in Developing Countries* (National Academy Press: Washington, 1986).

Bacillus anthracis was reported to have caused over 10 000 human cases of anthrax[21] and 82 deaths[22] in Zimbabwe between 1979 and 1980. Several viral DTAs cause natural disease outbreaks with very high incidence and/or mortality rates (see table 21.1). More than 2 billion people are at risk of becoming affected by dengue virus, a DTA. Between 1985 and 1989, 993 000 cases of dengue haemorrhagic fever/dengue shock syndrome (DHF/DSS) were reported.[23] In South-East Asia, DHF/DSS ranks as one of the leading causes of hospitalization and death among children.[24] Hantaan virus causes over 100 000 cases of Korean haemorrhagic fever per year in China alone.[25] Japanese encephalitis, caused by another DTA, is estimated to affect over 50 000 people annually and to cause 11 000 deaths annually.[26]

[21] Nass, M., 'Anthrax epizootic in Zimbabwe, 1978–1980: due to deliberate spread?', *Physicians for Social Responsibility Quarterly*, vol. 2, no. 6 (Dec. 1992), pp. 198–209.

[22] 'Rhodesia's chemical warfare against freedom fighters?: scientists to probe anthrax epidemic', *Zimbabwe Herald*, 25 Jan. 1993, p. 1.

[23] Halstead, S. B., 'Global epidemiology of dengue hemorrhagic fever', *Southeast Asian Journal of Tropical Medicine and Public Health*, vol. 21 (1990), pp. 636–37.

[24] Lederberg *et al.* (note 3), p. 50.

[25] Morse, S., 'Conference report, "Vaccines for Peace"', *Politics and the Life Sciences*, vol. 12, no. 1 (Feb. 1993), pp. 99–101.

[26] Tsal, T. F., 'Japanese encephalitis vaccines', eds S. A. Plotkin and E. A. Mortimer, *Vaccines* (W. B. Saunders: Philadelphia, 1988), quoted in Gubler, D. J., 'Emergent and resurgent arboviral diseases as public health problems', in eds B. W. J. Mahy and D. K. Lvov, *Concepts in Virology: From Ivanovsky to*

Table 21.2. Putative BW agents that cause emerging diseases and their mode of transmission

Agent	Mode of transmission
Chikungunya virus	Bite of infected mosquito
Crimean-Congo haemorrhagic fever virus	Aerosol, bite of infected tick
Dengue virus	Bite of infected mosquito
Ebola virus	Contact with infected blood, etc.
Hantaan virus	Aerosol
Influenza virus	Aerosol
Japanese encephalitis virus	Bite of infected mosquito
Lassa virus	Contact with infected urine, blood
Marburg virus	Contact with infected blood
Rift Valley fever virus	Bite of infected mosquito
Venezuelan encephalitis virus	Bite of infected mosquito
Vibrio cholerae	Ingestion of contaminated water, etc.
Yellow fever virus	Bite of infected mosquito

Sources: Geissler, E., 'Vaccines for Peace: an international program of development and use of vaccines against dual-threat agents', *Politics and the Life Sciences*, vol. 11, no. 2 (Aug. 1992), pp. 231–43; Lederberg, J., Shope, R. E. and Oaks, Jr, S. C. (eds), *Emerging Infections: Microbial Threats to Health in the United States* (National Academy Press: Washington, DC, 1992), pp. 36–40, 199–247.

There is also increasing concern in Northern countries that DTAs might cause 'emerging diseases'[27] (see table 21.2). Although emerging diseases cause illness and death in significant numbers, many of them are too restricted geographically or currently affect too few people to be attractive for commercial vaccine efforts. According to a recent evaluation by the US Committee on Emerging Microbial Threats to Health, 'there may be potentially catastrophic consequences [caused by emerging microbes] if the [vaccine] development process is left entirely to free enterprise'.[28] Therefore 'the committee recommends that the United States develop a means for generating stockpiles of selected vaccines and a "surge" capacity for vaccine development and production that could be mobilized to respond quickly to future infectious disease emergencies'.[29] The USA is not the only country faced with the possible threat of emerging diseases,[30] thus this may be another reason for selecting DTAs as targets of the

the Present, Proceedings of the Symposium 100 Years of Virology, Ivanovsky Institute International Symposium, St Petersburg, 21–25 Sep. 1992, pp. 257–73.

[27] See Morse, chapter 16, in this volume; Morse, S. (ed.), *Emerging Viruses* (Oxford University Press: Oxford, 1993); Zilinskas, R. A., 'Confronting biological threats to international security: a biological hazards early warning program', in Zilinskas (note 3), pp. 146–76, see especially pp. 147–51; see also Tsal (note 26).

[28] Lederberg *et al.* (note 3), p. 11.

[29] Lederberg *et al.* (note 3), pp. 11–12.

[30] An unusual outbreak of acute illness occurred in the first half of 1993 in the south-western USA. As of 16 Nov. 1993, 42 cases of the syndrome had been reported, 26 of whom died. See Marshall, E., 'Hantavirus outbreak yields to PCR', *Science*, vol 262 (5 Nov. 1993), pp. 832–36; Altman, L. K., 'Virus that caused deaths in New Mexico is isolated', *New York Times*, national edn, 21 Nov. 1993, p. 24. The disease, which has been called Hantavirus Pulmonary Syndrome, is caused by a thus far unknown hantavirus which has been named Muerto Canyon virus. Two cases owing to two new hantaviruses different from Muerto Canyon virus have recently been identified in Florida and Louisiana. See 'Emerging infectious diseases: newly identified hantaviruses–Florida, 1994', *Morbidity and Mortality Weekly Report*, vol. 43, no. 6 (18 Feb. 1994), pp. 99, 105. There was an epidemic due to a related hantavirus in Europe in 1993. See Kulzer, P. *et al.*, 'Haemorrhagic fever with renal syndrome, 1993: endemic or unrecognized pandemic?', *The Lancet*, vol. 342 (1993), p. 313.

VFP programme. Such an international programme would appear to provide the best means of building up vaccine stocks against emerging diseases. Vaccines must also be developed and produced to protect against natural outbreaks of diseases caused by DTAs, without regard to the possible military importance of such agents.

There are already programmes run by the WHO *inter alia* for the prevention of those diseases which most seriously affect developing nations. The Expanded Programme on Immunization (EPI), the Children's Vaccine Initiative (CVI), the Programme for Vaccine Development (PVD) and other international programmes have as their goal the research and production of vaccines against pathogens that pose natural health threats. An additional vaccine programme against *major health* threats need not be established. It is more important to implement the above programmes, especially since they have encountered some difficulties in the past.[31] Exclusive concentration on DTAs would create a clear distinction between VFP and BVI and other vaccine programmes.

Vaccines against DTAs should be developed under a comprehensive VFP programme not only to reduce the danger of BW proliferation, but also to 'provide transparency . . . in research, development, and production of vaccines, including vaccines developed for military purposes' and to 'contribute to health protection, especially in developing countries . . .'.[32] *Transparency* is needed to remove suspicion about the intentions of military vaccine research and production activities.[33]

An additional advantage of concentrating on vaccines against DTAs would be the possibility of obtaining funds from sources which are not interested in supporting the development of vaccines against non-DTAs. Fund-raising would be necessary because the VFP and the BVI must not compete with other WHO vaccine programmes for resources, and because there is already inadequate support for the other programmes.

V. Different vaccines for public health and military defence?

Various views have been expressed in this volume and elsewhere on the relationship of public health to military defence. The authors of this chapter agree with the notion that there is a synergy between BW control and public health[34] and that 'to protect our troops . . . from new biological threats, we [in the USA] need to use the same high levels of expertise that we utilize to address the infectious diseases that plague our populations'.[35] On the other hand, it has also been argued that vaccines for public health are different from those used for

[31] Kane, M., 'Introduction of new vaccines into public health use', Paper presented at the Biesenthal workshop Vaccines for Peace, 13 Sep. 1992; Russell, P., 'The Children's Vaccine Initiative: technologic challenges and management opportunities', Paper presented at the ICGEB Conference Biotechnology R&D Trends: Science Policy for Development, Trieste, 2 Oct., in ed G. T. Tzotzos, *Biotechnology R&D Trends: Science Policy for Development*, Annals of the New York Academy of Sciences, vol. 700 (New York Academy of Sciences: New York, 1993), pp. 1–8.

[32] Geissler, E., 'Vaccines for Peace: an international program of development and use of vaccines against dual-threat agents', *Politics and the Life Science*, vol. 11, no. 2 (Aug. 1992), pp. 231–43, see especially p. 231.

[33] See Geissler, chapter 3, in this volume.

[34] See Wheelis, chapter 17, in this volume.

[35] Halvorson, H. O., 'Civilian control of biological defense research', in Zilinskas (note 3), pp. 191–201, see especially p. 196.

biological defence.[36] This is correct, in principle, if it is assumed that a BW agent might be disseminated as an aerosol so that 'the resulting exposure would be far greater than encountered in a natural exposure'.[37] However, this argument does not hold true for DTAs if they are spread by arthropod or other vectors, such as the viruses of chikungunya, Crimean-Congo haemorrhagic fever, dengue, Japanese encephalitis, Rift Valley fever, Venezuelan equine encephalitis and yellow fever (see table 21.2). It has also been argued that military vaccines might be licensed for adults only.[38] For a disease that causes severe illness in both adults and children, would it not be better to vaccinate the (civilian) adults rather than to deprive the entire population of the benefits of a vaccine because it cannot be used for children? In fact, the large-scale use of such a vaccine for civilian adults would be valuable for later licensing for use by children.

The authors of this chapter agree with the Assistant to the US Secretary of Defense that scientific efforts to develop vaccines for military defence purposes *'are largely common with those used in the civilian biomedical research'* (emphasis added).[39]

Vaccines developed against putative BW agents should be made available to the civilian population in order that it be protected not only from naturally occurring pathogens but also from possible BW attack. Infectious agents do not recognize borders or discriminate between individuals,[40] and military experts admit that a BW threat also exists for the civilian population.[41] As early as 1983, US defence experts expressed concern about 'the uncertainty of how, where, and against whom biological warfare threat agents may be employed' and that 'military forces may not be the only, or even the primary, target of such an attack'.[42] Today, when the cold war between two blocs has been replaced by an increasing number of low-intensity conflicts, undeclared wars and an emerging threat of (state) terrorism, not only isolated areas and defined battlefields are endangered by BW attacks. Particularly because BW agents are frequently ineffective battlefield weapons, 'limited use of BW agents may be perceived as advantageous in a small-scale conflict'.[43] The authors of this chapter share the view that hostile use of biological agents might most likely be clandestine.[44] This holds true especially as regards the threat of terrorist use of BW and TW agents.[45]

[36] See Pearson, chapter 14, in this volume.

[37] Anderson, III, W. C. and King, J. M., *Vaccine and Antitoxin Availability for Defense against Biological Threat Agents*, US Army Health Care Studies Division, report, no. 83-002 (US Army Health Services Command: Fort Sam Houston, Texas, 1983), p. 33.

[38] See Melling, chapter 13, in this volume.

[39] Barker, R. B., Letter to the Hon. John Glenn with replies to questions regarding the US BDRP, 24 Aug. 1989, in *Global Spread of Chemical and Biological Weapons*, Hearings before the Committee on Governmental Affairs and its Permanent Subcommittee on Investigations, US Senate (US Government Printing Office: Washington, DC, 1990), pp. 474–84, see especially p. 478.

[40] King, J., 'Germ wars: biological weapons proliferation and the new genetics', 17 May 1989, testimony in *Global Spread of Chemical and Biological Weapons* (note 39), pp. 211–14, see especially p. 211.

[41] Richardson, B., Acting Deputy Assistant Secretary for Chemical Matters, US DOD, in *Global Spread of Chemical and Biological Weapons* (note 39), p. 196.

[42] Anderson and King (note 37), pp. 34–35.

[43] Poupard, J. A. and Miller, L. A., 'Biological warfare', ed. J. Lederberg, *Encyclopedia of Microbiology*, vol. 1, A-C (Academic Press: San Diego, 1992), pp. 297–308, see especially p. 305.

[44] See Wheelis, chapter 17, in this volume.

[45] Zilinskas, R. A., 'Terrorism and biological weapons: inevitable alliance?', *Perspectives in Biology and Medicine*, vol. 34, no. 1 (autumn 1990), pp. 44–71.

VI. Biological terrorism

The biological terrorist threat 'may be much higher now than it was at the time of the [1991 Persian Gulf] war'.[46] German[47] and US[48] open-air tests have demonstrated the vulnerability of airports and subway systems to terrorist biological attacks.[49] According to the US Special Inquiry into the Chemical and Biological Threat, 'in rear areas, used against unprotected military and civilian personnel, and because of the large areas that may be covered with small amounts of agents and the large number of casualties that may be produced, biological weapons may truly deserve the appellation "poor man's atomic bomb"'.[50]

Had the New York World Trade Center's ventilation system been used to spread BW or TW agents the consequences might have been more disastrous than those of the 1993 attack using explosives detonated in its garage. 'Hundreds of thousands, conceivably millions, of people could have died in a well-executed urban attack . . . The requisite technology, laboratory facilities, and aerosolization devices were already within the grasp of the weakest countries'.[51] According to Vladimir Pasechnik,[52] Soviet BW planners discussed the releasing of BW agents by special forces or terrorists in undeclared wars: 'Terrorists might introduce it in any city and than deny it'.[53] 'Illustrative scenarios' of conceivable terrorist biological attacks are described by Kupperman and Smith.[54]

Politicians and military leaders as well as the civilian population could be targets for terrorist BW and TW attacks. Joseph Stalin, for example, clearly considered having Marshal Tito assassinated by the use of BW agents.[55] The Soviet Security Service planned to disseminate *Pasteurella pestis* at a reception attended by Tito. The fact that the plan included protecting the potential assassin in advance by vaccination supports the argument that the development and use of vaccines could be done with hostile intent. It is impossible to protect humans against terrorist surprise attacks using BW or TW agents. However, vaccines against DTAs produced, stockpiled and immediately available under the VFP programme could provide a unique means to protect against infections transmitted by those exposed to terrorist BW or TW attack.

Other targets of BW and TW attacks might be *inter alia* arms production facilities, including facilities conducting BW-related R&D. While the level of

[46] Kupperman, R. H. and Smith, D. M., 'Coping with biological terrorism', in Roberts (note 3), pp. 35–46, see especially p. 36.

[47] According to a respected British journalist, in 1933 Germany carried out secret BW experiments using simulant bacteria both in the Berlin-Tegel airport and in the subway systems of London and Paris. See Wickham Steed, G., 'Aerial warfare: secret German plans', *The Nineteenth Century and After*, vol. 116, no. 689 (1934), pp. 1–16; Hugh-Jones, M., 'Wickham Steed and German biological warfare research', *Intelligence and National Security*, vol. 7, no. 4 (1992), pp. 379–402.

[48] Cole, L. A., 'Biological warfare tests over American cities: lessons from the past', eds E. Geissler and R. H. Haynes, *Prevention of a Biological and Toxin Arms Race and the Responsibility of Scientists* (Akademie-Verlag: Berlin, 1991), pp. 107–27.

[49] According to Hugh-Jones (note 47, p. 381), the disclosure of the German experiments triggered a restructuring of the ventilation and air filter system of the London subway.

[50] *Countering the Chemical and Biological Weapons Threat in the Post-Soviet World* (note 3), p. 9.

[51] Kupperman and Smith (note 46), p. 37.

[52] Pasechnik was one of the leading scientists of the Soviet BW programme; see Leitenberg, chapter 8, in this volume.

[53] Urban, M., 'The cold war's deadliest secret', *The Spectator*, 23 Jan. 1993, pp. 9–10; Barry, J., 'Planning a plague?', *Newsweek*, 1 Feb. 1993, pp. 40–41.

[54] Kupperman and Smith (note 46), pp. 41–43.

[55] Wolkogonow, D., 'The assassination which did not take place: how the Soviet agent Max prepared a terrorist attack against Tito', *Izvestia*, 11 June, 1993, p. 7 (in Russian).

security of military facilities is high, numerous non-military contractors of BDRPs could be convenient targets for such attacks.[56]

The authors of this chapter agree with Brad Roberts that 'the BW terrorism challenge . . . raises the question of whether BW defenses have been too narrowly confined to specifically battlefield concerns and whether it might not be prudent to expand protection to the civilian population more generally . . . Given the proliferation and terrorism factors . . . the United States would be well advised to rethink its degree of preparation for this contingency'.[57] Similarly, the US Special Inquiry into the Chemical and Biological Threat concluded that 'the vaccine production problem is significant *not only to the military*, but also to the US civilian community as well' (emphasis added),[58] and a subsection of their report is titled 'extending the biological defense program to the civilian sector'.

In the aftermath of the cold war no bloc or member state of a bloc is threatened by another bloc, but *all* countries observing the international norm against biological warfare are potentially threatened by a hitherto unknown hostile state or terrorist group.[59] The Geneva Protocol prohibits the use of chemical weapons (which include, according to the understanding of most experts, toxin weapons) '*in war*' as well as the 'use of bacteriological [biological] methods *of warfare*', while other hostile use of BW and TW agents is not covered by the Geneva Protocol.[60] Common protection against the use of such weapons of mass destruction in undeclared wars and for other hostile activities is therefore necessary and urgent.

VII. National vs. international biological defence

For the reasons discussed above, biological defence should be considered not only for the protection of members of the armed forces on the battlefield but also for all people (and livestock) which might be exposed to DTAs by natural means or hostile action. This could best be accomplished by an international initiative. Such a proposal is criticized by some experts because, despite the changed international situation, the USA and other countries, including some developing countries, still insist on their vested right of self-defence—including protection from BW and TW agents.

Without doubt such a right exists. It was established decades ago in a very different strategic climate. Today states should consider whether this right should be relinquished, at least in certain areas. Multilateral defence activities are currently conducted, not least in the field of biological defence, by Canada, the UK and the USA. The UK and the USA have also agreed to create working groups together with the Russian Federation to consider *inter alia* 'cooperation in developing biological weapons defence'.[61]

[56] Poupard and Miller (note 43), p. 306.

[57] Roberts (note 10), p. 83.

[58] *Countering the Chemical and Biological Weapons Threat in the Post-Soviet World* (note 3), p. 55.

[59] Barry (note 53).

[60] However, all use of TW agents is forbidden by the CWC.

[61] *Joint Statement on Biological Weapons by the Governments of the United Kingdom, the United States and the Russian Federation* (US Department of State, Office of the Assistant Secretary/Spokesman: Washington. DC, 14 Sep. 1992); see also *CBW News*, no. 11 (Jan. 1993), pp. 2–3.

Initiatives have also been taken to establish world-wide co-operation in the important area of missile defence. Russia and the USA have agreed, for example, to 'work with their allies and other interested states to develop a "concept" for a Global Protection System against ballistic missiles "as part of an overall strategy regarding the proliferation of ballistic missiles *and weapons of mass destruction*"' (emphasis added).[62]

Comments on the VFP proposal by defence experts from industrialized countries give the impression that these experts are concerned about possible weakening of *Northern* defence capabilities rather than of defence capabilities in general. The concern of the VFP programme, however, is *global* security. Critics appear more worried about the VFP programme than about the so-called 'defence research programs' which exist in some countries, especially those approximately 11 countries suspected to be interested in or conducting offensive BW programmes.[63] (Even Iraq's BW capabilities are still of concern in this context.[64]) If all States Parties to the BWC, could be persuaded to abolish any such national programmes and join a comprehensive VFP programme—while also participating in the Global Epidemiological Surveillance System (GESS) discussed in section XI below—it would contribute to international security as regards BW.[65]

States should be convinced of the need for a system of common security. Owing to the relative inferiority of BW and TW as compared to other battlefield weapon systems, a relatively easy first step would be to implement a common *biological security system* which would guarantee security to the armed forces and the civilian population from both natural pathogenic enemies and BW attack. Similar ideas were discussed at the First Review Conference of the BWC in 1980. Australia, for example, 'wondered whether consideration should not be given to the possibility of internationalizing research into means of defence against bacteriological weapons. For example, it might be possible . . . to place all research activities under international control'.[66]

US President Richard Nixon's decisions in 1969 and 1970 to stop the development and production of BW and TW created an opportunity to negotiate and conclude the BWC. The efficacy of the US BDRP is under evaluation,[67] and the Clinton Administration and governments of other Northern countries should again seize the initiative and establish a system of *common biological security*.

[62] Quoted in Arnett, E. A. and Kokoski, R., 'Military technology and international security: the case of the USA', SIPRI, *SIPRI Yearbook 1993: World Armaments and Disarmament* (Oxford University Press: Oxford, 1993), p. 319.

[63] *Countering the Chemical and Biological Weapons Threat in the Post-Soviet World* (note 3), p. 11.

[64] According to James Woolsey, Director of the US Central Intelligence Agency, 'Iraq's biological weapons capability is perhaps of greatest immediate concern. Baghdad had an advanced program before Desert Storm, and neither war nor inspections have seriously degraded this capability', in testimony before the Senate Governmental Affairs Committee on 'Proliferation threats of the 1990s', 24 Feb. 1993, quoted in *Arms Sales Monitor*, no. 19 (15 Mar. 1993), pp. 2–3.

[65] It goes without saying that the VFP programme cannot completely prevent violations of the international norm against biological warfare, but no treaty can guarantee the total absence of violations.

[66] Review Conference of the Parties to the Convention on the Prohibition of the Development, Production and Stockpiling of Bacteriological (Biological) and Toxin Weapons and on their Destruction, *Summary Record of the 8th Meeting*, BWC/CONF.I/SR.8, 12 Mar. 1980, pp. 7–8; see also Sims, chapter 6, in this volume.

[67] *Biological Warfare: Better Controls in DOD's Research Could Prevent Unneeded Expenditures*, Report to the Chairman, Committee on Governmental Affairs, US Senate, GAO/NSIAD-91-68 (US General Accounting Office: Washington, DC, Dec. 1990); *Biological Warfare: Role of Salk Institute in Army's Research Program*, Report to the Chairman, Committee on Governmental Affairs, US Senate GAO/NSIAD-92-33 (US General Accounting Office: Washington, DC, Dec. 1991).

VIII. Production and stockpiling of vaccines

For the reasons discussed above, and because some experts feared that the VFP programme might contribute to proliferation (see section XIII, below) and weaken deterrence (see section IX, below), it was concluded that 'defence vaccines will need to be produced by national facilities'.[68]

However, defence vaccines need not be developed and produced by national *military* facilities, a lesson which was learned about US biological defence preparedness during the Persian Gulf War. This is also demonstrated by the fact that some 100 non-military facilities participate in the US BDRP, including facilities in foreign countries and even some in China.[69]

The Persian Gulf War also demonstrated the problems raised by limitations on the amounts of vaccines available. According to the Commanding General of the 7th Corps of the Coalition forces 'one of the hardest calls he had to make was deciding who should be immunized'.[70] In addition, the threat of emerging diseases requires not only the production but also the stockpiling of vaccines against agents, including DTAs (see table 21.2), which pose possible health threats to the civilian population of industrialized countries.[71]

IX. Deterrence

The VFP proposal has been criticized as weakening defence: 'A defence that is freely available to the potential aggressor to examine and evaluate is no defence, as he will seek to and be able to circumvent that defence'. Hence, effective biological defence would not 'contribute to the web of deterrence which reduces the utility of biological warfare to a potential aggressor'.[72]

However, if a common biological defence system could be established on a global or at least regional basis, the likelihood of 'biological blackmail' by a state or terrorist group against a party to such a defence system would be diminished. As 'deterrence, in one sense, is simply the negative aspect of political power; it is the power to dissuade as opposed to the power to coerce or compel',[73] information on the availability of certain vaccines and the existence of a global biological defence system might act as a deterrent preventing a potential aggressor from using such agent(s). The VFP programme could constitute one aspect of the so-called 'fifth phase' of deterrence doctrine[74] because it would 'contribute to discouraging resort to biological warfare'.[75]

[68] See Pearson, chapter 14, in this volume.

[69] 'Appendix 3. Institutions performing BDRP research', *Biological Defense Research Program: Final Programmatic Environment Impact Statement* (Department of the Army, US Army Medical Research and Development Command: Fort Detrick, Frederick, Md., 1989), pp. A3-1–A3-9.

[70] US Army Chemical School, *NBC Lessons from Operation Desert Shield/Storm*, draft report, quoted in *Countering the Chemical and Biological Weapons Threat in the Post-Soviet World* (note 3), p. 56.

[71] Lederberg *et al.* (note 3).

[72] See Pearson, chapter 14, in this volume.

[73] Snyder, G. H., *Deterrence and Defense: Toward a Theory of National Security* (Princeton University Press: Princeton, N.J., 1991), p. 9.

[74] The fifth phase in deterrence doctrine had been reached, according to Stephenson and Weal when 'on 23 March 1983 President Reagan announced a major reversal in deterrence theory. His Star Wars defensive project aimed to neutralize attacking missiles before they reached the USA . . . In the words of Defense Secretary Caspar Weinberger (March 1983): "Deterrence would be strengthened because we would remove an aggressor's capability to attack us rather then merely threatening retaliation after an attack had taken place". Or as President Reagan put it: "We would protect our people, not avenge them"', see Stephenson, M. and Weal, J., *Nuclear Dictionary* (Longman: Harlow, Essex, 1985), pp. 47–48.

[75] See Sims, chapter 6, in this volume.

Additionally, the benefits which would derive from a strong international biological defence programme would outweigh any advantage a potential aggressor might gain from knowing which vaccines another state possesses.

X. Verification

The differing attitudes of countries to the feasibility of verification[76] seem influenced mainly by the 'philosophical' question of whether incomplete verification is better or worse than no verification. Verification of compliance with the BWC will never be complete because of the tremendous difficulties which exist, as recently described by Moodie [77] and Huxsoll.[78] Huxsoll asks important questions such as: 'Who pays the high cost of verification? Will poor, developing countries refuse to participate? Will they drop out of the treaty? Will additional nations not join? With the appearance of new nations and the newly gained independence of others, might they choose not to accede to the BWC because of the hassle and expense?'.[79]

These difficulties do not constitute adequate criticism of the VFP proposal, which is designed *inter alia* to attract developing countries, rather they are reasons to support VFP, especially because of its inclusion of DTAs and the participation of former military facilities.

Misuse of the VFP programme for purposes forbidden by the BWC and the CWC can be prevented to a large extent by the presence of international scientists and technicians as employees at the facilities which participate in the VFP programme. Such vaccine production experts would assist in the development of good manufacturing practices and in the establishment of the research and production programme of a facility. They would serve to increase transparency, as would trainees from developing countries who come to a facility to learn vaccine research techniques and the implementation of high-quality vaccine production. With international scientists working alongside the national staff, it would be very difficult to hide prohibited activities.

In addition, participation in the VFP programme would require: (*a*) membership both in the BWC and the CWC;[80] (*b*) full participation in the confidence-building measures (CBMs) agreed by the Second and Third Review Conferences;[81] and (*c*) readiness to participate in a strong verification system developed and established for the purpose of running the VFP programme.

As long as no general BWC verification system is in force,[82] establishment of a VFP verification system, restricted to participation in the international vaccine programme, would have *inter alia* the following advantages:

[76] Most European countries are in favour, while the USA and some developing countries doubt the verifiability of the Convention; see *Arms Control* (note 3), pp. 18–23.

[77] Moodie, M., 'Arms control programs and biological weapons', in Roberts (note 3), pp. 47–57.

[78] Huxsoll, D. L., 'The US Biological Defense Research Program', in Roberts (note 3) pp. 58–67.

[79] Huxsoll (note 78), p. 65.

[80] The VFP programme might also involve, though on a minor scale, the development of vaccines against toxins. Toxins covered by the BWC are—in contrast to statements released by several countries including Germany and the United States—chemical weapons because they are inanimate and not able to multiply. They are thus also covered by the CWC.

[81] See Thränert, chapter 5, in this volume.

[82] An *Ad Hoc* Group of Governmental Experts to Identify and Examine Potential Verification Measures from a Scientific and Technical Standpoint was established by the Third Review Conference, and a special conference will consider further actions. See Tóth, Geissler and Stock, chapter 7, in this volume.

1. Vaccine R&D, production and use are the most sensitive activities of those permitted by the BWC.

2. Development of and agreement on a vaccine verification system might be easier to accomplish than consensus on a general BWC verification regime. Such a system would be restricted to the facilities, techniques and personnel involved and to the DTAs dealt with in the vaccine programme, and only States Parties interested in participation in the vaccine programme would be required to accept this verification regime.

3. A VFP verification regime could be used as a model suitable for the development and improvement of a comprehensive BWC verification regime.

As originally proposed for verification of the BWC,[83] the compliance monitoring regime adopted to study Iraq's compliance with the obligations of UN Security Council resolution 687[84] could be the starting point for a VFP verification regime. The authors of this chapter agree with Senator John Glenn that VFP 'may help finesse a key verification problem of the BWC'.[85]

XI. The Global Epidemiological Surveillance System proposal

At the Third Review Conference, French delegate Pierre Cannone supported proposals[86] that a global surveillance system be set up to watch for unusual outbreaks of disease that might be caused by the hostile use of DTAs. This proposal was endorsed in the final report of the Third Review Conference, as follows:

> The Conference urges the United Nations and States Parties to take specific measures within their competence for the promotion of the fullest possible international cooperation in this field through their active intervention. Such measures could include, *inter alia*, . . . Cooperation in providing information on their national epidemiological surveillance and data reporting systems, and in providing assistance, on a bilateral level and/or in conjunction with WHO, regarding epidemiological surveillance, with a view to improvements in the identification and timely reporting of significant outbreaks of human and animal diseases.[87]

This proposal[88] was seen as a complement to the VFP proposal, and its supporters were invited to the Biesenthal meeting, where it was discussed further.

[83] Pearson, G. S., 'Verification of the Biological Weapons Convention', ed. O. Thränert, *The Verification of the Biological Weapons Convention: Problems and Perspectives* (Friedrich-Ebert-Stiftung: Bonn, 1992), pp. 83–99.

[84] 'Plan for future ongoing monitoring and verification of Iraq's compliance with relevant parts of section C of Security Council resolution 687', Report of the UN Secretary-General, S/22871/Rev.1, 2 Oct. 1991.

[85] Glenn, J. [Senator], 'Next steps in biological weapons disarmament', *Proliferation Watch*, vol. 3, no. 1 (Jan./Feb. 1992). p. 1.

[86] Wheelis, M., 'The role of epidemiology in strengthening the Biological Weapons Convention', Geissler and Haynes (note 48), pp. 277–85; Wheelis, M., 'Strengthening biological weapons control through global epidemiological surveillance' [with commentaries and response], *Politics and the Life Sciences*, vol. 11, no. 2 (Aug. 1992), pp. 179–97; Wheelis, chapter 17, in this volume; Morse, S., 'Epidemiologic surveillance for investigating chemical or biological warfare and for improving human health', *Politics and the Life Sciences*, vol. 11, no. 1 (Feb. 1992), pp. 28–29; Morse, chapter 16, in this volume.

[87] Final Document of the Third Review Conference of the Parties to the Convention on the Prohibition of the Development, Production and Stockpiling of Bacteriological (Biological) and Toxin Weapons and on their Destruction, Part II, *Final Declaration*, BWC/CONF.III /23, 27 Sep. 1991, pp. 21–22.

[88] A similar proposal was made by Zilinskas, who recommended establishment of an international 'Biological Hazards Early Warning Program' to investigate 'any unusual outbreaks of diseases to determine whether they are of natural origin, or are instead the products of laboratory development and attributable to accident or design', (note 27), p. 146.

A Steering Committee was then established, chaired by Dr Stephen S. Morse of Rockefeller University and composed of 12 scientists from the academic world, key US public health agencies, the Rockefeller Foundation, the Federation of American Scientists (FAS) and the Pan-American and World Health Organizations. The Steering Committee developed a preliminary Mission Statement.

The FAS set up a meeting of the Steering Committee in New York on 24 February 1993. The Mission Statement was finalized at that meeting.[89] The Steering Committee also proposed the establishment of five working groups to plan implementation of the project. These working groups cover surveillance and response for human and animal infectious disease and crop threats, national development issues and the BWC. The chairmen of the working groups, together with a Steering Committee expanded to include members from outside the Western hemisphere, will oversee the project, its implementation and funding.

A number of essential requirements for successful operation of the programme were identified. Hospital facilities in strategic locations are needed to provide clinical and pathological data on patients. Comprehensive training at the regional level to adequately identify and report unusual disease outbreaks is essential, as shown recently by the delay in identifying the outbreak of yellow fever in Kenya, which had the potential of spreading to urban centres in East Africa and eventually to the Indian subcontinent.[90] First-class laboratory facilities must be available down to the regional level to enable rapid identification of pathogens. Good communications are needed, including a surveillance and reporting system and regular contact among the personnel of participating institutions. A central managerial structure must be in place to co-ordinate programmes, compile and distribute information, and maintain a central reference laboratory (there is clearly a role here for the WHO). Finally, an international emergency response system is a key component. Without commitments of assistance in emergency situations from dependable sources there is little point in setting up the programme at all.

The Steering Committee also met on 4 June 1993 in Washington, DC, again under the auspices of the FAS. At the second meeting the title of the programme was changed from the Global Epidemiological Surveillance System to the Program for Monitoring Emerging Diseases (ProMED). The change was made in response to the perception that the term 'global surveillance' could have unfortunate connotations outside the strictly public health field. There was also a desire to stress that the programme would look for unusual outbreaks, such as the optic neuritis epidemic in Cuba and the Hantavirus outbreak on the Navajo reservation in the south-western USA,[91] rather than conduct routine surveillance for, say, childhood diseases.

A Conference on Global Control of Emerging Infectious Diseases was held on 11–12 September 1993 in Geneva, co-sponsored by the FAS and the WHO. It brought together 50 interested scientists and experts, and was also open to experts from the WHO and delegates from disarmament delegations based in Geneva. A background document for the conference was a draft monitoring plan by Dr Jim LeDuc of the WHO, who was invited to the Steering Committee

[89] See the GESS Mission Statement, annexe E, in this volume.

[90] World Health Organization, 'Yellow fever: Kenya', *Weekly Epidemiological Record*, vol. 68, no. 11 (1993), pp. 77–78.

[91] See note 30.

meeting. The draft envisages a central administrative centre to mobilize response to outbreaks anywhere in the world, rather than a set of regional centres. Monitoring would be based primarily on diseases rather than on a list of agents. All existing institutional networks, such as the WHO world-wide arbovirus and influenza surveillance networks, the chain of Pasteur institutes, and the Food and Agriculture Organization/WHO/International Office of Epizootics (OIE) animal health collaborating centres would be linked together. Facilities must be identified for banking agents and pathological specimens, and there is a need for epidemiological investigative capabilities linked to clinical facilities.

The benefits of a programme of this sort would be available to all countries. However, in order to provide an incentive for countries that have not already signed or ratified the BWC to do so, States Parties would receive preference in the support of facilities and in training opportunities.

XII. VFP and ProMED would avoid the need for definitions

It is correct that if *only* vaccine production and development are internationalized this would mean that 'the key problem of the verification [of the BWC] issue, namely [to define] what amount of which types of pathogens are necessary for peaceful or defensive military uses, still remains unresolved'.[92] However, the original VFP proposal suggested simultaneous establishment of ProMED (see above).

The development of additional means to defend against DTAs, namely the design of drugs, does not require a similar differentiation between remedies for the treatment of naturally caused infectious diseases and those caused by agents disseminated for hostile purposes.[93]

Simultaneous establishment of these measures under international control would significantly contribute to solving one of the key problems of verification and would avoid the need for definitions, especially if establishment of the VFP, and possibly of ProMED, leads to agreement on specific verification measures, as discussed above.

With the exception of the development of physical protection measures, if all of the activities permitted by the BWC ('prophylactic, protective, or other peaceful purposes') necessary for civilian and military defence against DTAs[94] are carried out under international control and under conditions of full transparency, there would no longer be a need to define what amounts of which types of agents are covered by Article I of the BWC. The latter would also be dealt with by a comprehensive VFP programme, a prerequisite of which would be the establishment of lists of DTAs (i.e., of putative BW and TW agents).

XIII. Proliferation

Several experts have expressed concern that an international programme of vaccine development against DTAs will enhance rather than reduce the danger of proliferation. This concern 'would necessitate the imposition of tight controls

[92] See Thränert, chapter 5, in this volume; see also Thränert (note 2).

[93] See Langen, chapter 15, in this volume.

[94] The mission objective of the US BDRP is described in Geissler, chapter 3, section III, in this volume.

on the VFP programme'.[95] The authors of this chapter agree with the need for tight control of the programme and refer to the verification possibilities discussed above (see section X). Export controls are also clearly needed in this area, and numerous micro-organisms and viruses—not just DTAs—are already subject to export controls in several countries, including the USA.[96] A regulatory system must be developed before establishment of the VFP programme. Such a system would contribute to making export controls more precise and specific, and might exclude those biological agents that are not DTAs from export controls on proliferation. The authors of this chapter welcome in this connection the statement of then US Deputy Secretary of Defense-designate William J. Perry that 'we have to draw a clear distinction between defence-unique systems and between dual use technology . . . By having too wide, too extensive, a list of technologies we try to control, we effectively trivialize the process and make it almost impossible to execute'.[97]

If a potential aggressor could obtain vaccines against DTAs under the VFP programme, this could clearly pose a problem. It might enable an aggressor not only to 'examine, evaluate and defeat' the action of these vaccines,[98] but also to make use of them for offensive purposes by protecting BW researchers and armed forces. This is an additional reason to demand that participation in a comprehensive VFP programme include adequate verification measures. A VFP verification system must also include precautionary measures designed to reduce the danger of military misuse of the VFP programme and its products. On the other hand, the programmes, personnel, equipment and facilities involved in the VFP programme should be more easily verified than any other item directly related to the BWC.

The authors of this chapter do not agree that the VFP programme would enhance the danger of proliferation rather than reduce it for the following reasons:

1. Putative BW agents are DTAs against which not only armed forces but all people have an equal right to be protected. The same holds true with respect to the techniques, equipment and facilities necessary for the development of vaccines. This is the main difference between the VFP programme and Atoms for Peace. There are limited personnel, facilities and funds available for the research and production of vaccines against even the major health threats covered by the CVI, the EPI and the PVD. It would appear both unwise and inhumane to fail to join forces to develop and produce vaccines against DTAs.

2. Article X of the BWC must be implemented whether or not all states welcome such an occurrence. The VFP and ProMED proposals seem to offer ways to implement Article X without increasing but instead decreasing the risk of proliferation. All developing countries should have access to biological agents including DTAs for peaceful (mainly medical) purposes. This access should include the corresponding dual-use know-how, technology and equipment unless the North can guarantee to provide these countries with the means to prevent,

[95] See Pearson, chapter 14, in this volume.

[96] 'Commodity interpretations, interpretation 24: microorganisms', *Export Administration Bulletin*, Mar./June 1990, supplement no. 1 to 799.2, pp. 11–24.

[97] Perry, W. J., testimony before the US Senate Armed Services Committee, 25 Feb. 1993, quoted in *Arms Sales Monitor*, no. 19 (15 Mar. 1993), p. 4.

[98] See Pearson, chapter 14, in this volume.

diagnose and treat infectious diseases and intoxinations. Even if the political will existed, it is obvious that the North cannot give such a guarantee.

3. Much has been published on the danger of biological warfare, including the information submitted in the course of the confidence-building exchange of information directly related to the BWC, and many States Parties to the BWC have expended great effort to convince non-parties to join the Convention. The assumption that the VFP programme 'would bring biological weapons to the attention of developing countries through the international organization having to consider the nature of biological weapons'[99] is therefore a gross overstatement.

XIV. Participation in the BWC

One of the reasons for proposing the VFP programme was to strengthen the BWC by increasing participation, since the statement that 'most of those countries who did not participate in the BWC didn't do so because of political-strategic reasons'[100] seems unfounded. Several states in the Middle East are not willing to become parties to the BWC while other countries in the region refuse to renounce possession of (other) weapons of mass destruction. Nevertheless, in order to strengthen the BWC universal participation is the declared goal of its States Parties. The Third Review Conference 'call[ed] upon States which have not yet ratified or acceded to the Convention to do so without delay and upon those States which have not signed the Convention to join the States Parties thereto thus contributing to the achievement of universal adherence to the Convention'.[101] Of course 'an increase in the number of States Parties . . . [*per se*] is unlikely to help automatically improve it'.[102] One of the major goals of the VFP and BVI programmes is therefore implementation of Article X.

Implementation of Article X has been strongly urged by the participants of the BWC Review Conferences. The Third Review Conference, for example,

> note[d] with concern the increasing gap between the developed and the developing countries in the field of biotechnology, genetic engineering, microbiology and other related areas. The Conference urge[d] all States Parties actively to promote international cooperation and exchange with States Parties in the peaceful uses of biotechnology, and urge[d] the developed countries possessing advanced biotechnology to adopt positive measures to promote technology transfer and international cooperation on an equal and non-discriminatory basis, in particular with the developing countries, for the benefit of all mankind.[103]

In addition, according to the Report of the Committee of the Whole of the Third Review Conference:

> some delegations [to the Third Review Conference] underlined the view that any restriction on cooperation in the field of peaceful bacteriological (biological) activities might not only be detrimental to the participants and run contrary to the humanitarian purposes of this Article [X] and the prevailing trends in the world, but would also have a negative effect on attaining the universality of the Convention. It was felt by those

[99] See Pearson, chapter 14, in this volume.
[100] Thränert (note 2).
[101] Final Document of the Third Review Conference (note 87), p. 24.
[102] Thränert (note 2).
[103] Final Document of the Third Review Conference (note 87), p. 21.

delegations that ever-widening and deepening cooperation is a key factor to increased adherence to the Convention by countries presently outside its framework.[104]

XV. Co-ordination

It will be important to co-ordinate the VFP programme with other vaccine initiatives in order to avoid duplication of work and competition for funds. The Children's Vaccine Initiative is operated by the WHO as part of a consortium (with UNICEF, the United Nations Development Programme (UNDP), the Rockefeller Foundation and the World Bank), and the Programme for Vaccine Development is a joint WHO/UNDP project. Given the congruence of the aims of the VFP, the CVI and the PVD, it is worth considering whether the VFP programme should be combined with the CVI or the PVD (a change from the original proposal).[105] This would limit the proliferation of competing vaccine initiatives; the existing initiatives share with the VFP and the BVI proposals the aim of promoting local vaccine production in developing countries and technology transfer.

None of the DTA vaccines are of interest to the CVI,[106] but they are relevant to the PVD. Therefore co-ordination with the WHO/UNDP Programme for Vaccine Development should be pursued.

XVI. Funding

Since vaccines are one of the most cost-effective means available for preventing disease,[107] the cost of launching the VFP programme would not be excessive, particularly when compared to the economic losses experienced or likely to be experienced if vaccines for DTAs are not available. Nevertheless significant funding would be required to launch and conduct the VFP programme.

The VFP and the BVI programmes should not and cannot compete for funds with other vaccine initiatives; additional funding is needed to launch these new programmes. The suggestion was made to approach foundations and agencies that do not work in the health field but which have an interest in promoting peace and disarmament.[108] This proposal seems reasonable not only because of the overall intention of the VFP programme but also owing to the anticipated contribution of the VFP to the conversion of former BW facilities, thereby preventing proliferation by avoiding the transfer of know-how (by the 'brain drain'

[104] Final Document of the Third Review Conference (note 87), p. 54.

[105] Woodall (note 2).

[106] Martinez, L., Personal communication with E. Geissler and J. P. Woodall, Mar. 1993.

[107] See Lederberg *et al.* (note 3), p. 150; Lederberg provides the following calculation: with the newly approved use of the *Haemophilus influenza* type B vaccine 'the total cost savings for vaccinating a one-year cohort of infants is estimated to be more than $359 million. Including the cost of providing and administering the vaccine, this works out to $106 million in vaccine costs versus $465.3 million in disease/morbidity/mortality costs'. This cost estimate applies to the USA alone; world-wide cost savings would be far greater. The cost, direct and indirect, of the 1977 dengue epidemic in Puerto Rico has been calculated in the range of $6.0–15.6 million, of which epidemic control measures comprised 7.8–20.2% (von Allmen, S. D. *et al.*, 'Epidemic dengue fever in Puerto Rico, 1977: a cost analysis', *American Journal of Tropical Medicine and Hygiene*, vol. 28, no. 6 (1979), pp. 1040–44). In Asia, where large numbers of children are hospitalized with dengue haemorrhagic fever and shock syndrome every year, the cost–benefit of a vaccine would be proportionately greater. The benefit to cost ratio of measles immunization in Mexico has been estimated at 27:1, or 100:1 if lost earnings are included. See the chapter by S. O. Foster, D. A. McFarland and A. M. John in eds D. T. Jamison and W. H. Mosley, *Disease Control Priorities in Developing Countries* (Oxford University Press for the World Bank: New York, 1993).

[108] Kane (note 31).

of scientists and technicians), equipment and agents from such facilities to other places and regions.

The conversion component of the VFP programme might be supported by the newly created International Science and Technology Center established in Moscow by the Commonwealth of Independent States and Georgia, the European Community, Japan, the Russian Federation and the USA, as well as by other agencies and foundations which are interested in promoting the conversion of former Soviet warfare facilities. The Center will assist the CIS states and Georgia; funds will become available when establishment of the Center is approved by the Russian Parliament. However, at present it is envisaged that funds for the Center will be available only for R&D; additional sources of funding would be required for vaccine production.

States Parties to the BWC should also be approached to provide funds for the VFP programme.

XVII. Conclusions and recommendations

In conclusion, the authors of this chapter recommend that:

1. The comprehensive VFP programme should be established, step by step, beginning with implementation of the Biesenthal Vaccine Initiative.
2. Immediate action should be taken to use the programme for assisting in conversion of BW facilities, especially in the former Soviet Union. Any other facility in the former Soviet Union suitable for participation in the programme should be invited to participate and should be supported accordingly.
3. All suitable facilities world-wide should be invited to participate in the VFP and the BVI programmes on the condition that the country in which they are located is a State Party to the BWC and takes part in the information transfer CBMs.
4. Participation in the VFP programme requires readiness to participate in a verification system. The system should be based on the considerations outlined in section X above.
5. To establish a system of common biological security, states should reconsider their biological defence policies with respect to: transferring all biological activities permitted by the BWC to international programmes such as the VFP and ProMED, abolishing any distinction between defence against natural outbreaks of disease and diseases caused by hostile application of BW and TW agents, and addressing differences in protection of the civilian population and troops.
6. The UN Secretary-General should be asked to consider whether support can be given to the VFP, the BVI and ProMED in the context of the discussion and examination of improving implementation of Article X of the BWC, as requested by the Third Review Conference.

Part VII. Annexes

Annexe A. The 1972 Biological Weapons Convention

CONVENTION ON THE PROHIBITION OF THE DEVELOPMENT, PRODUCTION AND STOCKPILING OF BACTERIOLOGICAL (BIOLOGICAL) AND TOXIN WEAPONS AND ON THEIR DESTRUCTION

Signed at London, Moscow and Washington on 10 April 1972
Entered into force on 26 March 1975
Depositaries: UK, US and Soviet governments

The States Parties to this Convention,

Determined to act with a view to achieving effective progress towards general and complete disarmament, including the prohibition and elimination of all types of weapons of mass destruction, and convinced that the prohibition of the development, production and stockpiling of chemical and bacteriological (biological) weapons and their elimination, through effective measures, will facilitate the achievement of general and complete disarmament under strict and effective international control,

Recognizing the important significance of the Protocol for the Prohibition of the Use in War of Asphyxiating, Poisonous or Other Gases, and of Bacteriological Methods of Warfare, signed at Geneva on June 17, 1925, and conscious also of the contribution which the said Protocol has already made, and continues to make, to mitigating the horrors of war,

Reaffirming their adherence to the principles and objectives of that Protocol and calling upon all States to comply strictly with them,

Recalling that the General Assembly of the United Nations has repeatedly condemned all actions contrary to the principles and objectives of the Geneva Protocol of June 17, 1925,

Desiring to contribute to the strengthening of confidence between peoples and the general improvement of the international atmosphere,

Desiring also to contribute to the realization of the purposes and principles of the Charter of the United Nations,

Convinced of the importance and urgency of eliminating from the arsenals of States, through effective measures, such dangerous weapons of mass destruction as those using chemical or bacteriological (biological) agents,

Recognizing that an agreement on the prohibition of bacteriological (biological) and toxin weapons represents a first possible step towards the achievement of agreement on effective measures also for the problem of the development, production and stockpiling of chemical weapons, and determined to continue negotiations to that end,

Determined, for the sake of all mankind, to exclude completely the possibility of bacteriological (biological) agents and toxins being used as weapons,

Convinced that such use would be repugnant to the conscience of mankind and that no effort should be spared to minimize this risk,

Have agreed as follows:

Article I

Each State Party to this Convention undertakes never in any circumstances to develop, produce, stockpile or otherwise acquire or retain:

1. Microbial or other biological agents, or toxins whatever their origin or method of production, of types and in quantities that have no justification for prophylactic, protective or other peaceful purposes;
2. Weapons, equipment or means of delivery designed to use such agents or toxins for hostile purposes or in armed conflict.

Article II

Each State Party to this Convention undertakes to destroy, or to divert to peaceful purposes, as soon as possible but not later than nine months after the entry into force of the Convention, all agents, toxins, weapons, equipment and means of delivery specified in article I of the Convention, which are in its possession or under its jurisdiction or control. In implementing the provisions of this article all necessary safety precautions shall be observed to protect populations and the environment.

Article III

Each State Party to this Convention undertakes not to transfer to any recipient whatsoever, directly or indirectly, and not in any way to assist, encourage, or induce any State, group of States or international organizations to manufacture or otherwise acquire any of the agents, toxins, weapons, equipment or means of delivery specified in article I of the Convention.

Article IV

Each State Party to this Convention shall, in accordance with its constitutional processes, take any necessary measures to prohibit and prevent the development, production, stockpiling, acquisition or retention of the agents, toxins, weapons, equipment and means of delivery specified in article I of the Convention, within the territory of such State, under its jurisdiction or under its control anywhere.

Article V

The States Parties to this Convention undertake to consult one another and to cooperate in solving any problems which may arise in relation to the objective of, or in the application of the provisions of, the Convention. Consultation and cooperation pursuant to this article may also be undertaken through appropriate international procedures within the framework of the United Nations and in accordance with its Charter.

Article VI

1. Any State Party to this Convention which finds that any other State Party is acting in breach of obligations deriving from the provisions of the Convention may lodge a complaint with the Security Council of the United Nations. Such a complaint should include all possible evidence confirming its validity, as well as a request for its consideration by the Security Council.
2. Each State Party to this Convention undertakes to cooperate in carrying out any investigation which the Security Council may initiate, in accordance with the provisions of the Charter of the United Nations, on the basis of the complaint received by the Council. The Security Council shall inform the States Parties to the Convention of the results of the investigation.

Article VII

Each State Party to this Convention undertakes to provide or support assistance, in accordance with the United Nations Charter, to any Party to the Convention which so requests, if the Security Council decides that such Party has been exposed to danger as a result of violation of the Convention.

Article VIII

Nothing in this Convention shall be interpreted as in any way limiting or detracting from the obligations assumed by any State under the Protocol for the Prohibition of the Use in War of Asphyxiating, Poisonous or Other Gases, and of Bacteriological Methods of Warfare, signed at Geneva on June 17, 1925.

Article IX

Each State Party to this Convention affirms the recognized objective of effective prohibition of chemical weapons and, to this end, undertakes to continue negotiations in good faith with a view to reaching early agreement on effective measures for the prohibition of their development, production and stockpiling and for their destruction, and on appropriate measures concerning equipment and means of delivery specifically designed for the production or use of chemical agents for weapons purposes.

Article X

1. The States Parties to this Convention undertake to facilitate, and have the right to participate in, the fullest possible exchange of equipment, materials and scientific and technological information for the use of bacteriological (biological) agents and toxins for peaceful purposes. Parties to the Convention in a position to do so shall also cooperate in contributing individually or together with other States or international organizations to the further development and application of scientific discoveries in the field of bacteriology (biology) for prevention of disease, or for other peaceful purposes.
2. This Convention shall be implemented in a manner designed to avoid hampering the economic or technological development of States Parties to the Convention or international cooperation in the field of peaceful bacteriological (biological) activities, including the international exchange of bacteriological (biological) agents and toxins and equipment for the processing, use or production of bacteriological (biological) agents and toxins for peaceful purposes in accordance with the provisions of the Convention.

Article XI

Any State Party may propose amendments to this Convention. Amendments shall enter into force for each State Party accepting the amendments upon their acceptance by a majority of the States Parties to the Convention and thereafter for each remaining State Party on the date of acceptance by it.

Article XII

Five years after the entry into force of this Convention, or earlier if it is requested by a majority of Parties to the Convention by submitting a proposal to this effect to the Depositary Governments, a conference of States Parties to the Convention shall be held at Geneva, Switzerland, to review the operation of the Convention, with a view to assuring that the purposes of the preamble and the provisions of the Convention, including the provisions concerning negotiations on chemical weapons, are being realized. Such review shall take into account any new scientific and technological developments relevant to the Convention.

Article XIII

1. This Convention shall be of unlimited duration.

2. Each State Party to this Convention shall in exercising its national sovereignty have the right to withdraw from the Convention if it decides that extraordinary events, related to the subject matter of the Convention, have jeopardized the supreme interests of its country. It shall give notice of such withdrawal to all other States Parties to the Convention and to the United Nations Security Council three months in advance. Such notice shall include a statement of the extraordinary events it regards as having jeopardized its supreme interests.

Article XIV

1. This Convention shall be open to all States for signature. Any State which does not sign the Convention before its entry into force in accordance with paragraph (3) of this Article may accede to it at any time.

2. This Convention shall be subject to ratification by signatory States. Instruments of ratification and instruments of accession shall be deposited with the Governments of the United States of America, the United Kingdom of Great Britain and Northern Ireland and the Union of Soviet Socialist Republics, which are hereby designated the Depositary Governments.

3. This Convention shall enter into force after the deposit of instruments of ratification by twenty-two Governments, including the Governments designated as Depositaries of the Convention.

4. For States whose instruments of ratification or accession are deposited subsequent to the entry into force of this Convention, it shall enter into force on the date of the deposit of their instruments of ratification or accession.

5. The Depositary Governments shall promptly inform all signatory and acceding States of the date of each signature, the date of deposit of each instrument of ratification or of accession and the date of the entry into force of this Convention, and of the receipt of other notices.

6. This Convention shall be registered by the Depositary Governments pursuant to Article 102 of the Charter of the United Nations.

Article XV

This Convention, the English, Russian, French, Spanish and Chinese texts of which are equally authentic, shall be deposited in the archives of the Depositary Governments. Duly certified copies of the Convention shall be transmitted by the Depositary Governments to the Governments of the signatory and acceding States.

Source: *Treaties and Other International Acts, Series 8062* (US Department of State: Washington, DC, 1975)

Annexe B. Final Declaration of the Third Review Conference of the BWC

FINAL DECLARATION

THE STATES PARTY TO THE CONVENTION ON THE PROHIBITION OF THE DEVELOPMENT, PRODUCTION AND STOCKPILING OF BACTERIOLOGICAL (BIOLOGICAL) AND TOXIN WEAPONS AND ON THEIR DESTRUCTION, WHICH MET IN GENEVA FROM 9 TO 27 SEPTEMBER 1991 TO REVIEW THE OPERATION OF THE CONVENTION, SOLEMNLY DECLARE:

– Their conviction that the Convention is essential to international peace and security;

– Their reaffirmation of their determination to act with a view to achieving effective progress towards general and complete disarmament, including the prohibition and elimination of all types of weapons of mass destruction, and their conviction that the prohibition of the development, production and stockpiling of chemical and bacteriological (biological) weapons and their elimination, through effective measures, will facilitate the achievement of general and complete disarmament under strict and effective international control;

– Their continued determination, for the sake of mankind, to exclude completely the possibility of the use of bacteriological (biological) agents and toxins as weapons, and their conviction that such use would be repugnant to the conscience of mankind;

– Their reaffirmation of their firm commitment to the purposes of the preamble and the provisions of the Convention, and of their belief that universal adherence to the Convention would enhance international peace and security;

– Their determination to enhance the implementation and effectiveness of the Convention and to further strengthen its authority, including through the confidence-building measures and organizational arrangements set out below;

– Their recognition that effective verification could reinforce the Convention;

– Their conviction that the full implementation of the provisions of the Convention should not hamper economic and technological development and international co-operation in the field of peaceful biological activities.

The State parties recognize that the important principles contained in this Solemn Declaration can also serve as a basis for further strengthening of the Convention.

Preamble

The Conference reaffirms the importance of the elements in the review of the Preamble to the Convention contained in the Final Declaration of the Second Review Conference of the States Parties to the Convention on the Prohibition of the Development, Production and Stockpiling of Bacteriological (Biological) and Toxin Weapons and on their Destruction.

Article I

The Conference notes the importance of Article I as the article which defines the scope of the Convention and reaffirms its support for the provisions of this Article.

The Conference reaffirms that the Convention prohibits the development, production, stockpiling, other acquisition or retention of microbial or other biological agents or toxins harmful to plants and animals, as well as humans, of types and in quantities that have no justification for prophylactic, protective or other peaceful purposes.

The Conference, conscious of apprehensions arising from relevant scientific and technological developments, *inter alia,* in the fields of microbiology, genetic engineering and biotechnology, and the possibilities of their use for purposes inconsistent with the objectives and the provisions of the Convention, reaffirms that the undertaking given by the States parties in Article I applies to all such developments. The Conference also reaffirms that the Convention unequivocally covers all microbial or other biological agents or toxins, naturally or artificially created or altered, whatever their origin or method of production.

The Conference notes that experimentation involving open-air release of pathogens or toxins harmful to man, animals or plants that has no justification for prophylactic, protective or other peaceful purposes is inconsistent with the undertakings contained in Article I.

The Conference stresses that States parties should take all necessary safety precautions to protect populations and the environment in relation to activities not prohibited by the Convention.

The Conference emphasizes the vital importance of full implementation by all States parties of all the provisions of the Convention and expresses concern at statements by some States parties that compliance with Articles I, II and III has been, in their view, subject to grave doubt in certain cases and that efforts since the Second Review Conference to resolve these problems have not been successful. The Conference agrees that the application by States parties of a positive approach in questions of compliance in accordance with the provisions of the Convention is in the interest of all States parties and that continued non-compliance with its provisions could undermine confidence in the Convention.

On the basis of the principle that sciences should support quality of life, the Conference appeals through the States parties to their scientific communities to continue to support only activities that have justification under the biological and toxin weapons Convention for prophylactic, protective or other peaceful purposes, and refrain from activities which are in breach of obligations deriving from provisions of the Convention.

Article II

The Conference notes the importance of Article II and welcomes the statements made by States which have become parties to the Convention since the Second Review Conference that they do not possess agents, toxins, weapons, equipment or means of delivery referred to in Article I of the Convention. The Conference believes that such statements contribute to enhancing confidence in the Convention.

The Conference stresses that States which become parties to the Convention, in implementing the provisions of this Article, shall observe all necessary safety precautions to protect populations and the environment.

Article III

The Conference notes the importance of Article III and welcomes the statements which States that have acceded to the Convention have made to the effect that they have not transferred agents, toxins, weapons, equipment or means of delivery, specified in Article I of the Convention, to any recipient whatsoever and have not furnished assistance, encouragement or inducement to any State, group of States or international organizations to manufacture or otherwise acquire them. The Conference affirms that Article III is sufficiently comprehensive to cover any recipient whatsoever at international, national or subnational levels. The Conference notes that a number of States parties have already taken concrete measures to give effect to their undertakings under this Article, and calls for appropriate measures by all States parties. Transfers relevant to the Convention should be authorized only when the intended use is for purposes not prohibited under the Convention. The implementation of this Article with respect to such transfers should continue to be the subject of multilateral consideration.

The Conference notes that the provisions of this Article should not be used to impose restrictions and/or limitations on the transfer for purposes consistent with the objectives and the provisions of the Convention of scientific knowledge, technology, equipment and materials under Article X.

Article IV

The Conference notes the importance of Article IV under which each State party shall, in accordance with its constitutional processes, take any necessary measures to prohibit or prevent any acts or actions which would contravene the Convention.

The Conference notes those measures already taken by some States parties in this regard, for example the adoption of penal legislation, and reiterates its call to any State party that has not yet taken any necessary measures to do so immediately, in accordance with its constitutional processes. Such measures should apply within the territory of a State party, under its jurisdiction or under its control anywhere. The Conference invites each State party to consider, if constitutionally possible and in conformity with international law, the application of such measures to actions taken anywhere by natural persons possessing its nationality.

The Conference notes the importance of:

– Legislative, administrative and other measures designed to enhance domestic compliance with the Convention;

– Legislation regarding the physical protection of laboratories and facilities to prevent unauthorized access to and removal of microbial or other biological agents, or toxins;

– Inclusion in textbooks and in medical, scientific and military educational programmes of information dealing with the prohibition of microbial or other biological agents or toxins and the provisions of the Geneva Protocol of 1925.

The Conference believes that such measures which States parties might undertake in accordance with their constitutional processes would strengthen the effectiveness of the Convention.

The Conference notes that some States parties, as requested by the Second Review Conference, have provided to the United Nations Department for Disarmament Affairs information on and the texts of specific legislation enacted or other measures taken to assure domestic compliance with the Convention. The Conference invites these States parties, and encourages all States parties, to provide such information and texts in the future. In this regard the Conference welcomes agreement by the States parties participating in the Third Review Conference to implement a new confidence-building measure entitled 'Declaration of legislation, regulations and other measures'. In addition, the Conference invites all States parties to provide any useful information on the implementation of such measures.

The Conference welcomes regional measures such as the Mendoza Declaration as well as other initiatives dealing with the renunciation of weapons of mass destruction, including biological weapons, as concrete positive steps towards the strengthening of the biological and toxin weapons Convention regime.

Article V

In accordance with the decision of the Second Review Conference, and taking into account views expressed concerning the need to strengthen the implementation of the provisions of Article V, the Conference reviewed the effectiveness of the provisions in Article V for consultation and cooperation and of the cooperative measures agreed in the Final Declaration of the Second Review Conference, and considered whether or not further actions were called for to create further cooperative measures. The Conference came to the following conclusions and recommendations:

The Conference notes the importance of the confidence-building measures agreed upon at the Second Review Conference, as well as the modalities elaborated by the Ad Hoc Meeting of Scientific and Technical Experts from States parties to the Convention held in 1987. The Conference recognizes the exchange of information that took place on this agreed basis between 1987 and 1991. The Conference urges all States parties to submit information to future rounds of information exchange.

With a view to promoting increased participation and strengthening further the exchange of information, the Conference agrees to reaffirm those measures established at the Second Review Conference with the following improvements: to add a declaration on 'Nothing to declare' or 'Nothing new to declare'; to amend and extend the exchange of data on research centres and laboratories; to amend the exchange of information on outbreaks of infectious diseases and similar occurrences caused by toxins; to amend the measure for the active promotion of contacts; and to add three new confidence-building measures entitled 'Declaration of legislation, regulations and other measures'; 'Declaration of past activities in offensive and/or defensive biological research development programmes'; and 'Declaration of vaccine production facilities'.

Accordingly, the Conference, mindful of the provisions of Article V and Article X, and determined to strengthen the authority of the Convention and to enhance confidence in the implementation of its provisions, agrees that the States parties are to implement, on the basis of mutual cooperation, the following measures set out in the annex to this Final Declaration, in order to prevent or reduce the occurrence of ambiguities, doubts and suspicions, and in order to improve international cooperation in the field of peaceful bacteriological (biological) activities:

1. Declaration form on 'Nothing to declare' or 'Nothing new to declare':

2. Confidence-building measure 'A':

– Part 1: Exchange of data on research centres and laboratories;

– Part 2: Exchange of information on national biological defence research and development programmes.

3. Confidence-building measure 'B':

– Exchange of information on outbreaks of infectious diseases and similar occurrences caused by toxins.

4. Confidence-building measure 'C':

– Encouragement of publication of results and promotion of use of knowledge.

5. Confidence-building measure 'D':

– Active promotion of contacts.

6. Confidence-building measure 'E':

– Declaration of legislation, regulations and other measures.

7. Confidence-building measure 'F':

– Declaration of past activities in offensive and/or defensive biological research and development programmes.

8. Confidence-building measure 'G':

– Declaration of vaccine production facilities.

The Conference also agrees that the exchange of information and data, using the revised forms, be sent to the United Nations Department for Disarmament Affairs no later than 15 April on an annual basis and should cover the previous calendar year.

The Conference recognizes that the new and the revised procedures which the States parties have agreed to implement will add further duties to, and will make even greater demands on the time of, the United Nations Department for Disarmament Affairs. The Conference therefore requests the United Nations Secretary-General to allocate the necessary staff resources and other requirements based in the United Nations Department for Disarmament Affairs in Geneva to assist the effective implementation of the relevant decisions of the Third Review Conference, in particular of the confidence-building measures. In that respect the Secretary-General is requested to receive, compile, and make available to States parties information related to the implementation of the Convention and of the decisions of the Third Review Conference. The use of the United Nations Department for Disarmament Affairs computer database system could facilitate this work. The States parties agree to review *inter alia* the requirement for, and the operation of, these additional arrangements at the Fourth Review Conference.

The Conference notes the importance of Article V and reaffirms the obligation assumed by States parties to consult and cooperate with one another in solving any problems which may arise in relation to the objective of, or in the application of the provisions of, the Convention.

The Conference reaffirms the agreement reached at the Second Review Conference, and agrees that in order to strengthen the implementation of the provisions of Article V the following procedures should be adopted:

- A formal consultative meeting could be preceded by bilateral or other consultations by agreement among those States parties involved in the problems which had arisen;
- Requests for the convening of a consultative meeting shall be addressed to the Depositaries, who shall immediately inform all States parties of the request and shall convene within 30 days an informal meeting of interested States parties to discuss the arrangements for the formal consultative meeting, which shall be convened within 60 days of receipt of the request;
- With regard to the taking of decisions, the consultative meeting shall proceed in accordance with rule 28 of the rules of procedure of the Review Conference;
- The costs of the consultative meeting shall be met by the States parties participating in accordance with the United Nations assessment scale prorated to take into account differences between the United Nations membership and the number of States parties participating in the meeting;
- A consultative meeting may consider any problems which may arise in relation to the objective of, or in the application of the provisions of, the Convention, suggest ways and means for further clarifying, *inter alia,* with assistance of technical experts, any matter considered ambiguous or unresolved, as well as initiate appropriate international procedures within the framework of the United Nations and in accordance with its Charter;
- The consultative meeting, or any State party, may request specialized assistance in solving any problems which may arise in relation to the objective of, or in the application of the provisions of, the Convention, through, *inter alia,* appropriate international procedures within the framework of the United Nations and in accordance with its Charter;
- The States parties agree that, should the consultative meeting, or any State party, make use of such procedures within the framework of the United Nations, including lodging a complaint with the Security Council under Article VI of the Convention, the Secretary-General may be kept informed;
- The Conference considers that States parties shall cooperate with the consultative meeting in its consideration of any problems which may arise in relation to the objective of, or in the application of the provisions of, the Convention, and in clarifying ambiguous and unresolved matters, as well as cooperate in appropriate international procedures within the framework of the United Nations and in accordance with its Charter.

The Conference reaffirms that consultation and cooperation pursuant to this Article may also be undertaken through appropriate international procedures within the framework of the United Nations and in accordance with its Charter.

The Conference, determined to strengthen the effectiveness and improve the implementation of the Convention and recognizing that effective verification could reinforce the Convention, decides to establish an Ad Hoc Group of Governmental Experts open to all States parties to identify and examine potential verification measures from a scientific and technical standpoint.

The Group shall meet in Geneva for the period 30 March to 10 April 1992. The Group will hold additional meetings as appropriate to complete its work as soon as possible, preferably before the end of 1993. In accordance with the agreement reached in the Preparatory Committee, the Group shall be chaired by Ambassador Tibor Tóth (Hungary), who shall be assisted by two Vice-Chairmen to be elected by the States parties participating in the first meeting.

The Group shall seek to identify measures which could determine:

- Whether a State party is developing, producing, stockpiling, acquiring or retaining microbial or other biological agents or toxins, of types and in quantities that have no justification for prophylactic, protective or peaceful purposes;

– Whether a State party is developing, producing, stockpiling, acquiring or retaining weapons, equipment or means of delivery designed to use such agents or toxins for hostile purposes or in armed conflict.

Such measures could be addressed singly or in combination. Specifically, the Group shall seek to evaluate potential verification measures, taking into account the broad range of types and quantities of microbial and other biological agents and toxins, whether naturally occurring or altered, which are capable of being used as means of warfare.

To these ends the Group could examine potential verification measures in terms of the following main criteria:

– Their strengths and weaknesses based on, but not limited to, the amount and quality of information they provide, and fail to provide;

– Their ability to differentiate between prohibited and permitted activities;

– Their ability to resolve ambiguities about compliance;

– Their technology, material, manpower and equipment requirements;

– Their financial, legal, safety and organizational implications;

– Their impact on scientific research, scientific cooperation, industrial development and other permitted activities, and their implications for the confidentiality of commercial proprietary information.

In examining potential verification measures, the Group should take into account data and other information relevant to the Convention provided by the States Parties.

The Group shall adopt by consensus a report taking into account views expressed in the course of its work. The report of the Group shall be a description of its work on the identification and examination of potential verification measures from a scientific and technical standpoint, according to this mandate.

The report of the Group shall be circulated to all States Parties for their consideration. If a majority of States Parties ask for the convening of a conference to examine the report, by submitting a proposal to this effect to the Depositary Governments, such a conference will be convened. In such a case the conference shall decide on any further action. The conference shall be preceded by a preparatory committee.

The Conference stresses the need for all States to deal seriously with compliance issues and emphasizes that failure to do so undermines the Convention and the arms control and disarmament process in general.

The Conference appeals to States Parties to make all possible efforts to solve any problems which may arise in relation to the objective of, or in the application of the provisions of, the Convention with a view towards encouraging strict observance of the provisions subscribed to. In this connection, the States Parties agree to provide a specific, timely response to any compliance concern alleging a breach of their obligations under the Convention. Such responses should be submitted through the procedures provided for under the Convention. The Conference further requests that information on such efforts be provided to the Fourth Review Conference.

The Conference welcomes the proposals set out in annex I of United Nations document A/44/561 developed by a group of qualified experts and endorsed by the United Nations General Assembly in 1990 in its resolution 45/57 C for technical guidelines and procedures to guide the United Nations Secretary-General in the timely and efficient investigation of reports of the possible use of chemical and bacteriological (biological) or toxin weapons. The Conference recalls, in this context, United Nations Security Council resolution 620 of 1988, which encouraged the United Nations Secretary-General to carry out prompt investigations, in response to allegations brought to his attention by any Member State concerning the possible use of chemical and bacteriological (biological) or toxin weapons. The States Parties agree to consult, at the request of any State Party, regarding allegations of use or threat of use of bacteriological (biological) or toxin weapons and to cooperate fully with the United Nations Secretary-General in carrying out such investigations. The Conference stresses that in the case of alleged use the United Nations is called upon to take appropriate measures, which could include a request to the Security Council to consider action in accordance with the Charter.

Taking into account the specific characteristics of each region, neighbouring States or States belonging to the same region may also adopt measures that are consistent with the aims and objectives of the Convention in order to facilitate or complement the implementation of the decisions of the Third Review Conference with respect to Article V.

Article VI

The Conference notes that the provisions of this Article have not been invoked.

The Conference reaffirms the importance of Article VI, which, in addition to the procedures contained in Article V, provides that any State Party which finds that any other State Party is acting in breach of its obligations under the Convention may lodge a complaint with the United Nations Security Council.

The Conference emphasized the provision of Article VI that such a complaint should include all possible evidence confirming its validity. It stressed that, as in the case of the implementation of all the provisions and procedures set forth in the Convention, the procedures foreseen in Article VI should be implemented in good faith and within the scope of the Convention.

The Conference invites the Security Council to consider immediately any complaint lodged under Article VI and to initiate any measures it considers necessary for the investigation of the complaint. The Conference reaffirms the undertaking of each State Party to cooperate in carrying out any investigations which the Security Council may initiate.

The Conference recalls, in this context, United Nations Security Council resolution 620 of 1988, which encouraged the United Nations Secretary-General to carry out prompt investigations, in response to allegations brought to his attention by any Member State concerning the possible use of chemical and bacteriological (biological) or toxin weapons.

The Conference invites the Security Council to inform each State Party of the results of any investigation initiated under Article VI and to consider promptly any appropriate further action which may be necessary.

Article VII

The Conference notes with satisfaction that these provisions have not been invoked.

The Conference reaffirms the undertaking made by each State Party to provide or support assistance in accordance with the Charter of the United Nations to any Party to the Convention which so requests, if the Security Council decides that such Party has been exposed to danger as a result of violation of the Convention.

The Conference takes note of desires expressed that, should a request for assistance be made, it be promptly considered and an appropriate response provided. In this context, pending consideration of a decision by the Security Council, timely emergency assistance could be provided by States Parties if requested.

The Conference considers that in the event that this Article might be invoked, the United Nations, with the help of appropriate intergovernmental organizations such as the World Health Organization (WHO), could play a coordinating role.

Article VIII

The Conference reaffirms the importance of Article VIII and stresses the importance of the Protocol for the Prohibition of the Use in War of Asphyxiating, Poisonous or Other Gases and of Bacteriological Methods of Warfare signed at Geneva on 17 June 1925.

The Conference reaffirms that nothing contained in the Convention shall be interpreted as in any way limiting or detracting from the obligations assumed by any State under the Protocol for the Prohibition of the Use in War of Asphyxiating, Poisonous or Other Gases and of Bacteriological Methods of Warfare. The Conference appeals to all States Parties to the Geneva Protocol of 1925 to fulfil their obligations assumed under that Protocol and urges all States not yet Parties to the said Protocol to accede to it without delay.

The Conference acknowledges that the 1925 Geneva Protocol, by prohibiting the use of bacteriological methods of warfare, forms an essential complement to the biological and toxin weapons Convention.

The Conference stresses the importance of the withdrawal of all reservations to the 1925 Geneva Protocol related to the biological and toxin weapons Convention.

The Conference notes that the United Nations has taken significant action in support of the Geneva Protocol of 1925 during the period under review, including through Security Council resolution 620 (1988) and General Assembly resolutions 41/58 C, 42/37 C, 43/74 A, 44/115 B and 45/57 C.

The Conference recalls that the participating States at the Conference of States Parties to the 1925 Geneva Protocol and Other Interested States, held in Paris from 7 to 11 January 1989, solemnly reaffirmed in its Final Declaration the prohibition as established in the Geneva Protocol of 1925 and urged all States which had not done so to accede to it.

Article IX

The Conference reaffirms the obligation assumed by States Parties to continue negotiations in good faith towards an early agreement on effective measures for the prohibition of the development, production and stockpiling of chemical weapons and for their destruction.

All States Parties participating in the Conference reiterate their strong commitment to this important goal.

The Conference notes with satisfaction the substantial progress made in the negotiations on a convention on chemical weapons in the Conference on Disarmament during the period under review. The Conference also takes note of the bilateral agreement, signed in June 1990, between the Union of Soviet Socialist Republics and the United States of America on destruction and non-production of chemical weapons.

The Conference urges the Conference on Disarmament to exert all possible efforts to implement the mandate for the chemical weapons negotiations as amended on 20 June 1991, and to achieve final agreement by 1992 on the convention on the complete and effective prohibition of the development, production, stockpiling and use of chemical weapons and on their destruction. The Conference notes the statements of intent by many States to become original parties to the chemical weapons convention and calls on all States to adhere early to the convention when concluded so as to ensure its early entry into force.

Article X

The Conference emphasizes the increasing importance of the provisions of Article X, especially in the light of recent scientific and technological developments in the field of biotechnology, bacteriological (biological) agents and toxins with peaceful applications, which have vastly increased the potential for cooperation between States to help promote economic and social development, and scientific and technological progress, particularly in the developing countries, in conformity with their interests, needs and priorities.

The Conference, while acknowledging what has already been done towards this end, notes with concern the increasing gap between the developed and the developing countries in the field of biotechnology, genetic engineering, microbiology and other related areas. The Conference urges all States Parties actively to promote international cooperation and exchange with States Parties in the peaceful uses of biotechnology, and urges the developed countries possessing advanced biotechnology to adopt positive measures to promote technology transfer and international cooperation on an equal and non-discriminatory basis, in particular with the developing countries, for the benefit of all mankind.

The Conference urges the United Nations and States Parties to take specific measures within their competence for the promotion of the fullest possible international cooperation in this field through their active intervention. Such measures could include, *inter alia:*

– Transfer and exchange of information concerning research programmes in biosciences, and greater cooperation in international public health and disease control;

– Wider transfer and exchange of information, materials and equipment among States on a systematic and long-term basis;

– Active promotion of contacts between scientists and technical personnel on a reciprocal basis, in relevant fields;

– Increased technical cooperation and assistance, including training programmes to developing countries in the use of biosciences and genetic engineering for peaceful purposes through active association with United Nations institutions, including the International Centre for Genetic Engineering and Biotechnology;

– Facilitating the conclusion of bilateral, regional and multiregional agreements providing, on a mutually advantageous, equal and non-discriminatory basis, for their participation in the development and application of biotechnology;

– Encouraging the coordination of national and regional programmes and working out in an appropriate manner the ways and means of cooperation in this field;

– Cooperation in providing information on their national epidemiological surveillance and data reporting systems, and in providing assistance, on a bilateral level and/or in conjunction with WHO, regarding epidemiological surveillance, with a view to improvements in the identification and timely reporting of significant outbreaks of human and animal diseases.

The Review Conference considers that the establishment of a world data bank under the supervision of the United Nations might be a suitable way of facilitating the flow of information in the field of genetic engineering, biotechnology and other scientific developments.

The Conference urges the use of existing institutional means within the United Nations system and the full utilization of the possibilities provided by the specialized agencies and other international organizations.

The Conference notes that existing institutional ways and means of ensuring multilateral cooperation between the developed and developing countries would need to be developed further in order to promote international cooperation in the field of peaceful activities in such areas as medicine, public health and agriculture.

The Review Conference calls upon the Secretary-General of the United Nations to propose for inclusion on the agenda of a relevant United Nations body, not later than 1993, a discussion and examination of the means of improving institutional mechanisms in order to facilitate the fullest possible exchange of equipment, materials and scientific and technological information regarding the use of bacteriological (biological) agents and toxins for peaceful purposes.

The Conference recommends that invitations to participate in this discussion and examination should be extended to all States Parties, whether or not they are members of the United Nations or concerned specialized agencies.

The Conference requests the States Parties and the United Nations Secretariat to include in the document materials prepared for the above-mentioned discussion of States Parties, information and suggestions on the implementation of Article X, taking into account the preceding paragraphs. Furthermore, it urges the specialized agencies, *inter alia,* FAO, WHO, UNESCO, WIPO and UNIDO, to participate in this discussion and fully cooperate with the Secretary-General of the United Nations, and requests the Secretary-General to send all relevant information on this Conference to these agencies.

The Conference requests that the Secretary-General collate on an annual basis, and for the information of States Parties, reports on how this Article is being implemented.

The Conference notes that one of the fields of cooperation in microbiology would be the study of the influence of enhanced radioactivity on microorganisms aimed at reducing its potentially harmful effects on humans, plants and animals, to be carried out within the United Nations programme for the minimization of the consequences of the Chernobyl accident.

The Conference welcomes efforts to elaborate an international programme of vaccine development for the prevention of diseases which would involve scientific and technical personnel from developing countries which are States Parties to the Convention. The Conference recognizes that such a programme might not only enhance peaceful international cooperation in biotechnology but will also contribute to improving health care in developing countries and provide transparency in accordance with the Convention.

Article XI

The Conference notes the importance of Article XI and that since the entry into force of the Convention the provisions of the article have not been invoked. In this context the Conference underlined that the provisions of Article XI should in principle be implemented in such a way as not to affect the universality of the Convention.

Article XII

The Conference decides that a Fourth Review Conference shall be held in Geneva at the request of a majority of States Parties not later than 1996.

The Conference decides that the Fourth Review Conference shall consider, *inter alia*:

– The impact of scientific and technological developments relating to the Convention;

– The relevance of the provisions of the chemical weapons convention on the effective implementation of the biological and toxin weapons Convention;

– The effectiveness of coordinated confidence-building measures as agreed in this Final Declaration;

– The report of the Ad Hoc Group of Governmental Experts on Verification, as well as the conclusions of a special conference, if it is convened earlier;

– The requirement for, and the operation of, the requested allocation by the United Nations Secretary-General of staff resources and other requirements to assist the effective implementation of the relevant decisions of the Third Review Conference, and in particular of the confidence-building measures;

– In the light of these considerations and of the provisions of Article XI, whether or not follow-up action is called for to create further cooperative measures in the context of Article V or legally binding improvements to the Convention, or a combination of both.

The Review Conference recommends that conferences of States Parties to review the operation of the Convention should be held at least every five years.

Article XIII

The Conference notes the provisions of Article XIII and expresses its satisfaction that no State Party to the Convention has exercised its right to withdraw from the Convention.

Article XIV

The Conference notes with satisfaction that a significant number of States have ratified or acceded to the Convention since the Second Review Conference and the 1989 Paris Conference of States Parties to the 1925 Geneva Protocol and Other Interested States, and that there are now more than 115 States Parties to the Convention, including all the permanent members of the Security Council of the United Nations.

The Conference calls upon States which have not yet ratified or acceded to the Convention to do so without delay and upon those States which have not signed the Convention to join the States Parties thereto thus contributing to the achievement of universal adherence to the Convention.

In this connection the Conference encourages States Parties to take action to persuade non-parties to accede to the Convention without delay.

The Conference particularly welcomes regional initiatives that would lead to wider accession to the Convention.

The Third Review Conference appeals to those States Parties to the Convention on the Prohibition of the Development, Production and Stockpiling of Bacteriological (Biological) and Toxin Weapons which have not taken part in the Conference to participate in the implementation of provisions contained in the Final Declaration of this Conference, and in particular to implement the agreed confidence-building measures.

Article XV

The Conference notes the provisions of Article XV.

Source: Final Document of the Third Review Conference of the Parties to the Convention on the Prohibition of the Development, Production and Stockpiling of Bacteriological (Biological) and Toxin Weapons and on their Destruction, Part III, *Final Declaration*, BWC/CONF.III/23, 1991, pp. 10–24.

Annexe C. The Biesenthal Vaccine Initiative (Vaccines for Peace) Biesenthal Consensus

Scientific, diplomatic, financial, and defence experts from Australia, France, Germany, Hungary, India, Peru, Russia, Sweden, the United Kingdom and the United States of America as well as representatives or observers from the World Health Organization (WHO), the United Nations Industrial Development Organization (UNIDO) and the United Nations Office for Disarmament Affairs[1] met in Biesenthal near Berlin, Germany,
9–14 September 1992 to discuss the proposed 'Vaccines for Peace' (VFP) program. The meeting was organized by the Max Delbrück Centre for Molecular Medicine (MDC), Berlin-Buch, and the Stockholm International Peace Research Institute (SIPRI) and was supported by the Volkswagen Foundation.

The meeting considered the original proposal for a VFP program[2] designed to strengthen the Convention on the Prohibition of the Development, Production and Stockpiling of Bacteriological (Biological) and Toxin Weapons and on their Destruction (BTWC), and to contribute to health care in developing countries, enhance international cooperation in molecular medicine and biotechnology, and reduce the dangers of weapons proliferation. The program would, with appropriate financial support, involve scientists, other personnel and facilities from States Parties to the BTWC, especially from developing countries and from the former Soviet Union.

The proposed VFP program was examined, modified, and further developed at the meeting.[3] The meeting took note of such urgent needs as improving health care and preventing disease in the developing countries, the limitations of existing vaccines, the importance of good manufacturing practice and quality control, the requirements for new and improved vaccines, the shortage of vaccine capacity worldwide and the

[1] Participants: Dr Félix *Calderón*, Deputy Head of the Special Delegation of Peru to the Conference on Disarmament, Geneva, Switzerland; Professor Sergey G. *Drozdov*, Director, Institute of Poliomyelitis and Viral Encephalitides, 142 782 Moscow Region, Russia; Professor Frank *Fenner*, John Curtin School of Medical Research, Australian National University, Canberra, A.C.T., Australia; Professor Detlev *Ganten*, Director, Max Delbrück Centre for Molecular Medicine (MDC), Berlin-Buch, Germany; Professor Erhard *Geissler*, Head, Bioethical Research Group, MDC; Professor Florian *Horaud*, Virologie Medicale, Institut Pasteur Paris, France, Vice President, International Association of Biological Standardization; Dr Mark *Kane*, Microbiology and Immunology Support Services, Division of Communicable Diseases, WHO, Geneva, Switzerland; Professor Johanna *L'age-Stehr*, Director, Yellow Fever Vaccine Production, Robert-Koch-Institut, Berlin; Professor Peter *Langen*, Coordinator, Cell Biology/Growth Control Research Program, MDC; Milton *Leitenberg*, Senior MacArthur Scholar, Center for International Security Studies at Maryland, College Park, Md.; Professor Jack *Melling*, Director, Centre for Applied Microbiology and Research, Porton Down, Salisbury, UK; Professor Stephen S. *Morse*, Rockefeller University, New York, N.Y.; Dr Sergey V. *Netesov*, Senior General Director, Institute of Molecular Biology, VECTOR Scientific and Production Association, Kol'tsovo, 633159 Novosibirsk Region, Russia; Professor Kathryn *Nixdorff*, Institut für Mikrobiologie, Technische Hochschule Darmstadt, Germany; Dr Graham *Pearson*, Director General, Chemical & Biological Defence Establishment, Porton Down, Salisbury, Wilts., UK; Dr Gunnar *Sandström*, Head, Division of Microbiology, Department of NBC Defence, National Defence Research Establishment (FOA), Umea, Sweden; Dr D. *Subrahmanyam*, UNIDO, Biotechnology and Genetic Engineering Unit, Vienna, Austria; Dr Oliver *Thränert*, Senior Researcher, Foreign Policy Research Division, Friedrich-Ebert-Stiftung, Bonn, Germany; Ambassador Tibor *Tóth*, Permanent Representative of the Republic of Hungary, Geneva, Switzerland, Chairman, *Ad Hoc* Group of Governmental Experts to Identify and Examine Potential Verification Measures; Dr Louis *Valette*, Scientific Director, Fondation Marcel Mérieux, Marnes-La-Coquette, France; Dr Mark Lewis *Wheelis*, Head, Department of Microbiology, University of California, Davis, Calif.; Dr John P. *Woodall*, Division of Epidemiological Surveillance and Health Situation & Trend Assessment, WHO, Geneva, Switzerland. Observer: Hannelore Hoppe, Political Affairs Officer, United Nations Office for Disarmament Affairs, New York, N.Y.

[2] Geissler, E., 'Vaccines for Peace: an international program of development and use of vaccines against dual-threat agents', *Politics and the Life Sciences*, vol. 11, no. 2 (Aug. 1992), pp. 231–43.

[3] The Biesenthal Consensus Steering Committee met on 29–30 November 1992 in Geneva and decided to designate the modified program the 'Biesenthal Vaccine Initiative (BVI)'.

benefits potentially available from the conversion of appropriate former biological weapons facilities to the production of vaccines and biological products for peaceful purposes. The meeting also considered the benefits available from a Global Epidemiological Surveillance System[4] especially in respect of the early identification of new or emerging disease outbreaks. Throughout, the meeting considered how the proposed program could best be used to strengthen the BTWC and increase participation in it whilst preventing misuse.

The participants at the Biesenthal meeting agreed that:

1. A Vaccines for Peace program should be established as welcomed by the Final Declaration of the Third Review Conference of the States Parties to the BTWC. The establishment of a Global Epidemiological Surveillance System, which was also welcomed in the Final Declaration of the Third Review Conference, was supported by the meeting as it would provide early identification of significant outbreaks of disease and of new or emerging diseases. These programs would both strengthen the BTWC and especially aid the implementation of Article X of the Convention.

2. Key objectives of the agreed VFP program should include

* strengthening the BTWC through implementation of Article X and increased mutual transparency in activities related to the Convention,

* prevention of diseases, especially in developing countries,

* enhancement of peaceful international cooperation in molecular medicine and biotechnology and prevention of misuse,

* conversion, where appropriate, of biological warfare (BW) facilities to peaceful purposes under civilian control,

* increasing world capacity to produce vaccines,

* expanding participation in the BTWC and its confidence-building measures.

3. The VFP should be achieved by a step-by-step approach utilizing to the fullest extent programs and facilities of existing international and national organizations such as WHO and UNIDO.

4. A steering committee has been formed under the chairmanship of Professor Jack Melling, CAMR, Porton Down, with Professor Erhard Geissler, MDC, Berlin-Buch, and Dr John P. Woodall, WHO, Geneva, acting as Vice Chairmen.[5] The steering committee is to set out the agreed VFP program and establish a schedule for its implementation to meet the above objectives, including identifying and suggesting mechanisms for funding.

5. In preparing the program and schedule the steering committee should, *inter alia,*

* consider the existing and emerging diseases in developing countries for which, under this program, improved or new vaccines are most required;

* consider the need for an inventory of existing relevant vaccine facilities;

* consider how to open up these facilities for international collaboration;

* consider the need for a communication network connecting existing relevant vaccine and public health facilities;

* consider good manufacturing practice (GMP) and quality control aspects to ensure that vaccine products meet appropriate standards;

* identify areas where assistance is needed for conversion of facilities;

* consult with other experts as appropriate;

[4] Wheelis, M., 'Strengthening biological weapons control through global epidemiological surveillance', *Politics and the Life Sciences*, vol. 11, no. 2 (Aug. 1992), pp. 179–89.

[5] Members of the BVI Steering Committee are: F. Calderón, E. Geissler, M. Kane, J. Melling, S. Morse, G. Pearson, T. Tóth, M. Wheelis and J. Woodall.

* consider how the program should be integrated into existing organisations, programs and activities within the context of the BTWC;

* consider how to prevent misuse of molecular medicine and biotechnology.

6. The meeting also urged that a convergent initiative be mounted to implement the Global Epidemiological Surveillance System. In this connection the steering committee should be encouraged to interface with groups developing this System.

7. The report of the steering committee will be forwarded to the States Parties to the BTWC and to the UN Secretary-General for their consideration in implementing the commitments set out in the Final Declaration of the Third Review Conference. The steering committee shall also prepare the final chapter of the forthcoming SIPRI book *Vaccines for Peace* which will include its report to the State Parties.

Biesenthal, 13 September 1992

Annexe D. The Biesenthal Vaccine Initiative Mission Statement

Article X of the Biological Weapons Convention states that 'Parties . . . shall . . . co-operate in . . . the further development and application of scientific discoveries in the field of bacteriology (biology) for prevention of disease'.

It is universally agreed that immunisation is one of the most effective measures against infectious disease. Indeed, for many diseases, vaccines constitute our only hope. Despite this, there are many weaknesses in global capabilities for vaccine research, development, production and distribution.

The cost of commercial vaccine development may prevent the availability of vaccines against many diseases, for which vaccines would be desirable, especially in developing countries. In addition, stability and dosing methods remain limitations to the use of many existing vaccines, again especially in developing countries.

Research leading to improvements in these aspects would greatly increase the effectiveness and availability of vaccines. There is also a shortage of facilities which can be used for vaccine R&D or production.

There are recently declared biological weapons facilities in some countries which could be converted to development and production of vaccines for diseases of significance to public health. In addition, there are benefits arising from defence programmes relating to improved development, production, stability, application and efficacy of vaccines that could, with advantage, be applied to vaccines for diseases of public health importance.

The Biesenthal Vaccine Initiative (BVI) aims to identify appropriate resources and facilities and to encourage and promote their conversion to solving problems in vaccine development, production and application of public health importance. It will also encourage and promote the transfer of technology, and training in its use, particularly to developing countries, from defence programmes which have sought new or improved vaccines and vaccine technologies.

The programme will operate within present and future measures for transparency of the BWC regime to avoid proliferation and will not assist in the transfer of technologies which might aid in the mass production of microorganisms, vaccines or products of biological warfare concern.

The benefits of conversion of appropriate biological weapons facilities and transfer of technologies arising from defence programmes into new and improved vaccines will be available to all countries especially the developing countries. Participation in this programme will be open to all States Parties to the Biological Weapons Convention to encourage increased membership.

Vaccine developments which could benefit from the initiative and which are also relevant to co-operative programmes under the BWC include Dengue, Hepatitis A, Japanese encephalitis, cholera and typhoid. These are also relevant to other vaccine programmes. The BVI will aim to co-operate with and complement other vaccine activities such as the Children's Vaccine Initiative (CVI) and the Expanded Programme on Immunization (EPI) and interact with other programmes such as the United Nations Industrial Development Organization (UNIDO) designed to achieve north/south technology transfer. It is intended to seek appropriate industrial participation.

BVI Steering Committee
Geneva, 30 November 1992

Annexe E. Mission Statement of the Federation of American Scientists (FAS) Project on the Global Control of Emerging Infectious Diseases*

Numerous recent episodes of emerging and re-emerging infections, including AIDS, the continuing spread of dengue viruses, multi-drug resistant tuberculosis and other antibiotic resistant bacteria, cholera in Africa and South America, and the resurgence of measles in US cities, attest to our continuing vulnerability to infectious diseases, both in the US and globally. Many experts, both within and outside government, have warned of the need to improve capabilities for dealing with emerging infectious diseases. A recent report from the Institute of Medicine of the National Academy of Sciences declared:

> Disease causing microbes have threatened human health for centuries. . . . [The Committee] believes that this threat will continue and may even intensify during the coming years. . . . Infectious diseases remain the major cause of death worldwide. . . . the next major infectious agent to emerge as a threat to health in the United States, may, like HIV, be a pathogen that has not been previously recognized. . . . The key to recognizing new or emerging infectious diseases, and to tracking the prevalence of more established ones, is surveillance.

The need to monitor and control the global spread of infectious diseases has become critical as new diseases or formerly obscure or geographically isolated diseases spread rapidly across the globe. These diseases often appear first in tropical countries and areas of civil conflict from which, if not recognized and contained, they may spread globally, aided by large scale population movements or environmental destruction. During the last two decades more than a dozen new viral diseases and drug-resistant pathogens affecting humans have been identified, yet during this same period of time, money for research, disease surveillance and reporting systems has been cut.

The development of a global infectious disease surveillance system has been the primary recommendation of expert analyses, including the Institute of Medicine report. A program to identify and quickly respond to unusual outbreaks of infectious diseases to prevent their spread would be highly beneficial, not only to the region of origin, but to the rest of the world as well. Unfortunately, existing international structures to monitor and contain infectious disease outbreak are poorly coordinated and understaffed. International structures are also inadequate for the containment and monitoring of animal and plant diseases, which could threaten food supplies and, in some cases, could infect humans.

The value of a cooperative international health project as an incentive for a strengthened Biological Weapons Convention has also been recognized by the parties to the

* Participants at the Preliminary Meeting of the FAS Project on Global Control of Infectious Diseases held 1 Mar. 1993: Ruth L. Berkelman, MD, Deputy Director, National Center for Infectious Diseases (NCID), Centers for Disease Control (CDC); Dr Scott Halstead, Associate Director, Health Services, The Rockefeller Foundation; D. A. Henderson, MD, Associate Director, Office of Science and Technology Policy (OSTP), Executive Office of the President; James M. Hughes, MD, Director, NCID, CDC; Dr John R. La Montagne, Director, Division of Microbiology & Infectious Diseases (DMID), National Institutes of Health; Dr Stephen S. Morse, Professor, Rockefeller University; Ciro A. de Quadros, MD, Pan American Health Organization; Dr Barbara Hatch Rosenberg, Director, FAS Chemical & Biological Weapons Verification Project, State University of New York, Purchase; Robert Shope, MD, Director, Yale Arbovirus Research, Department of Epidemiology & Public Health; Ann M. Walsh, Research Assistant, FAS; Dr Mark L. Wheelis, Department of Microbiology, University of California, Davis; and Dr Jack Woodall, World Health Organization (WHO).

Convention, which bans the development, production and stockpiling of biological weapons. The Final Declaration adopted by the third Biological Weapons Convention Review Conference in 1991 urged greater cooperation in international public health and disease control, the provision of training programs to developing countries, the coordination of international and regional programs and the pooling of information from national epidemiological surveillance and data reporting systems 'with a view to improvements in the identification and timely reporting of significant outbreaks of human and animal diseases'. However, no mechanisms were set up for achieving these lofty goals, and precedent indicates that they will, in all likelihood, be ignored. The consensus declaration also noted that existing international means are inadequate and must be developed further in order to promote international cooperation in medicine, public health and agriculture.

The timely conjunction of public health and arms control needs makes this an opportune time to mount a coordinated initiative. The working group will bring together international experts to develop a plan and encourage the implementation of a fully effective global program for infectious disease surveillance and response.

Annexe F. US House of Representatives Resolution H.R. 5241*

To require that all Federal research, development, testing, and evaluation of the use of biological agents in the development of defenses against biological warfare be conducted by the Director of the National Institutes of Health, and for other purposes.

In the House of Representatives, August 11, 1988 Mr. Owens of Utah introduced the following bill; which was referred jointly to the Committees on Energy and Commerce and Armed Services

A Bill

To require that all Federal research, development, testing, and evaluation of the use of biological agents in the development of defenses against biological warfare be conducted by the Director of the National Institutes of Health, and for other purposes.

Be it enacted by the Senate and House of Representatives of the United States of America in Congress assembled,

Section 1. Director of National Institutes of Health to conduct biological defense research programs

(*a*) In general—Except as provided in subsection (*b*), the Secretary of Health and Human Services, acting through the Director of the National Institutes of Health, shall conduct all Federal research, development, testing, and evaluation of the use of biological agents in the development of defenses against biological warfare, including the research, development, testing, and evaluation conducted as of the date of the enactment of this Act by the Secretary of the Army under the Biological Defense Research Program at the United States Army Medical Research Institute of Infectious Diseases.

(*b*) Exceptions—The Secretary of Health and Human Services may not conduct any research, development, testing, or evaluation under subsection (*a*) which involves—

(1) the field testing of biological agents, including the detection or containment of biological agents in the field or the testing of protective clothing or decontamination devices; or

(2) the use of classified information.

Section 2. Transfer of certain aspects of the Biological Defense Research Program

(*a*) In general—All functions and personnel of the Biological Defense Research Program conducted by the Secretary of the Army as of the date of the enactment of this Act are hereby transferred to the Secretary of Health and Human Services, except for those functions and personnel—

(1) relating to the field testing of biological agents, including the detection or containment of biological agents in the field or the testing of protective clothing or decontamination devices; or

(2) involving the use of classified information.

(*b*) Transfer and allocation of appropriations and civilian personnel—

(1) The civilian personnel employed, and the assets, liabilities, contracts, property, records, and unexpended balances of appropriations, authorizations, allocations, and other funds employed, used, held, arising from, available to, or to be made available, in

* H.R. 5241, 100th Congress, 2nd session, 11 Aug. 1988.

connection with functions and offices transferred under subsection (*a*) shall be transferred to the Secretary of Health and Human Services.

(2) Personnel transferred pursuant to paragraph (1) shall be transferred in accordance with applicable laws and regulations relating to the transfer of functions, except that the classification and compensation of such personnel shall not be reduced for 1 year after such transfer.

(3) Unexpected funds transferred pursuant to paragraph (1) may be used only for the purposes for which the funds were originally authorized and appropriated.

(*c*) Participation of members of the armed forces—

(1) The Secretary of Health and Human Services is authorized to provide for participation of members of the armed forces in carrying out the functions transferred under subsection (*a*) by entering into cooperative agreements with the Secretary concerned under which members of the armed forces may be detailed for service in the National Institutes of Health by the Secretary concerned.

(2) The detailing of a member of the armed forces pursuant to paragraph (1) shall not affect the status, office, rank, or grade which such member may occupy or hold or any right, privilege, or benefit incident to or arising out of such status, office, rank, or grade. Any member so detailed shall not be charged against any limitation on personnel strengths applicable to the armed forces but shall be charged against any appropriate personnel limitations applicable to the National Institutes of Health. Any member of the armed forces detailed pursuant to paragraph (1) shall not be subject to direction or control by the armed force of which he is a member with respect to such member's participation in carrying out the functions transferred under subsection (*a*).

(3) For purposes of this subsection, the term 'armed forces' and the term 'Secretary concerned' have the meaning given such terms under section 101 of title 10, United States Code.

Section 3. Restrictions on research projects and programs conducted by Secretary of Defense or Secretary of the Army.

(*a*) Authority of Secretary of Defense to engage in research projects—Section 2358 of title 10, United States Code, is amended—

(1) by striking out 'Subject to approval by the President,' and inserting in lieu thereof '(*a*) Subject to approval by the President and except as provided in subsection (*b*),'; and

(2) by adding at the end the following new subsection:

'(*b*) The Secretary of Defense may not engage in any research, development, testing, or evaluation of the use of biological agents in the development of defenses against biological warfare, other than research, development, testing, or evaluation which involves—

'(1) the field testing of biological agents, including the detection or containment of biological agents in the field or the testing of protective clothing or decontamination devices; or

'(2) the use of classified information in the development of defenses against biological warfare.'.

(*b*) Authority of Secretary of the Army to conduct and participate in research and development programs—Section 4503 of title 10, United States Code, is amended—

(1) by striking out 'The Secretary of the Army' and inserting in lieu thereof '(*a*) Except as provided in subsection (*b*), the Secretary of the Army'; and

(2) by adding at the end the following new subsection:

'(*b*) The Secretary of the Army may not conduct or participate in any research, development, testing, or evaluation of the use of biological agents in the development of defenses against biological warfare, other than research, development, testing, or evaluation which involves—

'(1) the field testing of biological agents, including the detection or containment of biological agents in the field or the testing of protective clothing or decontamination devices; or

'(2) the use of classified information in the development of defenses against biological warfare.'.

Section 4. Effective date

The provisions of this Act shall take effect 1 year after the date of the enactment of this Act.

SIPRI publications on CBW

• The Problem of Chemical and Biological Warfare, 6 vols

1. The Rise of CB Weapons. 1971. ISBN 91–85114–10–3.
2. CB Weapons Today. 1973. 91–85114–16–2.
3. CBW and the Law of War. 1974. 91–85114–17–0.
4. CB Disarmament Negotiations, 1920–1970. 1971. 91–85114–11–1.
5. The Prevention of CBW. 1971. 91–85114–13–8.
6. Technical Aspects of Early Warning and Verification. 1975. 91–85114–18–9.

• Chapters in the SIPRI Yearbooks

SIPRI Yearbook of World Armaments and Disarmament, 1968/69. 1969. 91–85114–03–0. pp. 112–34. Development in chemical and biological warfare.

SIPRI Yearbook of World Armaments and Disarmament, 1969/70. 1970. 91–85114–07–3. pp. 185–206. The CBW debate and other disarmament measures.

World Armaments and Disarmament: SIPRI Yearbook 1972. 1972. 91–85114–12–X. pp. 501–22. Chemical and biological disarmament.

World Armaments and Disarmament: SIPRI Yearbook 1973. 1973. 91–85114–19–7. pp. 383–91. Chemical disarmament.

World Armaments and Disarmament: SIPRI Yearbook 1974. 1974. 0–262–19129–6. pp. 370–84. Chemical disarmament.

World Armaments and Disarmament: SIPRI Yearbook 1975. 1975. 0–262–19140–7. pp. 426–32. Chemical disarmament.

World Armaments and Disarmament: SIPRI Yearbook 1977. 1977. 91–22–00116–6.
pp. 86–102. Dioxin: a potential chemical-warfare agent; and
pp. 364–67. Prohibition of biological and chemical weapons.

World Armaments and Disarmament: SIPRI Yearbook 1978. 1978. 0–85066–134–X. pp. 360–76. The destruction of chemical warfare agents.

World Armaments and Disarmament: SIPRI Yearbook 1979. 1979. 0–85066–181–1. pp. 470–89. Stockpiles of chemical weapons and their destruction.

World Armaments and Disarmament: SIPRI Yearbook 1980. 1980. 0–85066–201–X. pp. 365–79. Chemical disarmament.

World Armaments and Disarmament: SIPRI Yearbook 1982. 1982. 0–85066–230–3. pp. 317–61. The changing status of chemical and biological warfare: recent technical, military and political developments; and pp. 456–57. Chemical weapons.

World Armaments and Disarmament: SIPRI Yearbook 1983. 1983. 0–85066–247–8.
pp. 391–426. Chemical and biological warfare: developments in 1982; and
pp. 563–67. Chemical disarmament.

World Armaments and Disarmament: SIPRI Yearbook 1984. 1984. 0–85066–263–X.
pp. 319–49. Chemical and biological warfare: developments in 1983; and
pp. 421–54. Implications of genetic engineering for chemical and biological warfare.

World Armaments and Disarmament: SIPRI Yearbook 1985. 1985. 0–85066–297–4.
pp. 159–205. Chemical and biological warfare: developments in 1984; and
pp. 206–19. An analysis of the reports of Iraqi chemical warfare against Iran, 1980–84.

World Armaments and Disarmament: SIPRI Yearbook 1986. 1986. 0–19–829100–0. pp. 159–79. Chemical and biological warfare: developments in 1985.

SIPRI Yearbook 1987: World Armaments and Disarmament. 1987. 0–19–829114–0. pp. 97–115. Chemical and biological warfare: developments in 1986.

SIPRI Yearbook 1988: World Armaments and Disarmament. 1988. 0–19–829126–4. pp. 101–25. Chemical and biological warfare: developments in 1987.

SIPRI Yearbook 1989: World Armaments and Disarmament. 1989. 0–19–827751–2. pp. 99–130. Chemical and biological warfare: developments in 1988.

SIPRI Yearbook 1990: World Armaments and Disarmament. 1990. 0–19–827862–4.
pp. 107–40. Chemical and biological warfare: developments in 1989; and
pp. 521–44. Multilateral and bilateral talks on chemical and biological weapons.

SIPRI Yearbook 1991: World Armaments and Disarmament. 1991. 0–19–829145–0.
pp. 85–112. Chemical and biological warfare: developments in 1990; and
pp. 513–39. Multilateral and bilateral talks on chemical and biological weapons.

SIPRI Yearbook 1992: World Armaments and Disarmament. 1992. 0–19–829159–0.
pp. 147–86. Chemical and biological warfare and arms control developments in 1991; and
pp. 509–30. The United Nations Special Commission on Iraq.

SIPRI Yearbook 1993: World Armaments and Disarmament. 1993. 0–19–829166–3.
pp. 259–92. Chemical and biological weapons: developments and proliferation;
pp. 293–305. Benefits and threats of developments in biotechnology and genetic engineering;
pp. 691–703. The United Nations Special Commission on Iraq: activities in 1992;
pp. 705–34. The Chemical Weapons Convention: the success of chemical disarmament negotiations; and
pp. 735–56. The Convention on the Prohibition of the Development, Production, Stockpiling and Use of Chemical Weapons and on their Destruction.

• Other SIPRI publications

Chemical Disarmament: Some Problems of Verification. 1973. 91–85114–20–0.

The Effects of Developments in the Biological and Chemical Sciences on CW Disarmament Negotiations. SIPRI research report 13, SIPRI, 1974.

Delayed Toxic Effects of Chemical Warfare Agents. 1975. 91–85114–29–4.

Chemical Disarmament: New Weapons for Old. 1975. 91–85114–27–8.

Medical Protection against Chemical-Warfare Agents. 1976. 91–22000–44–5.

Ecological Consequences of the Second Indochina War. 1976. 91–22000–62–3, pp. 24–45, 53–55.

Weapons of Mass Destruction and the Environment. 1977. 0–85066–132–3, pp. 31–48.

The Fight against Infectious Diseases: A Role for Applied Microbiology in Military Redeployment. SIPRI, 1979, mimeo. 91–85114–26–X.

Chemical Weapons: Destruction and Conversion. 1980. 0–85066–199–4.

Herbicides in War. 1984. 0–85066–265–6.

Biological and Toxin Weapons Today. 1986. 0–19–829108–6.

SIPRI publications may be obtained through all main bookshops. In case of difficulty, please contact the publishers or SIPRI.

SIPRI Chemical & Biological Warfare Studies

No. 1 Effects of Chemical Warfare: A selective review and bibliography of British state papers, by Andy Thomas
No. 2 Chemical Warfare Arms Control: A framework for considering policy alternatives, by Julian Perry Robinson
No. 3 The Detoxification and Natural Degradation of Chemical Warfare Agents, by Ralf Trapp
No. 4 The Chemical Industry and the Projected Chemical Weapons Convention: Proceedings of a SIPRI/Pugwash Conference, volume I
No. 5 The Chemical Industry and the Projected Chemical Weapons Convention: Proceedings of a SIPRI/Pugwash Conference, volume II
No. 6 Chemical and Biological Warfare Developments: 1985, by Julian Perry Robinson
No. 7 Chemical Weapon Free Zones?, edited by Ralf Trapp
No. 8 International Organization for Chemical Disarmament, by Nicholas A. Sims
No. 9 Non-Production by Industry of Chemical-Warfare Agents: Technical Verification under a Chemical Weapons Convention, edited by S. J. Lundin
No. 10 Strengthening the Biological Weapons Convention by Confidence-Building Measures, edited by Erhard Geissler
No. 11 National Implementation of the Future Chemical Weapons Convention, edited by Thomas Stock and Ronald Sutherland
No. 12 Views on Possible Verification Measures for the Biological Weapons Convention, edited by S. J. Lundin
No. 13 Verification of Dual-use Chemicals under the Chemical Weapons Convention: The Case of Thiodiglycol, edited by S. J. Lundin
No. 14 Verification under the Chemical Weapons Convention: On-Site Inspection in Chemical Industry Facilities, by Ralf Trapp
No. 15 Control of Dual-Threat Agents: The Vaccines for Peace Programme, edited by Erhard Geissler and John P. Woodall

The manufacturer's authorised representative in the EU for product safety is Oxford University Press España S.A. of el Parque Empresarial San Fernando de Henares, Avenida de Castilla, 2 – 28830 Madrid (www.oup.es/en or product.safety@oup.com). OUP España S.A. also acts as importer into Spain of products made by the manufacturer.

www.ingramcontent.com/pod-product-compliance
Lightning Source LLC
Chambersburg PA
CBHW081122200926
51611CB00008B/33
* 9 7 8 0 1 9 8 2 9 1 7 2 5 *